Designing Hydrogels for Controlled Drug Delivery

Designing Hydrogels for Controlled Drug Delivery

Special Issue Editors

Sonia Trombino
Roberta Cassano

MDPI • Basel • Beijing • Wuhan • Barcelona • Belgrade • Manchester • Tokyo • Cluj • Tianjin

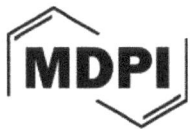

Special Issue Editors
Sonia Trombino
University of Calabria
Italy

Roberta Cassano
University of Calabria
Italy

Editorial Office
MDPI
St. Alban-Anlage 66
4052 Basel, Switzerland

This is a reprint of articles from the Special Issue published online in the open access journal *Pharmaceutics* (ISSN 1999-4923) (available at: https://www.mdpi.com/journal/pharmaceutics/special_issues/Hydrogels_Drug_Delivery).

For citation purposes, cite each article independently as indicated on the article page online and as indicated below:

LastName, A.A.; LastName, B.B.; LastName, C.C. Article Title. *Journal Name* **Year**, *Article Number*, Page Range.

ISBN 978-3-03928-356-9 (Pbk)
ISBN 978-3-03928-357-6 (PDF)

© 2020 by the authors. Articles in this book are Open Access and distributed under the Creative Commons Attribution (CC BY) license, which allows users to download, copy and build upon published articles, as long as the author and publisher are properly credited, which ensures maximum dissemination and a wider impact of our publications.

The book as a whole is distributed by MDPI under the terms and conditions of the Creative Commons license CC BY-NC-ND.

Contents

About the Special Issue Editors vii

Preface to "Designing Hydrogels for Controlled Drug Delivery" ix

Sonia Trombino and Roberta Cassano
Special Issue on Designing Hydrogels for Controlled Drug Delivery: Guest Editors' Introduction
Reprinted from: *Pharmaceutics* **2020**, *12*, 57, doi:10.3390/pharmaceutics12010057 1

Franklin Afinjuomo, Paris Fouladian, Ankit Parikh, Thomas G. Barclay, Yunmei Song and Sanjay Garg
Preparation and Characterization of Oxidized Inulin Hydrogel for Controlled Drug Delivery
Reprinted from: *Pharmaceutics* **2019**, *11*, 356, doi:10.3390/pharmaceutics11070356 5

Maria Cristina Cardia, Anna Rosa Carta, Pierluigi Caboni, Anna Maria Maccioni, Sara Erbì, Laura Boi, Maria Cristina Meloni, Francesco Lai and Chiara Sinico
Trimethyl Chitosan Hydrogel Nanoparticles for Progesterone Delivery in Neurodegenerative Disorders
Reprinted from: *Pharmaceutics* **2019**, *11*, 657, doi:10.3390/pharmaceutics11120657 27

Angela Fabiano, Anna Maria Piras, Lorenzo Guazzelli, Barbara Storti, Ranieri Bizzarri and Ylenia Zambito
Impact of Different Mucoadhesive Polymeric Nanoparticles Loaded in Thermosensitive Hydrogels on Transcorneal Administration of 5-Fluorouracil
Reprinted from: *Pharmaceutics* **2019**, *11*, 623, doi:10.3390/pharmaceutics11120623 39

Hsiu-Chao Lin, Madonna Rica Anggelia, Chih-Chi Cheng, Kuan-Lin Ku, Hui-Yun Cheng, Chih-Jen Wen, Aline Yen Ling Wang, Cheng-Hung Lin and I-Ming Chu
A Mixed Thermosensitive Hydrogel System for Sustained Delivery of Tacrolimus for Immunosuppressive Therapy
Reprinted from: *Pharmaceutics* **2019**, *11*, 413, doi:10.3390/pharmaceutics11080413 55

Narsimha Mamidi, Aldo González-Ortiz, Irasema Lopez Romo and Enrique V. Barrera
Development of Functionalized Carbon Nano-Onions Reinforced Zein Protein Hydrogel Interfaces for Controlled Drug Release
Reprinted from: *Pharmaceutics* **2019**, *11*, 621, doi:10.3390/pharmaceutics11120621 67

Saeid Mezail Mawazi, Sinan Mohammed Abdullah Al-Mahmood, Bappaditya Chatterjee, Hazrina AB. Hadi and Abd Almonem Doolaanea
Carbamazepine Gel Formulation as a Sustained Release Epilepsy Medication for Pediatric Use
Reprinted from: *Pharmaceutics* **2019**, *11*, 488, doi:10.3390/pharmaceutics11100488 83

Eleonora Russo and Carla Villa
Poloxamer Hydrogels for Biomedical Applications
Reprinted from: *Pharmaceutics* **2019**, *11*, 671, doi:10.3390/pharmaceutics11120671 97

Eleonora Russo and Carla Villa
Poloxamer Hydrogels for Biomedical Applications
Reprinted from: *Pharmaceutics* **2019**, *11*, 671, doi:10.3390/pharmaceutics11120671 115

Sonia Trombino, Camilla Servidio, Federica Curcio and Roberta Cassano
Strategies for Hyaluronic Acid-Based Hydrogel Design in Drug Delivery
Reprinted from: *Pharmaceutics* **2019**, *11*, 407, doi:10.3390/pharmaceutics11080407 . . . . **133**

About the Special Issue Editors

Sonia Trombino graduated in Pharmacy at the University of Calabria (Italy) in 1998 where, five years later, she also specialized in Clinical Pathology. From 2006 to 2016, she was a researcher in pharmaceutical technology, and, from 2016 onward, has been an associate professor in the Department of Pharmacy and Health and Nutrition Sciences at the same university. Her research activities include: drug delivery systems (DDS), biomaterials, multifunctional carriers, micro- and nano-particles, pro-drugs, polymeric matrices, natural fibers, antioxidants, membranes, and liquid crystals. Sonia Trombino is author or coauthor of 77 publications in international journals with good or excellent diffusion, 8 reviews published in books, and 65 conference proceedings.

Roberta Cassano graduated in Chemistry at the University of Calabria (Italy) in 2000 and where, five years later, she also obtained her Ph.D in Science and Technology of Mesophases and Molecular Materials. From 2010 to 2019, she was a researcher in pharmaceutical technology, and is an associate professor in the Department of Pharmacy and Health and Nutrition Sciences at the same university. Her research activities involve: drug delivery systems (DDS), biomaterials, multifunctional carriers, micro- and nano-particles, pro-drugs, polymeric matrices, natural fibers, antioxidants, membranes, and liquid crystals. Roberta Cassano is the author or coauthor of 66 publications in international journals with good or excellent diffusion, 12 reviews published in books, and 70 conference proceedings.

Preface to "Designing Hydrogels for Controlled Drug Delivery"

Hydrogels are interesting materials for pharmaceutical application and are particularly useful as drug delivery systems because they are biocompatible and nontoxic. They consist of three-dimensional, hydrophilic, and polymeric networks capable of absorbing large quantities of water or biological fluids in the presence of hydrophilic groups and releasing the drugs entrapped in them through slow diffusion. According to their features, they can be natural or synthetic and classified as neutral or ionic hydrogels, whereas the network can be composed of linear homopolymers, linear copolymers, and block or graft copolymers. Hydrogels provide a spatial and temporal control of various therapeutic agents, including both small molecules and macromolecular drugs. They possess modulable physical properties and the capability to protect labile drugs from degradation, controlling their release.

The purpose of this Special Issue book is provide an overview of recent advances in delivery of drugs using synthetic or natural hydrogels highlighting, through research articles and reviews, the significant role of these materials in the pharmaceutical field.

Sonia Trombino, Roberta Cassano
Special Issue Editors

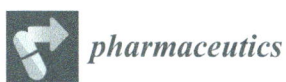

Editorial

Special Issue on Designing Hydrogels for Controlled Drug Delivery: Guest Editors' Introduction

Sonia Trombino * and Roberta Cassano *

Department of Pharmacy and Health and Nutrition Sciences, University of Calabria, Arcavacata di Rende, 87036 Cosenza, Italy
* Correspondence: sonia.trombino@unical.it (S.T.); roberta.cassano@unical.it (R.C.); Tel.: +39-984-493203 (S.T.); +39-984-493227 (R.C.)

Received: 7 January 2020; Accepted: 8 January 2020; Published: 10 January 2020

Hydrogels have received growing attention in recent years as materials for drug delivery systems (DDS), because they are biocompatible and nontoxic. They consist of three-dimensional, hydrophilic, polymeric networks capable of imbibing large quantities of water or biological fluids, due to the presence of hydrophilic groups, and releasing the drugs entrapped in them through slow diffusion. According to their features, they can be natural or synthetic and classified as neutral or ionic hydrogels, while the network can be made up of linear homopolymers, linear copolymers, and block or graft copolymers. Hydrogels can provide a spatial and temporal control over the release of various therapeutic agents, including both small molecules and macromolecular drugs. They possess modulable physical properties and the capability to protect labile drugs from degradation controlling their release. This special issue fits into this context and has the aim of describing, through seven research papers and two review articles, recent studies concerning the design, preparation and evaluation of the performance of hydrogels for the controlled delivery of drugs.

In the first article Cesar Torres-Luna and colloaborators evaluated the in vitro release of diclofenac sodium, an anionic drug useful for the treatment of pain and eye inflammation, from contact lenses based on poly-2-hydroxyethyl methacrylate hydrogels containing an embedded microemulsion. In particular, the aim of the work was to extend the release duration of the diclofenac sodium [1]. The oil in water microemulsion systems were prepared with two non-ionic surfactants, Brij 97 or Tween 80 and cetalkonium chloride as cationic surfactant. The results indicated that in such systems, microemulsions serves as a diffusion barrier that retards diclofenac sodium release, while cetalkonium chloride further extends drug release due to the ionic interactions between the positively charged-contact lenses and the negatively charged drug.

In their research paper Afinjuomo et al. have obtained new injectable inulin hydrogels by crosslinking oxidized inulin with adipic acid dihydrazide without the use of a catalyst or initiator [2]. In vitro releases of 5-fluorouracil (5FU) from the various inulin hydrogels was enhanced in acidic conditions (pH 5) respect to physiological ones (pH 7.4). It was also observed an initial burst release followed by a controlled release pattern. In addition, blank gels did not show any appreciable cytotoxicity, whereas 5-FU-loaded hydrogels demonstrated efficacy against a type of colon cancer cells, which further confirms the potential use of these delivery platforms for direct targeting of 5-FU to the colon.

Lin and collaborators have fabricated mixed heat-sensitive hydrogel systems to support the release of tacrolimus [3], an immunosuppressant agent useful for acute rejection after allograft. The copolymers used, which consist of poloxamer and poly(L-alanine) with L-lysine segments at both ends (P-Lys-Ala-PLX), were able to transport tacrolimus in a gelled form in situ with acceptable biocompatibility, biodegradability, and low gelation concentrations. F-127 Pluronic has been added to formulate a mixed hydrogel system and to maintain adequate drug levels in animals with transplants. In addition to the in situ gelling properties, the system has shown greater encapsulation efficiency, easy administration and applicability to various types of drugs. Therefore, using these mixed hydrogel systems for sustaining delivery of tacrolimus can give important advancements in immunosuppressive therapy.

Mawazi et al. developed a carbamazepine sustained release new dosage form for pediatric use [4]. In particular, the carbamazepine was first prepared as sustained release microparticles, and then these last were embedded in alginate beads, and finally, these beads were suspended in iota carrageenan gel as vehicle. The developed formulations showed the advantages of a suspension formulation such as a flexible dosing and being easy to swallow. It also could overcome the issue of carbamazepine precipitation that was seen in the suspension formulation, which can lead to overdose. Carbamazepine sustained release gel has the potential to make the advantages of a sustained release dosage form to pediatric patients accessible, especially children below six years old who have no current option for such a formulation.

In their study Mamidi and collaborators made poly 4-mercaptophenyl methacrylate-carbon nano-onions (PMPMA-CNOs = f-CNOs) reinforced natural protein (zein) composites (zein /f-CNOs) using the acoustic cavitation technique [5]. The cytotoxicity of hydrogels was tested with osteoblast cells. The results showed good cell viability and cell growth. To explore the efficacy of hydrogels as drug transporters, 5-fluorouracil release was measured under gastric and intestinal pHs. The results showed pH-responsive sustained drug release over 15 days of study, and pH 7.4 showed a more rapid drug release than pH 2.0 and 4.5. All obtained results suggested that zein/f-CNOs hydrogel could be a potential pH-responsive drug transporter for a colon-selective delivery system.

The aim of the work of Fabiano et al. was to study the impact of the surface characteristics of new nanoparticles contained in a thermosensitive hydrogel formulation based on chitosan or its derivatives, on ocular 5-fluorouracil bioavailability [6]. The chitosan derivatives used to prepare nanoparticles were quaternary ammonium-chitosan conjugate (QA-Ch), S-protected derivative thereof (QA-Ch-S-pro), and a sulphobutyl chitosan derivative (SB-Ch). The drug release from hydrogel formulation containing nanoparticles based on QA-Ch or QA-Ch-S-pro was virtually equal, whereas the hydrogel formulation containing nanoparticle based on SB-Ch was significantly slower. The authors demonstrated that negative charges on the nanoparticles surface slowed down 5-FU release from thermosensitive hydrogel formulation based on chitosan or its derivatives while positive charges increased nanoparticles contact with the negatively charged ocular surface. Either resulted in enhanced ocular bioavailability.

With the aim to deliver progesterone, a sex hormone with neuroprotective effects, to the brain, Cardia and coworkers have fabricated, characterized, and tested *in vivo* progesterone-loaded hydrogel nanoparticle formulations [7]. In particular, nanoparticles, loaded with different progesterone concentrations, have been obtained by polyelectrolyte complex formation between trimethyl chitosan and sodium alginate, followed by ionotropic gelation with sodium tripolyphosphate as a cross-linking agent. All formulations showed a mean diameter compatible with inhalable administration and a high progesterone encapsulation efficiency. The zeta potential values were set to ensure nanoparticles stability against aggregation phenomena as well as interaction with negative sialic residues of the nasal mucosa. Finally, in vivo studies on Sprague-Dawley male rats demonstrated a 5-fold increase in brain progesterone concentrations compared to basal progesterone level after 30 min of hydrogel nanoparticle inhalation.

The two review articles treated in this special issue concern the characteristics and performances of two types of hydrogels: the first of natural origin, based on hyaluronic acid and the second type a synthetic one based on poloxamers. In particular, Trombino et al. described the properties of hydrogels made with hyaluronic acid (HA) in the release of drugs [8]. HA is an interesting material for hydrogels design due to its biocompatibility, native biofunctionality, biodegradability, non-immunogenicity, and versatility. In the last years, different strategies for the design of physical and chemical HA hydrogels have been developed, such as click chemistry reactions, enzymatic and disulfide crosslinking, supramolecular assembly via inclusion complexation, and so on. HA-based hydrogels are widely investigated for biomedical applications like drug delivery, tissue engineering, regenerative medicine, cell therapy, and diagnostics. Furthermore, the overexpression of HA receptors on various tumor cells makes these materials promising drug delivery systems for targeted cancer therapy.

Finally, Russo and Villa focused on heat-resistant hydrogels consisting of poloxamers which are of great interest for the administration of ophthalmic, injectable, transdermal and vaginal drugs [9]. The particular characteristic of these hydrogels is that they remain fluid at room temperature and become more viscous gels when exposed to body temperature. In this way, the gelation system remains topical for a long time and the release of the drug is controlled and prolonged. Poloxamers can have different consistencies and be liquids, pastes and solids, with respect to the molecular weights and weight ratios of ethylene oxide-propylene oxide present in their structure. Concentrated aqueous solutions of poloxamers form heat-reversible gels that arouse interest in tissue engineering. Finally, the use of poloxamers as biosurfactants has been described since they are capable of forming micelles in an aqueous environment above a concentration threshold known as critical concentration of micelles. This property is interesting for drug delivery and various therapeutic applications.

The purpose of this special issue was to provide an overview of recent advances in delivery of drugs by synthetic or natural hydrogels. Based on the interesting results described in the research articles and reviews presented here, we can conclude that these types of DDS make a significant contribution to the pharmaceutical field.

Conflicts of Interest: The authors declare no conflict of interest.

References

1. Torres-Luna, C.; Hu, N.; Koolivand, A.; Fan, X.; Zhu, Y.; Domszy, R.; Yang, J.; Yang, A.; Wang, N.S. Effect of a Cationic Surfactant on Microemulsion Globules and Drug Release from Hydrogel Contact Lenses. *Pharmaceutics* **2019**, *11*, 262. [CrossRef] [PubMed]
2. Afinjuomo, F.; Fouladian, P.; Parikh, A.; Barclay, T.G.; Song, Y.; Garg, S. Preparation and Characterization of Oxidized Inulin Hydrogel for Controlled Drug Delivery. *Pharmaceutics* **2019**, *11*, 356. [CrossRef] [PubMed]
3. Lin, H.-C.; Anggelia, M.R.; Cheng, C.-C.; Ku, K.-L.; Cheng, H.-Y.; Wen, C.-J.; Wang, A.Y.L.; Lin, C.-H.; Chu, I.-M. A Mixed Thermosensitive Hydrogel System for Sustained Delivery of Tacrolimus for Immunosuppressive Therapy. *Pharmaceutics* **2019**, *11*, 413. [CrossRef] [PubMed]
4. Mawazi, S.M.; Al-Mahmood, S.M.A.; Chatterjee, B.; Hadi, H.A.; Doolaanea, A.A. Carbamazepine Gel Formulation as a Sustained Release Epilepsy Medication for Pediatric Use. *Pharmaceutics* **2019**, *11*, 488. [CrossRef] [PubMed]
5. Mamidi, N.; González-Ortiz, A.; Lopez Romo, I.; Barrera, E.V. Development of Functionalized Carbon Nano-Onions Reinforced Zein Protein Hydrogel Interfaces for Controlled Drug Release. *Pharmaceutics* **2019**, *11*, 621. [CrossRef] [PubMed]
6. Fabiano, A.; Piras, A.M.; Guazzelli, L.; Storti, B.; Bizzarri, R.; Zambito, Y. Impact of Different Mucoadhesive Polymeric Nanoparticles Loaded in Thermosensitive Hydrogels on Transcorneal Administration of 5-Fluorouracil. *Pharmaceutics* **2019**, *11*, 623. [CrossRef] [PubMed]
7. Cardia, M.C.; Carta, A.R.; Caboni, P.; Maccioni, A.M.; Erbì, S.; Boi, L.; Meloni, M.C.; Lai, F.; Sinico, C. Trimethyl Chitosan Hydrogel Nanoparticles for Progesterone Delivery in Neurodegenerative Disorders. *Pharmaceutics* **2019**, *11*, 657. [CrossRef] [PubMed]
8. Trombino, S.; Servidio, C.; Curcio, F.; Cassano, R. Strategies for Hyaluronic Acid-Based Hydrogel Design in Drug Delivery. *Pharmaceutics* **2019**, *11*, 407. [CrossRef] [PubMed]
9. Russo, E.; Villa, C. Poloxamer Hydrogels for Biomedical Applications. *Pharmaceutics* **2019**, *11*, 671. [CrossRef] [PubMed]

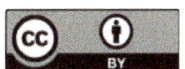

© 2020 by the authors. Licensee MDPI, Basel, Switzerland. This article is an open access article distributed under the terms and conditions of the Creative Commons Attribution (CC BY) license (http://creativecommons.org/licenses/by/4.0/).

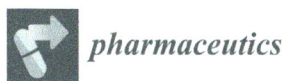

Article

Preparation and Characterization of Oxidized Inulin Hydrogel for Controlled Drug Delivery

Franklin Afinjuomo, Paris Fouladian, Ankit Parikh, Thomas G. Barclay, Yunmei Song and Sanjay Garg *

School of Pharmacy and Medical Sciences, University of South Australia, Adelaide, South Australia 5001, Australia
* Correspondence: sanjay.garg@unisa.edu.au

Received: 21 June 2019; Accepted: 17 July 2019; Published: 22 July 2019

Abstract: Inulin-based hydrogels are useful carriers for the delivery of drugs in the colon-targeted system and in other biomedical applications. In this project, inulin hydrogels were fabricated by crosslinking oxidized inulin with adipic acid dihydrazide (AAD) without the use of a catalyst or initiator. The physicochemical properties of the obtained hydrogels were further characterized using different techniques, such as swelling experiments, in vitro drug release, degradation, and biocompatibility tests. The crosslinking was confirmed with Fourier transform infrared spectroscopy (FTIR), thermal gravimetric analysis (TGA), and differential scanning calorimetry (DSC). In vitro releases of 5-fluorouracil (5FU) from the various inulin hydrogels was enhanced in acidic conditions (pH 5) compared with physiological pH (pH 7.4). In addition, blank gels did not show any appreciable cytotoxicity, whereas 5FU-loaded hydrogels demonstrated efficacy against HCT116 colon cancer cells, which further confirms the potential use of these delivery platforms for direct targeting of 5-FU to the colon.

Keywords: hydrogels; oxidized inulin; periodate oxidation; colon targeting

1. Introduction

Inulin is an important fructan found in plants and vegetables, such as garlic, leeks, bananas, and Jerusalem artichokes [1]. Inulin belongs to the fructan class of polysaccharides typically containing about 2–60 fructose units in linear chains with $\beta(2\rightarrow1)$ glycosidic linkages and typically linked to a terminal glucose unit [2]. There is a growing interest in inulin because of the key role that fructans play in both food and the pharmaceutical industry. Inulin is only digested by colon bacteria and not in the small intestine, promoting its health benefits as a prebiotic and in food [3–5]. Inulin also serves as a replacement for fat and sugar in the food industry [6,7]. Inulin is Food and Drug Administration (FDA) approved Generally Recognized As Safe (GRAS) polysaccharide with excellent biodegradability, biocompatibility, water solubility, renewability, and non-toxicity, making it very attractive as a drug delivery carrier targeting colon delivery and pulmonary delivery [8–13]. Other important applications include use as a flocculant for wastewater treatment [14] and in tissue engineering scaffolds [15]. The modification of inulin hydroxyl groups allows the introduction of new functional groups into the polymer. In addition to the multiple hydroxyl groups, the flexible furanose backbone, as well as its increased solubility compared with other polysaccharides, means that it can be readily modified chemically. This allows the use of inulin derivatives as carriers for a variety of pharmaceutical applications. Inulin is considered to be a very attractive polysaccharide for colon targeting, because it is only degraded by specific inulinase enzymes found in the colon [9].

For this reason, we hope to exploit the variation in the microflora concentration of various segments of the gastrointestinal tract for site-specific delivery of drugs to the colon. The chemical modification or derivatization of hydrophilic inulin results in new materials with hydrophobic characters making them suitable for drug delivery systems (DDSs), including hydrogels [16–19], micelles [20–22], liposomes [23], nanoparticles [24–26], vaccine adjuvants [27–29], solid dispersion [30,31], microparticles [8,12,32], and macromolecular bioconjugates/prodrugs [33,34]. To develop hydrogel drug delivery systems, different chemical strategies and techniques have been utilized for hydrogel synthesis. Reported methods of preparation include radical polymerization of inulin derivatives [10,11], Michael-addition crosslinking [35], condensation reaction [36], chemical crosslinking using crosslinkers [5,16,37], or chemical crosslinking followed by UV radiation [19] with subsequent formation of pH-sensitive inulin hydrogels. The limitations with the methods reported above include the use of a toxic catalyst [10,16], initiators [36,38], several reaction steps during synthesis, and long gelation period [37]. The use of modified polysaccharides with aldehyde functionality crosslinked with adipic acid hydrazide has been reported for biodegradable polysaccharides, such as pectin [39,40], dextran [41], chitosan [42], alginate [43,44], xanthan, hyaluronic acid [45–48], and gum with potential application as injectable hydrogel. Periodate oxidation of inulin is a well-known method of functionalizing inulin with an aldehyde group [33,49]. This enables the use of oxidized inulin as a macromolecular bioconjugate to couple a cardiac depressant and antiarrhythmic agent procainamide [33], as well as an enzyme immobilizing agent [49].

However, the use of oxidized inulin for hydrogel fabrication by crosslinking the polyaldehyde inulin with adipic acid hydrazide (AAD) has yet to be reported. To the best of our knowledge, there are no prior studies on the use of oxidized inulin in the formation of a hydrogel via crosslinking with non-toxic AAD. In this work, sodium periodate was used as an oxidizing agent to attack the hydroxyl group of inulin between C_3–C_4, breaking the C–C bond and producing two aldehyde groups (Scheme 1A,B). The resulting intermediate obtained from periodate oxidation is highly reactive toward nucleophilic compounds, such as carbazates, amines, and hydrazines. This oxidized inulin reacts with AAD to form a crosslink without the use of a catalyst. It is worth mentioning that this inulin hydrogel was fabricated in physiologic pH conditions (pH 7.4) in phosphate-buffered saline (PBS) as compared with the organic solvents used in most reported inulin hydrogels. Other clear advantages include (1) the fact that the oxidized inulin/AAD hydrogels were formed within 2–4 min and (2) the potential to control their mechanical and degradation properties with the amount of crosslinker used.

We hypothesized that the chemical crosslinking of oxidized inulin with different ratios of AAD would result in hydrogels with different degrees of crosslinking density, which can allow the controlled release of 5-fluorouracil (5FU). The aim of this study was to crosslink oxidized inulin with AAD to obtain a hydrogel with a hydrazone bond. The oxidized inulin was characterized using ^{1}H NMR and FTIR, as well as colorimetric titration. The three hydrogels formed were evaluated using different techniques, such as swelling experiments, rheological measurement, FTIR, TGA, differential scanning calorimetry (DSC), SEM, and degradation as well as biocompatibility and cytotoxicity studies using 33-(4,5-dimethylthiazol-2-yl)-2,5-diphenyl-tetrazolium bromide blue-indicator dye (MTT) assay.

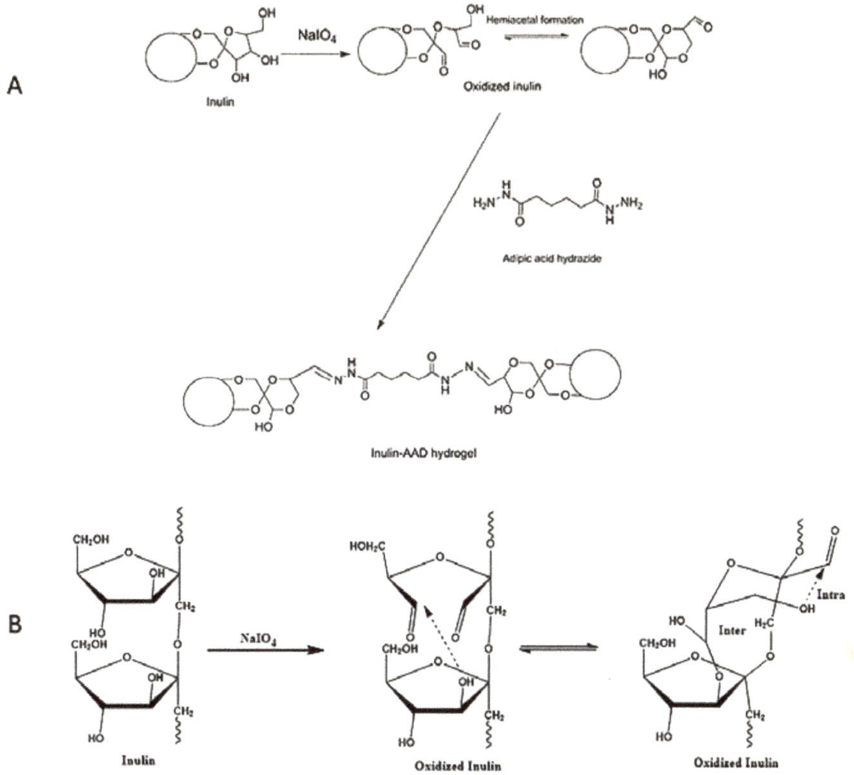

Scheme 1. (**A**) Periodate oxidation of inulin and subsequent crosslinking with adipic acid dihydrazide (AAD) and (**B**) periodate oxidation of inulin with cleavage at C_3–C_4.

2. Materials and Methods

2.1. Materials

Inulin polysaccharide from a Dahlia plant was purchased from Sigma-Aldrich (Castle Hill, New South Wales, Australia), and the average chain length (DPn) 39.2 and MWn = 6381.7 was determined by using end-group analysis via an 1H NMR spectroscopy method previously reported by Barclay et al. [50]. Adipic acid dihydrazide, phosphate-buffered saline tablets, 5-fluorouracil, hydrochloride acid 32%, trichloroacetic acid, sodium metaperiodate, tert-butyl carbazate (tBC), ethylene glycol, hydroxylamine hydrochloride, trinitrobenzenosulfonic acid, methyl orange, McCoy's 5A (Modified) Medium, L-glutamine, potassium bromide (KBr), inulinase and sodium bicarbonate were all acquired from Sigma–Aldrich. Sodium hydroxide was obtained from Ajax FineChem (Taren Point, New South Wale, Australia). CelluSep T4 25-mm flat width 12,000 MWCO Dialysis membranes were purchased from Fisher Biotec Australia (Wembley, Western Australia, Australia). Acetonitrile from Merck Pty Ltd. (Baywaters, Victoria, Australia). Deuterated water (D_2O) and DMSO (DMSO-d_6) for 1H NMR were obtained from Cambridge Isotope Laboratories (Tewksbury, MA, USA). For the MTT assay, 3-(4,5-dimethylthiazol-2-yl)-5-(3-carboxymethoxyphenyl)-2-(4-sulfophenyl)-2H-tetrazolium; 96-well plates; media ingredients including penicillin, streptomycin, and trypsin; and fetal bovine serum (FBS) were purchased from Thermo Fisher Scientific (Thebarton, Adelaide, Australia). All chemicals were of analytic grade and used as received without any further modification or purification.

2.2. Oxidation of Inulin to Inulin Aldehyde Derivative

Preparation and Characterization of Oxidized Inulin

Inulin was modified to obtain an aldehyde derivative by using the method previously reported [51]. Briefly, 1.2 g of inulin (12.3 mmol fructose units) was dissolved in 25 mL of distilled water, and a half equimolar amount of $NaIO_4$ sodium periodate (0.6 g, 6 mmol) to fructose-repeating unit of inulin was added to the inulin suspension and stirred at 25 °C. The molar ratio of fructose-repeating units of raw inulin to $NaIO_4$ was 2:1, which was expected to give a theoretical degree of oxidation (DO) of 50%. The periodate oxidation reaction was protected from light by carrying out the reaction in the dark and at room temperature. The reaction was allowed to proceed for different times (2 h, 3 h, 4 h, 15 h, and 20 h) in order to investigate the effect of reaction time on the oxidation process. The reaction was terminated by adding an excess quantity of ethylene glycol (molar ratio of 3:1 to $NaIO_4$). Then, the reaction mixture was purified using a simple dialysis membrane bag in milliQ water for 3 days [52]. During the dialysis process, the water was changed daily, and the final oxidized inulin product (a white fluffy product) was obtained after freeze-drying the resulting solution.

2.3. Determination of the Degree of Oxidation (Aldehyde Content Analysis)

2.3.1. Determination of Degree of Oxidation

The number of aldehyde functional groups obtained from the periodate oxidation reaction, referred to as the degree of oxidation, was quantified using hydroxylamine titration [53] and ^{1}H NMR spectroscopy after reaction with tBC [41,54].

Hydroxylamine Titration

The reaction of hydroxylamine with oxidized inulin results in the formation of oximes and hydrochloric acid [53]. The released HCl was then quantified by titration with sodium hydroxide. For the hydroxylamine hydrochloride titration method, an accurately weighed amount of about 50.0 mg of each freeze-dried oxidized inulin sample was dissolved in 20 mL of 0.25 N hydroxylamine hydrochloride solution–methyl orange solution, and the pH was adjusted to 4.5 before use. The resulting mixture was allowed to react for 24 h with continuous stirring, resulting in the formation of oximes and hydrochloric acid. The released hydrochloric acid was then titrated with a standardized 0.5 mol/L NaOH solution, while the progress of the titration was monitored with a pH meter and visual observation of the color change until a red-to-yellow endpoint was achieved. The change in pH and the volume of sodium hydroxide consumed was recorded. Inulin oxidation using periodate produces two equivalent aldehyde groups for each mole of periodate consumed [51]. The related reactions and calculation formulas are as follows:

$$INU\text{-}(CHO)n + NH_2OH \cdot HCL \rightarrow INU\text{-}(CH=N\text{-}OH)n + nH_2O + nHCL$$

$$HCL + NaOH \rightarrow NaCL + H_2O.$$

The degree of oxidation can be calculated from the formula below:

$$\frac{\text{The volume of NaOH consumed} \times \text{Concentration (NaOH)} \times 10^{-3}}{\text{Weight of the sample (g)} \times \text{Molecular Weight of inulin}} = \frac{\text{Mol of aldehyde}}{\text{Mol of inulin}} \quad (1)$$

^{1}H NMR Spectroscopy after Titration with tBC

The degree of oxidation was also characterized using the ^{1}H NMR spectroscopy method previously reported by Maia et al. [41]. In this method, a mixture of about 20 mg of oxidized inulin samples dissolved in about 3 mL of sodium acetate buffer with pH 5.0 (acidic condition) was reacted with excess tBC (81.278 mg) at room temperature for 24 h. Thereafter, the unreacted tBC was removed using dialysis. The resulting solution was then freeze-dried, and the ^{1}H NMR spectroscopy spectrum was obtained using DMSO-d_6 solvent. The ^{1}H NMR spectroscopy method used in this experiment enables the quantification of the degree of oxidation (aldehyde content of the oxidized inulin) by comparing the ratio of the integral peak (δ) at 7.2 ppm belonging to the proton of the carbazone group to the glucose anomeric proton from inulin at δ 5.2 ppm. This method provides a similar result to that of colorimetric titration in the case of oxidized dextran. However, the formation of precipitates with highly oxidized sugar may limit the application of this method [41]. Using ^{1}H NMR, the degree of oxidation of inulin can be determined using the equation below:

$$\text{The degree of oxidation} = \frac{A \times 100}{B} \qquad (2)$$

where A represents the integral peak (δ) at 7.2 ppm from the carbazone proton and B is the integral of the glucose anomeric proton at 5.2 ppm.

2.4. Preparation and Characterization of Hydrogels (Wissembourg, France)

The oxidized inulin (Oxi-4h) was dissolved in PBS (pH 7.4) to obtain a 6% (w/v) polysaccharide concentration [47]. AAD was also dissolved in PBS solution (pH 7.4) in order to obtain 2.5%, 5%, and 10% concentration. Finally, 800 µL of oxidized inulin solution was mixed with 200 µL of each different concentration of the AAD solution to form hydrogels [47]. The crosslinking of the hydrogels was allowed to proceed at 37 °C. Three hydrogels were formed using a different amount of crosslinker, namely INUAAD2.5, INUAAD5, and INUAAD10, corresponding to the gel obtained with 2.5%, 5% and 10% of crosslinker, respectively. The synthesized hydrogels were soaked in de-ionized water for 1 day in order to remove any unbound crosslinker and other unreacted reagents before freeze-drying.

2.5. Characterization of Oxidized Polymer and Hydrogels: FTIR and ^{1}H NMR

The modification of the vicinal hydroxyl groups in inulin into aldehyde functional groups was confirmed by ^{1}H NMR (Bruker Avance III 500 NMR, Wissembourg, France) and FTIR spectrophotometer (Shimadzu IRPrestige-21 FTIR 8400 spectrophotometer, Kyoto, Japan). The FTIR spectra of all the oxidized samples and hydrogels were acquired using a Schimadzu FTIR spectrophotometer in the region of 4000–400 cm^{-1} by recording 128 scans with a resolution of 4 cm^{-1}. Briefly, about 2 mg of the freeze-dried samples and hydrogels were ground into powder before being mixed with about 100 mg of KBr and pressed into pellets using a hydraulic press. The ^{1}H NMR spectra were acquired with a Brucker NMR spectrometer using a 5-mm broadband NMR probe, and DMSO was used as the solvent for all the samples except where stated otherwise.

2.6. Characterization of Hydrogels: TGA

Based on preliminary characterization, oxidized inulin obtained after 4 h of oxidation time was selected for further characterization and for hydrogel fabrication. About 6 ± 0.1 mg of each freeze-dried sample of oxidized inulin, crosslinker (AAD), and the hydrogels (INUAAD2.5, INUAAD5, and INUAAD10) were accurately weighed, and thermal gravimetric analysis was carried out in a TA Instrument (Thermogravimetric Analyzer Discovery TGA 550, New Castle, DE, USA) by heating the sample from 25 to 500 °C at a heating rate of 10 °C/min under a nitrogen atmosphere (10 mL min^{-1}).

2.7. Characterization of Hydrogels: DSC

Differential scanning (DSC) of the synthesized inulin hydrogels (INUAAD2.5, INUAAD5, and INUAAD10), AAD, and the modified inulin was investigated using a Discovery DSC TA Instrument (model Discovery DSC 2920, New Castle, DE, USA). Briefly, ~2 ± 0.1 mg of each freeze-dried sample was weighed accurately in a platinum cup before being heated from 25 to 250 °C in a nitrogen atmosphere at a rate of 10 °C/min.

2.8. Rheological Evaluation

The rheological measurement of the synthesized inulin hydrogel was carried out using a rheometer (Malvern Kinexus pro+ Rotational, Worcestershire, UK) with parallel plates (diameter, 25-mm steel). In order to investigate the viscoelastic behavior of the hydrogels, the procured hydrogel was placed between the parallel plates with a gap of 1 mm in oscillatory mode while maintaining the temperature at 37 °C. Prior to rheological analysis, the inulin hydrogel was procured at 37 °C and allowed to stand for 30 min before testing. In order to ensure that all measurement was within the viscoelastic region, prior to the start of the frequency sweep experiments, a strain sweep was conducted using 1.0-Hz frequency and 0.1% strain. Thereafter, storage modulus (G') and loss modulus (G'') of the inulin hydrogels were determined using a frequency sweep test from 0.1 to 10 Hz and controlled strain (γ = 0.01).

2.9. Scanning Electron Microscope (SEM) Analysis

SEM imaging was conducted using FEI Quanta 450 FEG Environmental SEM (FEI, Hillsboro, OR, USA). Before the imaging process, the fully swollen hydrogels in sodium acetate buffer (pH 5.0) and PBS buffer (pH 7.4) were frozen using liquid nitrogen before freeze-drying to ensure that the morphology of the hydrogels was preserved. The freeze-dried hydrogels (INUAAD2.5, INUAAD5, and INUAAD10) were then transferred to double-sided tape before being sputter-coated with 10 mm of palladium, and the morphology was viewed using FEI Quanta 450 FEG Environmental SEM at an accelerated voltage of 10 KV. Furthermore, the pore size was determined from the SEM micrographs using image J software 1.49 v from the National Institutes of Health, Bethesda, MD, USA.

2.10. Dynamic Swelling Experiments: Swelling Analysis

The swelling properties of the hydrogels (INUAAD2.5, INUAAD5, and INUAAD10) were determined by the gravimetry method. Briefly, dry inulin hydrogel was weighed (Wd) before being immersed in deionized water and PBS buffer solution (pH 7.4) until the equilibrium swelling was reached, after which the hydrogels were removed. Excess surface water on the hydrogels was then blotted with the use of tissue paper before the swollen hydrogel was finally weighed. All the swelling experiments were performed in triplicate and at 37 °C. Finally, the equilibrium swelling ratio and percentage of swelling were calculated from Equations (3) and (4), respectively:

$$\text{Equilibrium swelling ratio of the hydrogel} = \frac{(Ws - Wd)}{Wd} \quad (3)$$

$$\%S = \frac{(Ws - Wd) \times 100}{Wd} \quad (4)$$

where Ws represents the final weight of the fully swollen hydrogel and Wd is the dry weight of the hydrogel before swelling.

2.11. Release Kinetics of 5FU from Crosslinked Hydrogels

The encapsulation of 5FU to the hydrogels was accomplished during the crosslinking of the hydrogels. Briefly, 0.8 mL of oxidized inulin solution was mixed with 1 mg of 5FU before crosslinking this mixture with 0.2 mL of AAD, and subsequently, the mixture was incubated at 37 °C. The 5FU in the hydrogels was fixed at 1 mg/mL, and subsequently, the hydrogels were freeze-dried to obtain dried powder. Furthermore, the in vitro release experiment was carried out using the obtained freeze-dried powder. The release experiment was performed at physiological body temperature 37 °C in a 50-mL falcon tube. Then, 10 mL of release medium (phosphate buffer at pH 7.4 or sodium acetate buffer at pH 5.0) was added with constant stirring at 50 RPM. At scheduled time intervals, about 500 µL of the release aliquot was collected from the release medium, and the 5FU concentration in this aliquot was assayed using the HPLC method previously reported [55]. The HPLC system (Shimadzu Corporation, Kyoto, Japan) consisted of a pump (LC-20ADXR), an autosampler, a photodiode array (PDA) detector set to 268 nm, and a column for separation (Agilent Zorbax 300–SCX C18, 250 mm × 4.6 mm, 5 μm, Agilent Technologies Australia, Mulgrave, Victoria, Australia). The mobile phase for the HPLC assay was 10% acetonitrile and 90% water, and the flow rate was maintained at 0.9 mL/min in isocratic mode [55]. The injection volume of 5FU into the HPLC was 20 μL, the run time was 6 min, and the retention time for the 5FU peak was 3.061 min. The concentration of analytes was diluted to ensure that they fall within the standard calibration curve concentration range. A linear calibration curve of 5FU was plotted in the concentration range of 0.1–10 μg/mL ($R^2 > 0.999$). All measurements were conducted in triplicate.

2.12. Degradation Studies

The degradation studies of the fabricated inulin hydrogels (INUAAD2.5, INUAAD5, and INUAAD10) were conducted in PBS (pH 7.4) without inulinase enzyme [49]. In addition, the in vitro degradation of the inulin hydrogels in the presence of inulinase was also investigated by immersing the three different hydrogels (INUAAD2.5, INUAAD5, and INUAAD10) into sodium acetate buffer (pH 5.0) containing 10 units inulinase/mL [36]. Inulinase was chosen because this enzyme is specifically expressed by the colon and is capable of degrading inulin polysaccharide [56–58]. In brief, dry inulin hydrogels (0.050 g) were added into 5 mL of the medium (PBS or acetate), followed by incubation at 37 °C with and without inulinase enzyme. At a predetermined time interval, the hydrogels were removed from the falcon tube and washed with water to remove any remnant of the enzyme. Finally, the remaining hydrogels were dried and weighed, and the weight was recorded as Wdt. All the experiments were performed in triplicate.

The degradation of the hydrogels was determined using Equation (5) below:

$$\% \text{ Degradation} = \frac{(Wd - Wdt) \times 100}{Wd} \quad (5)$$

where Wd and Wdt are the initial starting weights before and after degradation, respectively.

2.13. MTT Assay

The cytotoxicity of the synthesized inulin hydrogels and drug-loaded hydrogels were investigated against HCT116 human colorectal carcinoma cell lines (a gift from Professor Shudong of Wang Laboratory) using 3-(4,5-dimethylthiazol-2-yl)-2,5-diphenyl-tetrazolium bromide blue-indicator dye (MTT assay). First, HCT116 cancer cell lines were seeded in 96-well plates at 3×10^3 cells per well, maintained under the expected standard growth condition (37 °C, 5% CO_2, 10% FBS containing McCoy's 5A (Modified) Medium), and incubated for 24 h to allow for proper cell attachment. Subsequently, the drug-loaded hydrogels and blank inulin hydrogels were sterilized for 15 min using an ultraviolet ray. This was followed by rinsing with sterile PBS. Then, 5 mL of McCoy's 5A (Modified) Medium was added into the sterile hydrogel, and it was shaken for 24 h. Thereafter, the hydrogel was removed, and the resulting extracts were filtered using a 0.22-mm syringe. For the MTT assay, cells were incubated for 24 h with a free 5FU solution and the sterilized extracts from the hydrogels after diluting with McCoy's 5A (Modified) Medium to obtain concentrations of 10, 50, and 100 μg/mL [59–61]. This incubation process was followed by washing with PBS, and then, the cells were further treated with 5 mg/mL of MTT solution at 37 °C for 4 h. The culture medium containing MTT reagent was removed, and 0.1 mL of DMSO was added. Finally, the absorbance of the resulting solution was measured at 570 nm using a microplate reader.

3. Results and Discussion

The vicinal hydroxyl groups on inulin were oxidized using sodium periodate, resulting in a highly reactive hemiacetal aldehyde derivative that subsequently reacted with adipic acid dihydrazide to form an inulin hydrogel via a hydrazone bond. Scheme 1 shows the oxidation of inulin by $NaIO_4$ to create two aldehyde functional groups. Note that there is a chance of double oxidation from the glucose end group with the subsequent release of formic acid. However, this would likely represent a small portion of the polyaldehyde formed. This periodate oxidation occurred in an aqueous medium without utilizing any catalyst or any chemical initiator. The oxidation involved breaking the C3–C4 bond, resulting in two aldehyde groups [51], which then crosslinked with AAD to form a hydrogel. Prior studies suggest that one of the reactive aldehyde functional groups at C_3 can undergo a reaction with the neighboring C_6 hydroxyl group, which ultimately leads to the formation of stable intra-residue and inter-residue hemiacetals [62,63]. The stable hemiacetal could restrict the aldehyde functional groups available for nucleophilic reaction to one per fructose residue [51].

During the early stages of the reaction (the first 10 min), an aldehyde functional group peak with very low intensity was observed around 9.5 ppm (Supplementary Materials Figure S1). This peak was not observed at the end of the reaction, possibly suggesting that a masked aldehyde group was involved in the formation of hemiacetals as the reaction progressed. The formation of hemiacetals was further supported by the appearance of a new peak in the ^{1}H NMR spectra of the oxidized samples, with several distinctive peaks in the region of 3.5–5.0 ppm that were not present in the original raw inulin sample (Figure 1A,B). This result helps confirm that raw inulin was modified. (Supplementary Materials Figures S2 and S3A–E). The ^{1}H NMR spectra of the oxidized inulin samples show visible change with the increase in time of the reaction from 2 to 20 h. (Supplementary Materials Figure S3A–E). The formation of hemiacetals, as shown in Figure 1B, is consistent with reports in the literature regarding some oxidized polysaccharides, such as dextran [41,64], cellulose [65], hyaluronic acid [48], alginate [66], starch, pectin, and chitosan [67]. There was rapid release of formic acid, possibly from the oxidation of the reducing end glucose as the reaction proceeded, resulting in a pH drop from 4.15 to 3.88; however, as the reaction proceeded the pH of the reaction medium remained stable at 3.88 for the remaining part of the reaction process (Figure 1D and Supplementary Materials Figure S1). The hemiacetals are behind the disappearance of the aldehyde functional group formed during oxidation.

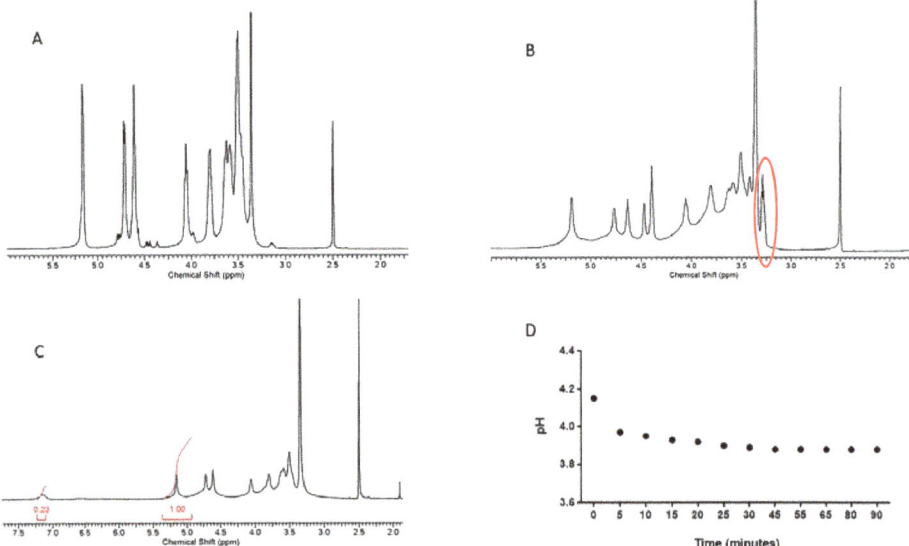

Figure 1. The ^{1}H NMR spectra of (**A**) raw inulin, (**B**) oxidized inulin 2 h (Oxi-2h), and (**C**) oxidized inulin after titration with tert-butyl carbazate (tBC) using DMSO solvent; (**D**) the variation of pH during the oxidation of inulin with periodate. (Red circle show appearance of new peaks after oxidation).

3.1. Oxidized Inulin Characterization

The oxidized inulin derivative was also characterized using ^{1}H NMR spectroscopy. From Figure 1C showing the ^{1}H NMR spectrum of raw inulin, peaks between δ 3.0–4.80 ppm were assigned to fructose and glucose carbon-attached protons except for the anomeric proton from glucose that occurs at 5.2 ppm. The quantification of aldehyde groups, i.e., degree of oxidation (DO), was evaluated using tBC. The aldehyde content of the modified inulin was also investigated using ^{1}H NMR spectroscopy by taking advantage of the reaction of the aldehydes with carbazate to form stable carbazones in same way as in hydrazone formation [41].

As shown in Figure 1C, the formation of carbazone shows that the reactive aldehyde portion of the oxidized inulin reacted with the amine portion of the tBC with evidence of a peak around 7.2 ppm. It is suggested that this peak resulted from the proton attached to the carbon atom modified by reacting the oxidized sample with tBC. Furthermore, there was evidence of the disappearance of peaks attributed to some of the hemiacetals after the formation of the final product. Comparing the carbazone integral's peak δ at 7.2 ppm to that of the glucose anomeric proton at δ 5.2 ppm allowed DO quantification using ^{1}H NMR spectroscopy (Figure 1A and Supplementary Materials Figure S5A–C). The DO of oxidized inulin (oxi-inu) 15 h and 20 h was not assayed by ^{1}H NMR because of the slight oxidation of the anomeric glucose after the long oxidation period, making quantification difficult and inaccurate. Hydroxylamine titration converted the aldehydes into oximes with the release of acid quantified via a titrimetric method. The volume of sodium hydroxide at the endpoint was determined using the first derivative curve of the titration between sodium hydroxide and hydrochloric acid. The result of the ^{1}H NMR spectroscopy for the oxidized inulin samples was lower than the result obtained from the hydroxylamine titration. The slight difference in the DO for the oxidized inulin samples (Table 1) can possibly be attributed to precipitation of the samples by the bulky tBC, as well as the pH of the reaction medium [51,68].

Table 1. The aldehyde content determination using ^{1}H NMR spectroscopy and hydroxylamine titration.

Oxidized Inulin	The Degree of Oxidation by Hydroxylamine (%) [a]	The Degree of Oxidation by NMR (%) [b]
Oxi-2h	25.6 ± 0.6	23 ± 0.9
Oxi-3h	31 ± 0.8	26 ± 0.7
Oxi-4h	34 ± 0.3	31 ± 1.2
Oxi-15h	38 ± 0.4	n
Oxi-20h	43.6 ± 0.5	n

[a] The results of all titration experiments were the average of three titrations; [b] ^{1}H NMR results calculated from four independent integrations with Advanced Chemistry Development (ACD) software; [n] not estimated.

3.2. FTIR

In order to investigate the changes and alterations to the inulin structure as a result of the periodate oxidation, both the raw inulin and modified samples were analyzed using FTIR. Despite the oxidation reaction, the inulin structure was partly preserved. Figure 2A shows the FTIR spectra of the raw inulin and modified inulin samples with different degrees of oxidation based on the reaction time. In Figure 2A, it is difficult to see any difference between the oxidized and raw inulin. However, for the highly oxidized inulin samples (oxi-15h and oxi-20h) there was a low-intensity signal at 1730 cm^{-1} ascribed to the stretching of the carbonyl group from an aldehyde [69]. In addition, there were several changes in the position of the bands, especially in the region of 1300–800 cm^{-1} for the oxidized inulin compared with the raw inulin (Supplementary Materials Figure S6A). The formation of hemiacetals made it difficult to notice any aldehyde groups in the oxidized sample [41], and this is consistent with the reported FTIR of oxidized polysaccharides, such as dextran [41] and alginates [52,70].

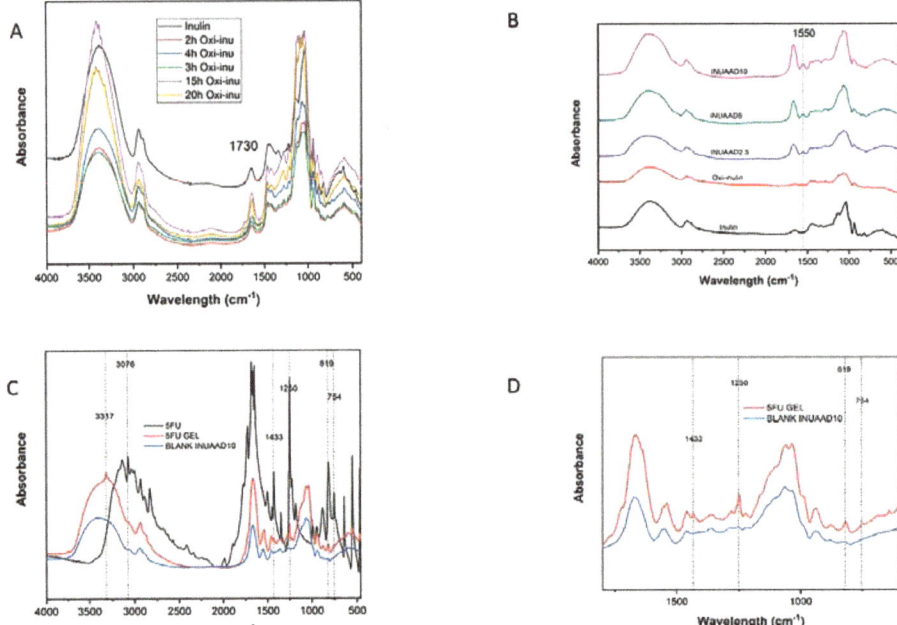

Figure 2. (**A**) The spectra of all the oxi-inulin and raw inulin samples. (**B**) The spectra of inulin, oxidized inulin (oxi-inulin), and the hydrogels. (**C**) Spectra of pure 5-fluorouracil (5FU), blank INUAAD10 gel, and 5FU-loaded hydrogel. (**D**) spectra of blank INUAAD10 and 5FU-loaded hydrogel.

The formation of the hydrogels by crosslinking oxidized inulin with AAD was confirmed by FTIR spectroscopy (Figure 2B). The spectra of the hydrogels show the appearance of the new band at 1550 cm^{-1}, which can be attributed to the NH bending from the crosslinker (AAD). The 5FU-loaded inulin hydrogels were also characterized using FTIR (Figure 2C,D). The FTIR spectra of the 5FU-loaded inulin hydrogels reveal small changes compared with the blank inulin hydrogels, including new bands at 3076, 1433, 1246, 819, and 754 cm^{-1} [71], which were attributed to the incorporation of 5FU. Furthermore, the change in the broad peak of the blank gels compared with that of the 5FU-loaded gels was presumably due to the hydrogen bonding interaction between the OH of the hydrogel and the NH stretching of 5FU, resulting in the formation of a sharp peak around 3317 cm^{-1} [71,72] (Figure 2C). The disappearance of some typical 5FU peaks can also be attributed to the strong hydrogen bond interactions between the blank gels and 5FU (Figure 2C,D and Supplementary Materials Figure S6B,C).

3.3. SEM

The interior morphologies of the fabricated inulin hydrogels, as well as their porous structures, were evaluated by SEM. Figure 3A,B clearly shows that the freeze-dried hydrogels (INUAAD2.5, INUAAD5, and INUAAD10) had irregular, interconnecting inner pores. It is evident that the pore size of the hydrogels decreased with the increase in AAD, as higher concentrations of AAD resulted in higher crosslink density, producing gels with smaller pore size. SEM was also able to show the pore size variation and hydrolysis of the hydrazone bond when the gels were immersed in acetate buffer (pH 5.0) as compared with PBS (pH 7.4) for 2 days. The SEM images confirm the slight degradation of the hydrogels in acetate buffer due to the hydrolysis of the bonds, as well as the increase in pore size (Figure 3A). The formation of porous materials has also been reported for other oxidized polysaccharides crosslinked with AAD in the literature [41,50], and pore formation with controllable pore size is important for drug encapsulation and delivery of drugs such as 5FU.

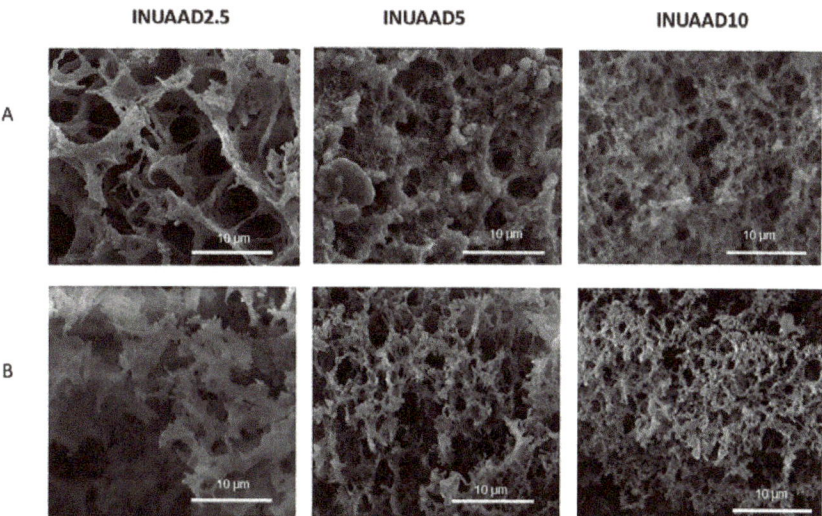

Figure 3. (**A**) SEM images of hydrogels (INUAAD2.5, INUAAD5, and INUAAD10) after immersion in acetate buffer for 2 days. (**B**) SEM images of hydrogels (INUAAD2.5, INUAAD5, and INUAAD10) after immersion in phosphate-buffered saline (PBS) for 2 days.

3.4. TGA/First derivative of the TGA Curve (DTG)

The thermal stability of the raw inulin, oxidized inulin, AAD, and hydrogels was assessed using TGA/DTG. As shown in Figure 4A,B, the crosslinker showed higher thermal stability compared with oxidized inulin. The TGA curve for AAD shows an onset of degradation at 282 °C, and raw inulin showed slight weight loss due to the elimination of water at a temperature below 100 °C and major weight loss occurring between 225 and 325 °C, which was attributed to inulin backbone degradation [73]. There was a clear shift in the onset temperature for degradation from 215 °C for raw inulin to 192 °C for oxidized inulin (reduced by 25 °C), and there was a different character of the thermogram that can be attributed to the damage to the raw inulin chain caused by its oxidation [74–77]. After crosslinking the oxidized inulin with AAD, the thermal stability of the synthesized hydrogels was enhanced and improved compared with the oxidized inulin, as seen in the TGA and DTG curve (Figure 4C). This was due to formation of a stable hydrazone bond and strong hydrogen bonding interactions introduced onto the molecular chain [78–80]. As expected, the hydrogels exhibited three stage mass loss. Below 100 °C, there was the removal of bound and free water in the hydrogels (about 7% weight loss). The second weight loss was due to the decomposition of the inulin backbone, and finally, the third stage was due to the degradation of the AAD. Increasing the AAD concentration during crosslinking resulted in hydrogels with higher decomposition temperature. The maximum thermal decomposition temperature for the hydrogels was found to be 218.4, 225.9, and 227.5 °C for the three hydrogel samples, INUAAD2.5, INUAAD5, and INUAAD10, respectively. The corresponding residual weight at 600 °C for the INUAAD2.5, INUAAD5, and INUAAD10 hydrogels was 17.2%, 3.02%, and 1.55% respectively. It is important to mention that all the oxi-inu hydrogels showed a similar degradation profile (Figure 4D). Proof of crosslinking between the modified oxidized inulin and AAD was confirmed by the change in the maximum temperature of degradation of the hydrogels when compared with that of the oxidized inulin.

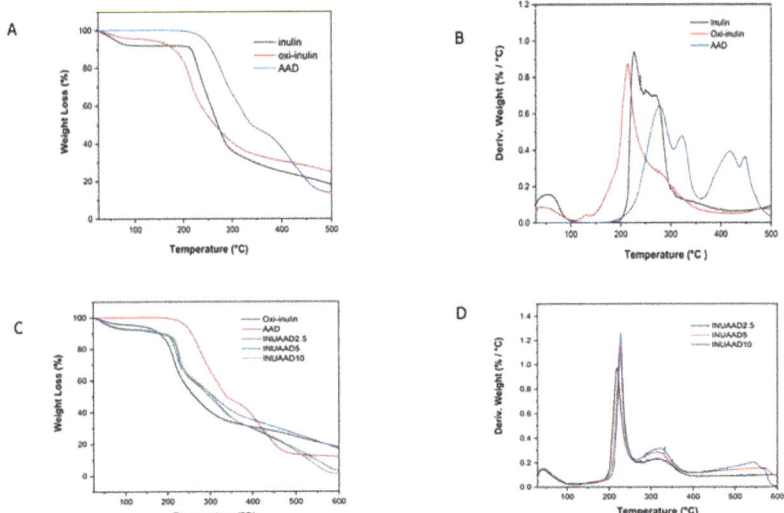

Figure 4. (**A**) Thermograms of the raw inulin, oxidized inulin, and AAD. (**B**) DTG thermograms of the raw inulin, oxidized inulin, and AAD. (**C**) Thermograms of the raw inulin, oxidized inulin, AAD, and hydrogels. (**D**) DTG thermograms of the hydrogels.

3.5. DSC

The DSC of the oxidized inulin, AAD, and hydrogels was also investigated (Figure 5A,B). As shown in the DSC thermogram, the melting point peak of the oxidized inulin was 161.3 °C, and the melting point of AAD was 183.22 °C. However, these peaks were absent in the final hydrogels, indicating the formation of new crosslinked polymeric material. In Figure 5B, the hydrogels exhibited endothermic peaks at 166, 164, and 160 °C for INUAAD2.5, INUAAD5.0, and INUAAD10 respectively, due to degradation of the hydrazone bond [16,81]. Interestingly, as the amount of AAD increased, the temperature of the endothermic peak decreased. In addition, there was a broad exothermic transition for all the hydrogels after the degradation of the hydrazone bond. Another endothermic peak at 196.96, 199.42, and 200.26 °C for INUAAD2.5, INUAAD5.0, and INUAAD10, respectively, can be seen in Figure 5B, which was attributed to the start of the hydrogel degradation. It is very clear that the degradation temperature was dependent on the crosslinking density.

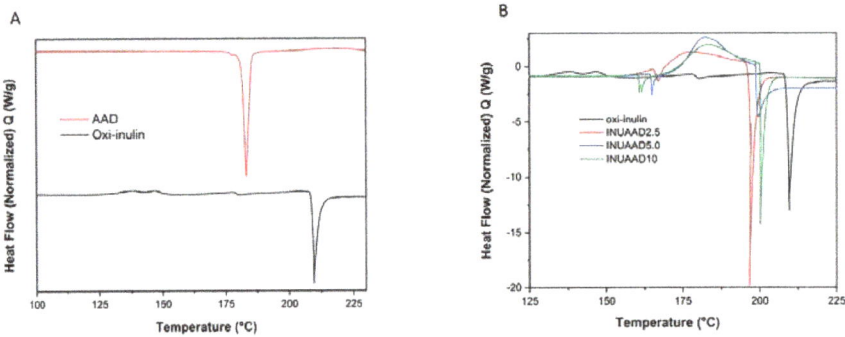

Figure 5. (**A**) Differential scanning calorimetry (DSC) thermograms of the oxidized inulin and AAD; (**B**) thermograms of the oxidized inulin and hydrogels.

3.6. Rheological Properties

As shown in Figure 6A,B, all three fabricated inulin hydrogels, INUAAD2.5, INUAAD5, and INUAAD10, showed higher G' compared with the G" for all the frequencies tested using the frequency sweep mode. As shown in Figure 5A, it is obvious that the G' increased with the increase in the concentration of the crosslinker from 2.5% to 10%, whereas there was little change with respect to G". By increasing the crosslinker from 2.5% to 10%, the G' increased from ca. 711 to 3015 (Pa) at a frequency of 1 Hz (Supplementary Materials Table S1). This increase in G' indicates that a stiff and highly crosslinked gel was formed at high AAD concentration [48]. These results indicate that the fabricated hydrogels possessed viscoelastic properties [52,82]. All the hydrogels exhibited high G' value, which was independent of the frequency that is indicative of a gel with stable viscoelastic solid-like behavior [52]. In addition, all the synthesized inulin hydrogels had similar loss moduli. The difference in elastic moduli also shows that the crosslinking density for the gels differed. This result corroborates the finding that, by varying crosslinker concentration, we can synthesize hydrogels with different degrees of crosslinking. The rheology measurements, particularly the elastic moduli of all the hydrogels, as well as the crosslink density, had a direct correlation to the content of AAD used during crosslinking.

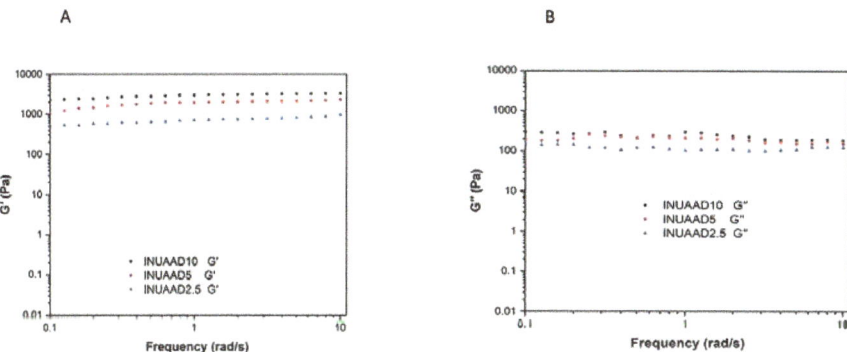

Figure 6. (A) Rheological properties of the INUAAD hydrogels showing the storage moduli (G') and (B) the loss moduli (G") of the different crosslinked inulin hydrogels.

3.7. Gelation and Swelling Studies

The swelling ratio of the fabricated inulin hydrogels in de-ionized water and PBS (pH 7.4) (Supplementary Materials Figure S7) shows a higher swelling ratio (SR) in de-ionized water compared with PBS, as expected. The gels showed moderate swelling in water, with a swelling ratio of 6.95, 5.61, and 3.8 for INUAAD2.5, INUAAD5, and INUAAD10, respectively. The result demonstrates that the swelling ratio of the hydrogels was inversely related to the degree of crosslinking. Furthermore, all the hydrogels reached equilibrium before 24 h, which can help facilitate the diffusion and release of drug molecules from such hydrogels. The SR obtained was comparable to pH-sensitive inulin hydrogels with reported values from 3.5 to 6.5 [19,37] but lower than inulin hydrogels made from pyromellitic dianhydride crosslinker [16]. The SR was also lower than the values reported for oxidized dextran crosslinked with AAD (4.3–8.7) [41] and polyaldehyde guluronate (12.6–15.3) [69]. The gelation time for the fabricated hydrogels obtained by the tube inversion method was directly related to the concentration of AAD used during hydrogel synthesis. The gelation time was reduced from 178 to 128 s with an increase in AAD concentration, which was very close to those reported for oxidized hyaluronic acid/adipic acid dihydrazide hydrogels (143–175 s) [48] and oxidized dextran/AAD gels (117–230 s) [41]. By controlling the amount of AAD used, we can easily tune the gelation time. As the concentration of AAD used during the hydrogel fabrication increases, the time required for the formation of the hydrogel decreases, which is attributed to the higher percentage of hydrazide available for effective crosslinking.

3.8. Release Kinetics of 5FU from Crosslinked Hydrogels

The drug delivery capability of the fabricated inulin hydrogels was further evaluated using 5FU as the model drug for in vitro release. The in vitro release results show that the amount of 5FU released can be tuned by varying the crosslinker ratio. The release of 5FU was initially characterized by burst release, which was subsequently followed by sustained release, as expected. In this study, the hydrogels with hydrazone linkages allowed faster cleavage at low acidic pH. The inulin hydrogel system exploited acidic pH around colon cancer tissues to achieve better drug release properties. Overall the release profile of 5FU from the crosslinked hydrogels was governed by both the pH of the release medium and the crosslinking density. As shown in Figure 7A,B, as expected, all the hydrogels demonstrated faster drug release in pH 5.0 than in pH 7.4. The hydrazone bond of the inulin hydrogels was relatively stable in physiological pH but was cleaved in acidic pH. As shown in Figure 7A,B, there was a burst release in both pH 5 and 7.4 on the first day, which was followed by a very slow release of 5FU. In the release study, 50%, 38%, and 35% of 5FU was released from INUAAD2.5, INUAAD5.0, and INUAAD10, respectively, in pH 7.4 after 24 h. In contrast, in the acidic media with pH 5.0, after 24 h, 68%, 47%, and 38% of 5FU was released from INUAAD2.5, INUAAD5.0, and INUAAD10, respectively. Moreover, after the initial burst release in pH 5.0, there was a continuous release of 5FU, with about 85% of 5FU released within 2 days for INUAAD2.5. The gels showed higher release in pH 5.0 compared with physiological pH 7.4.

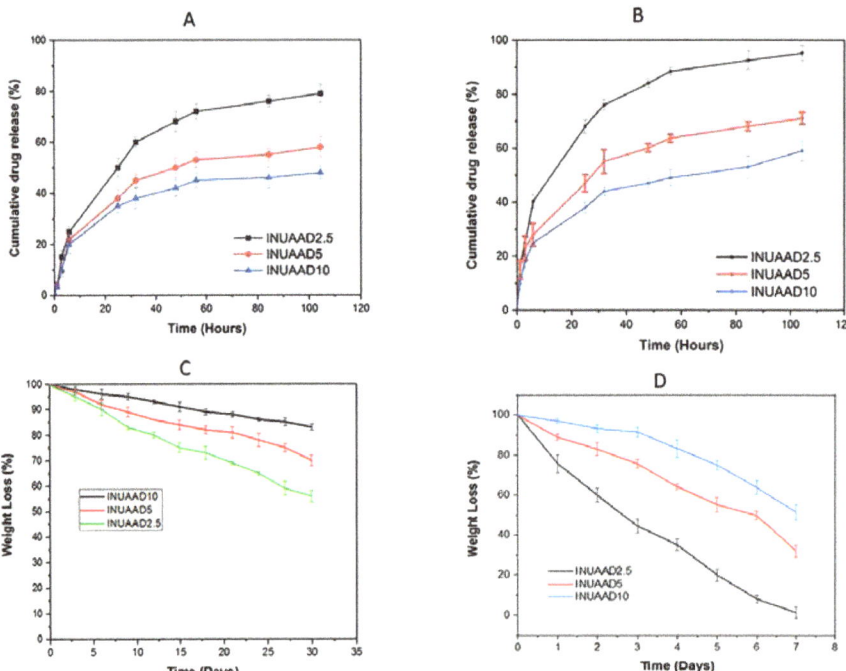

Figure 7. (**A**) The in vitro release rate of 5FU from the hydrogel batches in pH 7.4; (**B**) the in vitro release rate of 5FU from the hydrogel batches in pH 5.0; (**C**) the degradation of the hydrogels in pH 7.4; (**D**) the degradation of the hydrogels in pH 5.0 with the addition of inulinase.

The release of 5FU from the hydrogels was dependent on the crosslinking density and pH of the release media. The FTIR result for the 5FU-loaded hydrogels show that the 5FU amine group and inulin polymer hydroxyl may have formed a hydrogen bond interaction [71,83,84]. This polymer–drug interaction may have resulted in slow drug release from the hydrogel due to entrapment of the remaining drug in the gel network (Figure 2C,D). The smaller pore size allowed the encapsulation of structurally smaller drug moieties, such as 5FU, into the hydrogels [71]. The difference in the stability of the hydrazone bond in pH 7.4 compared with pH 5.0 was exploited for selective and localized targeting of 5FU between colon normal and cancers cells. The difference performance with respect to pH enables the use of this hydrogel as a useful strategy for delivering 5FU to the colon. This result clearly suggests that the acidic environment within colon cancer cells would trigger the degradation of the crosslinked hydrogel, which would result in a higher drug release from the hydrogel. This hydrogel system can potentially maintain a higher concentration of drugs around cancer cells and can possibly reduce adverse side effects on healthy tissue. In order to achieve successful colon targeting, the inulin drug delivery system will require enteric coating to prevent gastric degradation and premature release of drugs as the hydrogel passes through the stomach and small intestine.

3.9. Degradation

The degradation rate of the hydrogels was investigated by examining the weight loss in both PBS and acetate buffer, as shown in Figure 7C,D. INUAAD10, INUAAD5.0, and INUAAD2.5 experienced weight loss of 17%, 30%, and 44%, respectively, in PBS after 30 days of incubating, implying that a higher concentration of the crosslinker results in higher resistance to biodegradability. In addition, the in vitro degradation of the inulin hydrogels in the presence of inulinase incubated in sodium acetate buffer (pH 5.0) after one week was 49%, 68%, and 95% degradation for INUAAD10, INUAAD5, and INUAAD2.5, respectively (Figure 7D). Inulinase is known to degrade inulin in the colon and function better around pH 4.7, which is close to pH 5.0 [56]. As shown in Figure 7C,D, the degradation rate decreased with the increase in AAD concentration. This finding could be attributed to the increase in degree of crosslinking, making it harder for the inulinase to attack the hydrogel, as well as the higher hydrazone bond, which tends to be resistant to hydrolytic cleavage. The degradation behavior in acetate buffer was related to the cleavage of the hydrazone bond due to the acidic pH of the medium, as well as partial activity from the enzyme. The hydrogels' degradation was pronounced in acetate buffer with inulinase but slow in physiologic pH conditions. The in vitro degradation data clearly show that it is possible to tune the degradation rate by varying the ratio of the crosslinker. The prolonged degradation profile of these hydrogels make them useful for controlled delivery of drugs to the colon.

3.10. Cytotoxicity

The blank crosslinked inulin hydrogels were assayed against the HCT116 cancer cell line using MTT assay, because the application of the synthesized inulin hydrogel as a drug delivery carrier requires the biomaterials to be non-toxic and the 5FU-loaded inulin hydrogels were expected to cause high cytotoxicity to tumor cells. The cell cytotoxicity of different concentrations of extracts from the crosslinked inulin hydrogels, oxidized inulin, and crosslinker was evaluated. As shown in Figure 8A, the viabilities of HCT116 with different extracts of empty inulin hydrogel samples were all above 85% after 24 h of incubation, which clearly demonstrates that these hydrogels were biocompatible with negligible cytotoxicity at concentrations between 10 and 100 µg/mL and that they can be utilized as a delivery platform to deliver drugs to the colon.

In Figure 8A, we can clearly observe, as expected, a dose-dependent decrease in the cell viability as the concentration of the sample increased from 10 to 100 µg/mL with respect to the hydrogel extracts. The blank crosslink hydrogels did not have any appreciable cytotoxicity towards the HCT116 cancer cells. As expected, after 24 h of incubation, both the modified inulin with the aldehyde functional group and AAD showed reduced cell viability with a viability of 77.1% and 88%, respectively (Supplementary Materials Figure S8). This can be attributed to the reactive aldehyde group in the oxidized inulin, which tends to react to the nucleophilic portion of the cells. In addition, the 5FU-loaded hydrogels were assayed for its antitumor activity against the HCT116 cancer cells via MTT assay, and the free 5FU solution was employed as a control. After 24 h of incubation, the 5FU-loaded hydrogels showed a dose-dependent antitumor effect. Furthermore, the gel with the lowest concentration of crosslinker swelled better in the medium, causing a greater release of 5FU and more activity. As shown in Figure 8B, the cell viability of the 5FU-loaded gels against the HCT116 cell line was 65.2%, 71.1%, and 75.2%, respectively, compared with free 5FU, which was 35.9% at 100 µg/mL concentration. The difference in cell viability between the pure and loaded hydrogels was due to the slow release of 5FU from the hydrogel structure. The free 5FU exhibited more antitumor activity compared with the 5FU-loaded hydrogels. This was expected, because the fabricated hydrogel releases 5FU slowly as and a pH of 7.0 does not break the hydrazone bond of the gel. These results support the finding that inulin hydrogel could be utilized as a delivery platform. Based on these results, we can conclude that extracts obtained from the blank inulin hydrogels did not show any significantly difference from the control in terms of cell viability.

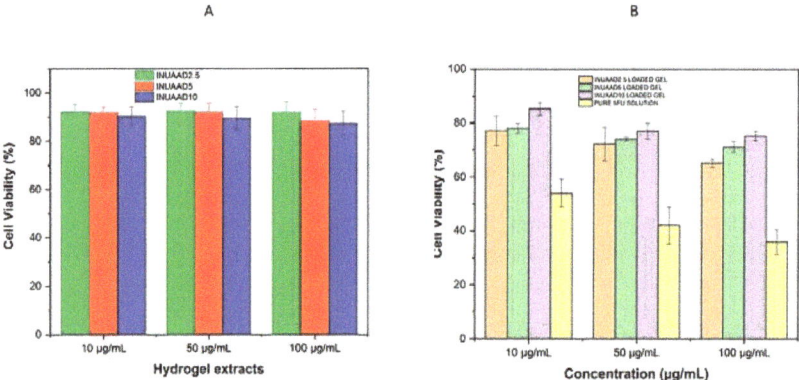

Figure 8. (**A**) Cell viability of the HCT116 cancer cells after treatment with the blank hydrogel extracts, and (**B**) cell viability of HCT116 cancer cells after treatment with the 5FU-loaded hydrogel extracts.

4. Conclusions

New injectable inulin hydrogels based on hydrazone crosslinking for potential use as drug delivery vehicles were fabricated by reacting oxidized inulin with AAD without the use of a catalyst. The novel hydrogels were formed within 2–3 min at 37 °C. The initial degree of oxidation was determined by hydroxylamine titration and ^{1}H NMR spectroscopy, whereas FTIR spectroscopy was used to confirm the covalent crosslinking by AAD with a new band at 1550 cm^{-1}. Changes in thermal properties was detected using DSC and TGA. By varying, the amount of AAD crosslinker used during hydrogel synthesis, the swelling, rheological properties, pore size, degradation, and 5FU release of the hydrogels can be tuned. The in vitro release rate of 5FU from all the hydrogels tested exhibited initial burst release followed by a controlled release pattern. The hydrogels are degradable both hydrolytically in physiologic conditions and by inulinase. In addition, the MTT results confirm that, at a concentration of 10–100 µg/mL, the INUAAD hydrogels showed no appreciable cytotoxicity. These findings demonstrate that these novel hydrogels could serve as delivery systems for anticancer drugs in the treatment of colon cancer.

Supplementary Materials: The Supplementary Materials are available online at http://www.mdpi.com/1999-4923/11/7/356/s1.

Author Contributions: Conceptualization—S.G., T.G.B., and F.A.; method—F.A., T.G.B., S.G., A.P., and Y.S.; investigation–synthesis, characterization, release, and in vitro work—F.A. and P.F.; writing original draft—F.A., P.F., and S.G.; Review and editing and result interpretation—F.A., T.G.B., A.P., Y.S., and S.G.; supervision—Y.S., T.G.B., and S.G., and project administration—S.G.

Acknowledgments: The authors would like to thank Ken Neubauer for help with SEM imaging and Karen Teague for assistance with laboratory set-up.

Conflicts of Interest: This research did not receive any specific grants from funding agencies in the public, commercial, or not-for-profit sectors.

References

1. Mensink, M.A.; Frijlink, H.W.; Maarschalk, K.V.; Hinrichs, W.L. Inulin, a flexible oligosaccharide I: Review of its physicochemical characteristics. *Carbohydr. Polym.* **2015**, *130*, 405–419. [CrossRef] [PubMed]
2. Barclay, T.; Ginic-Markovic, M.; Cooper, P.; Petrovsky, N. Inulin—A versatile polysaccharide with multiple pharmaceutical and food chemical uses. *J. Excip. Food Chem.* **2010**, *1*, 27–50.
3. Flamm, G.; Glinsmann, W.; Kritchevsky, D.; Prosky, L.; Roberfroid, M. Inulin and oligofructose as dietary fiber: A review of the evidence. *Crit. Rev. Food Sci. Nutr.* **2001**, *41*, 353–362. [CrossRef] [PubMed]
4. Roberfroid, M.B.; Delzenne, N.M. Dietary fructans. *Annu. Rev. Nutr.* **1998**, *18*, 117–143. [CrossRef] [PubMed]
5. Maris, B.; Verheyden, L.; van Reeth, K.; Samyn, C.; Augustijns, P.; Kinget, R.; van den Mooter, G. Synthesis and characterisation of inulin-azo hydrogels designed for colon targeting. *Int. J. Pharm.* **2001**, *213*, 143–152. [CrossRef]
6. Keenan, D.F.; Resconi, V.C.; Kerry, J.P.; Hamill, R.M. Modelling the influence of inulin as a fat substitute in comminuted meat products on their physico-chemical characteristics and eating quality using a mixture design approach. *Meat Sci.* **2014**, *96*, 1384–1394. [CrossRef] [PubMed]
7. Furlan, L.T.R.; Padilla, A.P.; Campderros, M.E. Development of reduced fat minced meats using inulin and bovine plasma proteins as fat replacers. *Meat Sci.* **2014**, *96*, 762–768. [CrossRef] [PubMed]
8. Poulain, N.; Dez, I.; Perrio, C.; Lasne, M.C.; Prud'homme, M.P.; Nakache, E. Microspheres based on inulin for the controlled release of serine protease inhibitors: Preparation, characterization and in vitro release. *J. Control Release* **2003**, *92*, 27–38. [CrossRef]
9. Lopez-Molina, D.; Chazarra, S.; How, C.W.; Pruidze, N.; Navarro-Peran, E.; Garcia-Canovas, F.; Garcia-Ruiz, P.A.; Rojas-Melgarejo, F.; Rodriguez-Lopez, J.N. Cinnamate of inulin as a vehicle for delivery of colonic drugs. *Int. J. Pharm.* **2015**, *479*, 96–102. [CrossRef]
10. Vervoort, L.; van den Mooter, G.; Augustijns, P.; Busson, R.; Toppet, S.; Kinget, R. Inulin hydrogels as carriers for colonic drug targeting: I. Synthesis and characterization of methacrylated inulin and hydrogen formation. *Pharm. Res.* **1997**, *14*, 1730–1737. [CrossRef]
11. Vervoort, L.; Vinckier, I.; Moldenaers, P.; van den Mooter, G.; Augustijns, P.; Kinget, R. Inulin hydrogels as carriers for colonic drug targeting. Rheological characterization of the hydrogel formation and the hydrogel network. *J. Pharm. Sci.* **1999**, *8*, 209–214. [CrossRef] [PubMed]
12. Jain, A.K.; Sood, V.; Bora, M.; Vasita, R.; Katti, D.S. Electrosprayed inulin microparticles for microbiota triggered targeting of colon. *Carbohydr. Polym.* **2014**, *112*, 225–234. [CrossRef] [PubMed]
13. Zijlstra, G.S.; Ponsioen, B.J.; Hummel, S.A.; Sanders, N.; Hinrichs, W.L.; De Boer, A.H.; Frijlink, H.W. Formulation and process development of (recombinant human) deoxyribonuclease I as a powder for inhalation. *Pharm. Dev. Technol.* **2009**, *14*, 358–368. [CrossRef] [PubMed]
14. Rahul, R.; Jha, U.; Sen, G.; Mishra, S. Carboxymethyl inulin: A novel flocculant for wastewater treatment. *Int. J. Biol. Macromol.* **2014**, *63*, 1–7. [CrossRef] [PubMed]
15. Palumbo, F.S.; Fiorica, C.; Di Stefano, M.; Pitarresi, G.; Gulino, A.; Agnello, S.; Giammona, G. In situ forming hydrogels of hyaluronic acid and inulin derivatives for cartilage regeneration. *Carbohydr. Polym.* **2015**, *122*, 408–416. [CrossRef] [PubMed]
16. Afinjuomo, F.; Barclay, T.G.; Song, Y.; Parikh, A.; Petrovsky, N.; Garg, S.; Parikh, A. Synthesis and characterization of a novel inulin hydrogel crosslinked with pyromellitic dianhydride. *React. Funct. Polym.* **2019**, *134*, 104–111. [CrossRef]
17. Mooter, G.V.D.; Vervoort, L.; Kinget, R. Characterization of methacrylated inulin hydrogels designed for colon targeting: In vitro release of BSA. *Pharm. Res.* **2003**, *20*, 303–307. [CrossRef]
18. Tripodo, G.; Pitarresi, G.; Cavallaro, G.; Palumbo, F.S.; Giammona, G. Controlled release of IgG by novel UV induced polysaccharide/poly(amino acid) hydrogels. *Macromol. Biosci.* **2009**, *9*, 393–401. [CrossRef]

19. Castelli, F.; Sarpietro, M.G.; Micieli, D.; Ottimo, S.; Pitarresi, G.; Tripodo, G.; Carlisi, B.; Giammona, G. Differential scanning calorimetry study on drug release from an inulin-based hydrogel and its interaction with a biomembrane model: pH and loading effect. *Eur. J. Pharm. Sci.* **2008**, *35*, 76–85. [CrossRef]
20. Licciardi, M.; Scialabba, C.; Sardo, C.; Cavallaro, G.; Giammona, G. Amphiphilic inulin graft co-polymers as self-assembling micelles for doxorubicin delivery. *J. Mater. Chem. B* **2014**, *2*, 4262–4271. [CrossRef]
21. Muley, P.; Kumar, S.; El Kourati, F.; Kesharwani, S.S.; Tummala, H. Hydrophobically modified inulin as an amphiphilic carbohydrate polymer for micellar delivery of paclitaxel for intravenous route. *Int. J. Pharm.* **2016**, *500*, 32–41. [CrossRef] [PubMed]
22. Mandracchia, D.; Rosato, A.; Trapani, A.; Chlapanidas, T.; Montagner, I.M.; Perteghella, S.; Di Franco, C.; Torre, M.L.; Trapani, G.; Tripodo, G. Design, synthesis and evaluation of biotin decorated inulin-based polymeric micelles as long-circulating nanocarriers for targeted drug delivery. *Nanomed. Nanotechnol. Biol. Med.* **2017**, *13*, 1245–1254. [CrossRef] [PubMed]
23. Essien, H.; Lai, J.Y.; Hwang, K.J. Synthesis of diethylenetriaminepentaacetic acid conjugated inulin and utility for cellular uptake of liposomes. *J. Med. Chem.* **1988**, *31*, 898–901. [CrossRef] [PubMed]
24. Volsi, A.L.; de Aberasturi, D.J.; Henriksen-Lacey, M.; Giammona, G.; Licciardi, M.; Liz-Marzan, L.M.Y. Inulin coated plasmonic gold nanoparticles as a tumor-selective tool for cancer therapy. *J. Mater. Chem. B* **2016**, *4*, 1150–1155. [CrossRef] [PubMed]
25. Zhang, L.; Li, Y.; Wang, C.; Li, G.; Zhao, Y.; Yang, Y. Synthesis of methylprednisolone loaded ibuprofen modified inulin based nanoparticles and their application for drug delivery. *Mater. Sci. Eng. C* **2014**, *42*, 111–115. [CrossRef] [PubMed]
26. Licciardi, M.; Volsi, A.L.; Mauro, N.; Scialabba, C.; Cavallaro, G.; Giammona, G. Preparation and characterization of inulin coated gold nanoparticles for selective delivery of doxorubicin to breast cancer cells. *J. Nanomater.* **2016**, *2016*, 1–12. [CrossRef]
27. Silva, D.G.; Cooper, P.D.; Petrovsky, N. Inulin-derived adjuvants efficiently promote both Th1 and Th2 immune responses. *Immunol. Cell Biol.* **2004**, *82*, 611–616. [CrossRef] [PubMed]
28. Cooper, P.D.; Petrovsky, N. Delta inulin: A novel, immunologically active, stable packing structure comprising beta-D-[2 -> 1] poly(fructo-furanosyl) alpha-D-glucose polymers. *Glycobiology* **2011**, *21*, 595–606. [CrossRef] [PubMed]
29. Kumar, S.; Tummala, H. Development of soluble inulin microparticles as a potent and safe vaccine adjuvant and delivery system. *Mol. Pharm.* **2013**, *10*, 1845–1853. [CrossRef] [PubMed]
30. Srinarong, P.; Hamalainen, S.; Visser, M.R.; Hinrichs, W.L.; Ketolainen, J.; Frijlink, H.W. Surface-active derivative of inulin (Inutec(R) SP1) is a superior carrier for solid dispersions with a high drug load. *J. Pharm. Sci.* **2011**, *100*, 2333–2342. [CrossRef] [PubMed]
31. Fares, M.M.; Salem, M.S.; Khanfar, M. Inulin and poly(acrylic acid) grafted inulin for dissolution enhancement and preliminary controlled release of poorly water-soluble Irbesartan drug. *Int. J. Pharm.* **2011**, *410*, 206–211. [CrossRef] [PubMed]
32. Robert, P.; Garcia, P.; Reyes, N.; Chávez, J.; Santos, J. Acetylated starch and inulin as encapsulating agents of gallic acid and their release behaviour in a hydrophilic system. *Food Chem.* **2012**, *134*, 1–8. [CrossRef]
33. Schacht, E.; Ruys, L.; Vermeersch, J.; Remon, J.P.; Duncan, R. Use of polysaccharides as drug carriers. Dextran and inulin derivatives of procainamide. *Ann. N. Y. Acad. Sci.* **1985**, *446*, 199–212. [CrossRef] [PubMed]
34. Hartzell, A.L.; Maldonado-Gómez, M.X.; Yang, J.; Hutkins, R.W.; Rose, D.J. In vitro digestion and fermentation of 5-formyl-aminosailcylate-inulin: A potential prodrug of 5-aminosalicylic acid. *Bioact. Carbohydr. Diet. Fibre* **2013**, *2*, 8–14. [CrossRef]
35. Sahiner, N.; Sagbas, S.; Yoshida, H.; Lyon, L.A. Synthesis and properties of inulin based microgels. *Coll. Interface Sci. Commun.* **2014**, *2*, 15–18. [CrossRef]
36. Mandracchia, D.; Denora, N.; Franco, M.; Pitarresi, G.; Giammona, G.; Trapani, G. New biodegradable hydrogels based on inulin and alpha,beta-polyaspartylhydrazide designed for colonic drug delivery: In vitro release of glutathione and oxytocin. *J. Biomater. Sci. Polym. Ed.* **2011**, *2*, 313–328. [CrossRef] [PubMed]
37. Pitarresi, G.; Tripodo, G.; Calabrese, R.; Craparo, E.F.; Licciardi, M.; Giammona, G. Hydrogels for potential colon drug release by thiol-ene conjugate addition of a new inulin derivative. *Macromol. Biosci.* **2008**, *8*, 891–902. [CrossRef]
38. Chiu, H.; Hsu, Y.; Lin, P. Synthesis of pH-sensitive inulin hydrogels and characterization of their swelling properties. *J. Biomed. Mater. Res.* **2002**, *61*, 146–152. [CrossRef]

39. Chen, S.; Cui, S.; Zhang, H.; Pei, X.; Hu, J.; Zhou, Y.Z.; Liu, Y. Cross-linked pectin nanofibers with enhanced cell adhesion. *Biomacromolecules* **2018**, *19*, 490–498. [CrossRef]
40. Gupta, B.; Tummalapalli, M.; Deopura, B.; Alam, M.S. Functionalization of pectin by periodate oxidation. *Carbohydr. Polym.* **2013**, *98*, 1160–1165. [CrossRef]
41. Maia, J.; Ferreira, L.; Carvalho, R.; Ramos, M.A.; Gil, M.H. Synthesis and characterization of new injectable and degradable dextran-based hydrogels. *Polymer* **2005**, *46*, 9604–9614. [CrossRef]
42. Cai, M.; Gong, J.; Cao, J.; Chen, Y.; Luo, X. In situ chemically crosslinked chitosan membrane by adipic acid. *J. Appl. Polym. Sci.* **2013**, *128*, 3308–3314. [CrossRef]
43. Maiti, S.; Singha, K.; Ray, S.; Dey, P.; Sa, B. Adipic acid dihydrazide treated partially oxidized alginate beads for sustained oral delivery of flurbiprofen. *Pharm. Dev. Technol.* **2009**, *14*, 461–470. [CrossRef] [PubMed]
44. Paşcalău, V.; Popescu, V.; Popescu, G.L.; Dudescu, M.C.; Borodi, G.; Dinescu, A.M.; Moldovan, M. Obtaining and characterizing alginate/k-carrageenan hydrogel cross-linked with adipic dihydrazide. *Adv. Mater. Sci. Eng.* **2013**, *2013*, 1–12. [CrossRef]
45. Hu, M.H.; Yang, K.C.; Sun, Y.H.; Chen, Y.C.; Yang, S.H.; Lin, F.H. In situ forming oxidised hyaluronic acid/adipic acid dihydrazide hydrogel for prevention of epidural fibrosis after laminectomy. *Eur. Cells Mater.* **2017**, *34*, 307–320. [CrossRef] [PubMed]
46. Shoham, N.; Sasson, A.L.; Lin, F.-H.; Benayahu, D.; Haj-Ali, R.; Gefen, A. The mechanics of hyaluronic acid/adipic acid dihydrazide hydrogel: Towards developing a vessel for delivery of preadipocytes to native tissues. *J. Mech. Behav. Biomed. Mater.* **2013**, *28*, 320–331. [CrossRef]
47. Su, W.-Y.; Chen, K.-H.; Chen, Y.-C.; Lee, Y.-H.; Tseng, C.-L.; Lin, F.-H. An injectable oxidized hyaluronic acid/adipic acid dihydrazide hydrogel as a vitreous substitute. *J. Biomater. Sci. Polym. Ed.* **2011**, *22*, 1777–1797. [CrossRef]
48. Su, W.-Y.; Chen, Y.-C.; Lin, F.-H. Injectable oxidized hyaluronic acid/adipic acid dihydrazide hydrogel for nucleus pulposus regeneration. *Acta Biomater.* **2010**, *6*, 3044–3055. [CrossRef]
49. Tabandeh, M.R.; Aminlari, M. Synthesis, physicochemical and immunological properties of oxidized inulin–l-asparaginase bioconjugate. *J. Biotechnol.* **2009**, *141*, 189–195. [CrossRef]
50. Barclay, T.; Ginic-Markovic, M.; Johnston, M.R.; Cooper, P.D.; Petrovsky, N. Analysis of the hydrolysis of inulin using real time 1H NMR spectroscopy. *Carbohydr. Res.* **2012**, *352*, 117–125. [CrossRef]
51. Schacht, E.; Vermeersch, J.; Vandoorne, F.; Vercauteren, R.; Remon, J. Synthesis and characterization of some modified polysaccharides containing drug moieties. *J. Control. Release* **1985**, *2*, 245–256. [CrossRef]
52. Zhang, K.; Yan, S.; Wang, T.; Feng, L.; Zhu, J.; Chen, X.; Cui, L.; Yin, J. Injectable in situ self-cross-linking hydrogels based on poly(l-glutamic acid) and alginate for cartilage tissue engineering. *Biomacromolecules* **2014**, *15*, 4495–4508.
53. Zhao, H.; Heindel, N.D. Determination of degree of substitution of formyl groups in polyaldehyde dextran by the hydroxylamine hydrochloride method. *Pharm. Res.* **1991**, *8*, 400–402. [CrossRef] [PubMed]
54. Jia, X.; Burdick, J.A.; Kobler, J.; Clifton, R.J.; Rosowski, J.J.; Zeitels, S.M.; Langer, R. Synthesis and characterization of in situ cross-linkable hyaluronic acid-based hydrogels with potential application for vocal fold regeneration. *Macromolecules* **2004**, *37*, 3239–3248. [CrossRef]
55. De Mattos, A.C.; Khalil, N.M.; Mainardes, R. Development and validation of an HPLC method for the determination of fluorouracil in polymeric nanoparticles. *Braz. J. Pharm. Sci.* **2013**, *49*, 117–126. [CrossRef]
56. Vervoort, L.; Rombaut, P.; van den Mooter, G.; Augustijns, P.; Kinget, R. Inulin hydrogels. II. In vitro degradation study. *Int. J. Pharm.* **1998**, *172*, 137–145. [CrossRef]
57. Damian, F.; Mooter, G.V.D.; Samyn, C.; Kinget, R. In vitro biodegradation study of acetyl and methyl inulins by Bifidobacteria and inulinase. *Eur. J. Pharm. Biopharm.* **1999**, *47*, 275–282. [CrossRef]
58. Pitarresi, G.; Tripodo, G.; Cavallaro, G.; Palumbo, F.S.; Giammona, G. Inulin–iron complexes: A potential treatment of iron deficiency anaemia. *Eur. J. Pharm. Biopharm.* **2008**, *68*, 267–276. [CrossRef]
59. Prabaharan, M.; Grailer, J.J.; Pilla, S.; Steeber, D.A.; Gong, S. Amphiphilic multi-arm block copolymer based on hyperbranched polyester, poly(L-lactide) and poly(ethylene glycol) as a drug delivery carrier. *Macromol. Biosci.* **2009**, *9*, 515–524. [CrossRef]
60. Seeli, D.S.; Prabaharan, M. Guar gum oleate-graft-poly(methacrylic acid) hydrogel as a colon-specific controlled drug delivery carrier. *Carbohydr. Polym.* **2017**, *158*, 51–57. [CrossRef]

61. Parikh, A.; Kathawala, K.; Li, J.; Chen, C.; Shan, Z.; Cao, X.; Zhou, X.-F.; Garg, S. Curcumin-loaded self-nanomicellizing solid dispersion system: Part II: In vivo safety and efficacy assessment against behavior deficit in Alzheimer disease. *Drug Deliv. Transl. Res.* **2018**, *8*, 1406–1420. [CrossRef] [PubMed]
62. Stevens, C.V.; Meriggi, A.; Booten, K. Chemical modification of inulin, a valuable renewable resource, and its industrial applications. *Biomacromolecules* **2001**, *2*, 1–16. [CrossRef] [PubMed]
63. Ishak, M.F.; Painter, T. Kinetic evidence for hemiacetal formation during the oxidation of dextran in aqueous periodate. *Carbohydr. Res.* **1978**, *64*, 189–197.
64. Pan, J.-F.; Yuan, L.; Guo, C.-A.; Geng, X.-H.; Fei, T.; Fan, W.-S.; Li, S.; Yuan, H.-F.; Yan, Z.-Q.; Mo, X.-M. Fabrication of modified dextran–gelatin in situ forming hydrogel and application in cartilage tissue engineering. *J. Mater. Chem. B* **2014**, *2*, 8346–8360. [CrossRef]
65. Kim, U.-J.; Kuga, S.; Wada, M.; Okano, T.; Kondo, T. Periodate oxidation of crystalline cellulose. *Biomacromolecules* **2000**, *1*, 488–492. [CrossRef] [PubMed]
66. Gomez, C.; Rinaudo, M.; Villar, M.; Gomez, C. Oxidation of sodium alginate and characterization of the oxidized derivatives. *Carbohydr. Polym.* **2007**, *67*, 296–304. [CrossRef]
67. Kristiansen, K.A.; Potthast, A.; Christensen, B.E. Periodate oxidation of polysaccharides for modification of chemical and physical properties. *Carbohydr. Res.* **2010**, *345*, 1264–1271. [CrossRef] [PubMed]
68. Maia, J.; Ribeiro, M.P.; Ventura, C.; Carvalho, R.A.; Correia, I.J.; Gil, M.H. Ocular injectable formulation assessment for oxidized dextran-based hydrogels. *Acta Biomater.* **2009**, *5*, 1948–1955. [CrossRef]
69. Bouhadir, K.H.; Hausman, D.S.; Mooney, D.J. Synthesis of cross-linked poly(aldehyde guluronate) hydrogels. *Polymer* **1999**, *40*, 3575–3584. [CrossRef]
70. Li, X.; Xu, A.; Xie, H.; Yu, W.; Xie, W.; Ma, X. Preparation of low molecular weight alginate by hydrogen peroxide depolymerization for tissue engineering. *Carbohydr. Polym.* **2010**, *79*, 660–664. [CrossRef]
71. Villanueva-Carcia, D.N.; Rangel-Vazquez, N.A.; Kalla, J. Structural analysis of adsorption processes of 5FU and imiquimod on hydrogels using AMBER/PM3 hybrid model. *Rev. Colomb. Quím.* **2018**, *47*, 28–35.
72. Miralinaghi, P.; Kashani, P.; Moniri, E.; Miralinaghi, M.; Monir, E.; Miralinaghi, M. Non-linear kinetic, equilibrium, and thermodynamic studies of 5-fluorouracil adsorption onto chitosan–functionalized graphene oxide. *Mater. Res. Express* **2019**, *6*, 65305. [CrossRef]
73. Dan, A.; Ghosh, S.; Moulik, S.P. Physicochemical studies on the biopolymer inulin: A critical evaluation of its self-aggregation, aggregate-morphology, interaction with water, and thermal stability. *Biopolymers* **2009**, *91*, 687–699. [CrossRef] [PubMed]
74. Bouhadir, K.; Lee, K.; Alsberg, E.; Damm, K.; Anderson, K.; Mooney, D. Degradation of partially oxidized alginate and its potential application for tissue engineering. *Biotechnol. Prog.* **2001**, *17*, 945–950. [CrossRef] [PubMed]
75. Maia, J.; Carvalho, R.A.; Coelho, J.F.; Simões, P.N.N.; Gil, M.H. Insight on the periodate oxidation of dextran and its structural vicissitudes. *Polymer* **2011**, *52*, 258–265. [CrossRef]
76. Balakrishnan, B.; Jayakrishnan, A. Self-cross-linking biopolymers as injectable in situ forming biodegradable scaffolds. *Biomaterials* **2005**, *26*, 3941–3951. [CrossRef] [PubMed]
77. Rinaudo, M. Periodate oxidation of methylcellulose: Characterization and properties of oxidized derivatives. *Polymer* **2010**, *2*, 505–521. [CrossRef]
78. Mitra, T.; Sailakshmi, G.; Gnanamani, A.; Mandal, A.B. Adipic acid interaction enhances the mechanical and thermal stability of natural polymers. *J. Appl. Polym. Sci.* **2012**, *125*. [CrossRef]
79. Chen, Y.-C.; Su, W.-Y.; Yang, S.-H.; Gefen, A.; Lin, F.-H. In situ forming hydrogels composed of oxidized high molecular weight hyaluronic acid and gelatin for nucleus pulposus regeneration. *Acta Biomater.* **2013**, *9*, 5181–5193. [CrossRef]
80. Zhu, R.; Chen, R.; Duo, Y.; Zhang, S.; Xie, D.; Mei, Y. An industrial scale synthesis of adipicdihydrazide (ADH)/polyacrylate hybrid with excellent formaldehyde degradation performance. *Polymer* **2019**, *11*, 86. [CrossRef]
81. Larrañeta, E.; Henry, M.; Irwin, N.J.; Trotter, J.; Perminova, A.A.; Donnelly, R.F. Synthesis and characterization of hyaluronic acid hydrogels crosslinked using a solvent-free process for potential biomedical applications. *Carbohydr. Polym.* **2018**, *181*, 1194–1205. [CrossRef] [PubMed]
82. Song, F.; Zhang, L.-M.; Li, N.-N.; Shi, J.-F. In situ crosslinkable hydrogel formed from a polysaccharide-based hydrogelator. *Biomacromolecules* **2009**, *10*, 959–965. [CrossRef] [PubMed]

83. Mohana, M.; Muthiah, P.; McMillen, C. Supramolecular hydrogen-bonding patterns in 1:1 cocrystals of 5-fluorouracil with 4-methylbenzoic acid and 3-nitrobenzoic acid. *Acta Crystallogr. Sect. C Struct. Chem.* **2017**, *73*, 259–263. [CrossRef] [PubMed]
84. Anirudhan, T.S.; Nima, J.; Divya, P.L. Synthesis, characterization and in vitro cytotoxicity analysis of a novel cellulose based drug carrier for the controlled delivery of 5-fluorouracil, an anticancer drug. *Appl. Surf. Sci.* **2015**, *355*, 64–73. [CrossRef]

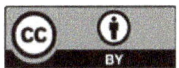

© 2019 by the authors. Licensee MDPI, Basel, Switzerland. This article is an open access article distributed under the terms and conditions of the Creative Commons Attribution (CC BY) license (http://creativecommons.org/licenses/by/4.0/).

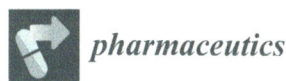

Article

Trimethyl Chitosan Hydrogel Nanoparticles for Progesterone Delivery in Neurodegenerative Disorders [†]

Maria Cristina Cardia [1], Anna Rosa Carta [2], Pierluigi Caboni [1], Anna Maria Maccioni [1], Sara Erbì [1], Laura Boi [2], Maria Cristina Meloni [1], Francesco Lai [1,*] and Chiara Sinico [1]

1. Department of Life and Environmental Sciences, Unit of Drug Sciences, University of Cagliari, 09124 Cagliari, Italy; cardiamr@unica.it (M.C.C.); caboni@unica.it (P.C.); maccion@unica.it (A.M.M.); erbisara@gmail.com (S.E.); mariacristina.meloni@unica.it (M.C.M.); sinico@unica.it (C.S.)
2. Department of Biomedical Sciences, University of Cagliari, 09124 Cagliari, Italy; acarta@unica.it (A.R.C.); laurettaboi@hotmail.it (L.B.)
* Correspondence: frlai@unica.it; Tel.: +39-070-6758514
† This work is dedicated to the memory of Prof. Sandro Fenu and Prof. Sandra Dessì.

Received: 31 October 2019; Accepted: 3 December 2019; Published: 6 December 2019

Abstract: Progesterone is a sex hormone which shows neuroprotective effects in different neurodegenerative disorders, including Parkinson's disease, stroke, and Alzheimer's disease. However, the pharmacokinetic limitations associated with the peripheral administration of this molecule highlight the need for more efficient delivery approaches to increase brain progesterone levels. Since the nose-to-brain administration of mucoadhesive hydrogel nanoparticles is a non-invasive and convenient strategy for the delivery of therapeutics to the central nervous system, in this work, progesterone-loaded hydrogel nanoparticle formulations have been prepared, characterized, and tested in vivo. Nanoparticles, loaded with different progesterone concentrations, have been obtained by polyelectrolyte complex formation between trimethyl chitosan and sodium alginate, followed by ionotropic gelation with sodium tripolyphosphate as a cross-linking agent. All formulations showed a mean diameter ranging from 200 nm to 236 nm, a polydispersity index smaller than 0.23, and a high progesterone encapsulation efficiency (83–95%). The zeta potential values were all positive and greater than 28 mV, thus ensuring nanoparticles stability against aggregation phenomena as well as interaction with negative sialic residues of the nasal mucosa. Finally, in vivo studies on Sprague–Dawley male rats demonstrated a 5-fold increase in brain progesterone concentrations compared to basal progesterone level after 30 min of hydrogel nanoparticle inhalation.

Keywords: trimethyl chitosan; progesterone; brain; hydrogel nanoparticles

1. Introduction

In recent years, research has focused on the potential repurposing of sex hormones, particularly progesterone (PG), for the treatment of neurodegenerative disorders, including Parkinson's disease (PD), stroke, and Alzheimer's disease [1,2]. Use of PG in PD initially raised interest following evidence of the higher incidence in men than in women [3,4]. PD is a complex pathology comprising multiple pathological events; therefore, molecules with several mechanisms of action, such as PG, are valuable options as neuroprotective agents [5]. Preclinical studies have suggested a neuroprotective effect of low doses of PG administered in several models of PD [6,7]. Similarly, the neuroprotective action of PG was also found in models of traumatic brain injury in both human and experimental animals [8–10] and is under investigation for cognitive impairment in Alzheimer's disease [11]. Therefore, while current evidence points to PG as a valid and promising therapeutic approach for several CNS disorders, the pharmacokinetic limitations associated with the peripheral administration of this molecule highlight a need for more efficient delivery approaches to increase its brain levels.

In particular, oral administration of PG is characterized by low bioavailability. Indeed, its rapid absorption is associated with an elevated clearance rate due to intestine and first-pass metabolism [12,13]. Moreover, PG absorption is influenced by food intake, formulation excipients, and drug crystal diameter [14]. Several PG derivatives with a higher stability have been synthetized, but their use often relates to different undesirable effects, such as a decrease in total high-density lipoprotein cholesterol and an increased risk of fetal malformations [12,14]. For these reasons, in order to overcome low oral bioavailability, parenteral PG administration routes have been explored. Intravenous and intramuscular administrations determine high serum PG concentrations [12,13]; however, in the case of chronic therapy, daily injections can be uncomfortable and are characterized by low patient compliance.

Therefore, as several high-molecular-weight drugs have shown promising results in the treatment of CNS disorders, alternative routes for brain delivery are steadily investigated [15,16]. Nose-to-brain administration is a non-invasive and convenient strategy for the delivery of therapeutics to the CNS, bypassing the blood-brain barrier (BBB). Indeed, the nasal cavity can be employed not only for local administration, but also for the systemic delivery of different therapeutic agents (e.g., peptides, proteins, stem cells, etc.) due to its large surface area and high degree of vascularization. Drug administered by this route can enter the brain principally using olfactory or trigeminal nerve pathways. Moreover, other pathways involving vasculature, cerebrospinal fluid, and the lymphatic system have been individuated [17,18].

Even though it is often not easy to identify the exact pathways that an intranasally administered molecule follows to penetrate the CNS, it has been observed that different experimental factors can influence the amount and rate of brain accumulation. Usually, an increase in the drug contact time (residence time) with the nasal mucosa enhances the overall nose-to-brain drug delivery. In particular, it has been demonstrated that the use of mucoadhesive hydrogel nanoparticles (NPs) can increase the residence time and, consequently, the brain bioavailability of loaded drugs [19,20].

N,N,N-Trimethyl chitosan (TMC) is a hydrophilic polymer obtained by chitosan methylation which is able to form a stable gel in presence of sodium alginate (SA), an anionic water-soluble polysaccharide composed of alternating blocks of a-L-guluronic and b-D-mannuronic acid (b 1–4 linked) [21]. Similarly to chitosan, it is characterized by low toxicity, good biodegradability, and biocompatibility. However, compared to chitosan, TMC shows a higher positive charge and consequently, good solubility at all physiological pH values. Moreover, TMC shows excellent mucoadhesive properties as well as the ability to improve the paracellular permeation of hydrophilic compounds by means of interactions with the tight junctions [22,23].

With the aim of both identifying a more effective route for PG administration and clarifying whether the mucoadhesive properties of TMC can affect its brain accumulation, in this work we prepared PG-loaded TMC hydrogel NPs for PG brain delivery.

PG-loaded hydrogel NPs were prepared by polyelectrolyte complex formation between TMC and SA followed by ionotropic gelation with sodium tripolyphosphate (TPP) as a cross-linking agent. NPs were characterized in terms of size, size distribution, surface charge, and encapsulation efficiency. Moreover, NP stability and in vitro PG release were assessed. Finally, brain PG accumulation was evaluated in vivo on Sprague–Dawley male rats after PG hydrogel NP inhalation.

2. Materials and Methods

2.1. Materials

Low-molecular-weight chitosan, sodium iodide, N-methyl-pyrrolidinone, methyl iodide, sodium chloride, sodium hydroxide, sodium alginate, sodium tripolyphosphate, and deuterated PG (D9-PG) were purchased from Sigma Aldrich. PG was purchased from Galeno (Carmignano, Italy). For the in vivo experiments Sprague–Dawley rats were purchased from Envigo (Huntingdon, England, UK).

2.2. TMC Synthesis and Characterization

The synthesis of TMC was performed starting with low-molecular-weight chitosan, slightly revising already reported procedures [21]. Chitosan (2 g) and sodium iodide (4.8 g) were dispersed in N-methylpyrrolidinone (80 mL) into a three empty flasks immersed in a water bath. The suspension was stirred vigorously with a paddle stirrer at a controlled temperature (60 °C) for 20 min. After stabilization of the temperature, an NaOH solution (11 mL, 15% w/w) and methyl iodide (12 mL) were added to the mixture, keeping the temperature at 60 °C (± 5 °C) for 60 min. Then, methyl iodide (5 mL) and NaOH solution (10 mL, 15% w/w) were added again to the mixture, and the suspension was stirred at 60 °C for 6 h. The mixture was allowed to reach room temperature under stirring overnight, and the resulting brown colored suspension was concentrated under vacuum and dialyzed against bidistilled water. To replace the I^- counterions with Cl^- counterions, the obtained polymer was treated with an NaCl solution (10% w/w, room temperature, overnight) and lyophilized. The dried polymer is stable at room temperature until the time of use and no further purification is needed. TMC was characterized by Proton Magnetic Resonance (^{1}H-NMR) spectroscopy to assess the degree of quaternization. TMC samples were prepared solubilizing freeze-dried TMC in D_2O (5 mg/1 mL). Spectra were determined on a Varian INOVA500 (Palo Alto, CA, USA) spectrometer at 27 °C and were recorded with the water suppression technique. Chemical shifts are expressed as δ value.

2.3. NP Preparation and Characterization

A water dispersion of SA (1 mg/mL) was added to a TMC dispersion (2 mg/mL) containing D9-PG or PG at different concentrations to obtain six different formulations (PGNP0, PGNP0.1, PGNP0.5, PGNP0.7, PGNP1, PGNP1D) as reported in Table 1. The mixture was kept under constant magnetic stirring (~1000 rpm) at room temperature for one hour and then sodium tripolyphosphate (TPP, 1 mg/mL) was added as cross-linking agent (~1000 rpm for 30 min). The volumetric ratio between TMC/SA/TPP was fixed to 6:1:2. A light opalescence revealed NP formation. PG concentrations in the final formulations were (0, 0.1, 0.5, 0.7, and 1 mg/mL).

The average diameter (nm ± SD) and polydispersity index (PDI) of all the formulations were determined by Photon Correlation Spectroscopy (PCS), using a Zetasizer nano-ZS (Malvern Instruments, Worcestershire, UK) Then, 0.2 mL of each formulation were diluted with bidistilled water up to 10 mL and backscattered by a helium-neon laser (633 nm) at an angle of 173° and a constant temperature of 25 °C.

ζ potential (ZP) was determined using the same instrument by means of the M3-PALS (Mixed Mode Measurement-Phase Analysis Light Scattering) technique, which measures the particle electrophoretic mobility. All the measurements were made in triplicate.

Morphology of freeze-dried nanoparticles was examined by scanning electron microscope (SEM).

The samples were fixed on a brass stub using carbon double-sided tape. Pictures were then taken at an excitation voltage of 20 kV using a Dual-beam Fei Nova Nano Lab 600 (Hillsboro, OR, USA), equipped with a high-brightness FEG source reaching resolutions up to 5 nm.

2.4. Stability Studies

Stability studies were carried out for 28 days on NP dispersions stored at 4 °C. At preselected time intervals, the refrigerated formulations were allowed to warm to room temperature under magnetic stirrer for 30 min and then the average diameter, polydispersity index, and ζ potential were determined as previously described. All the measurements were taken in triplicate.

2.5. Evaluation of Encapsulation Efficiency

The encapsulation efficiency of the PG containing NPs was estimated by means of an indirect method. NP dispersions were centrifuged at 15,000 rpm for 15 min at 4 °C (Scilogex mod. D3024R,

Rocky Hill, CT, USA) and the PG amount in the supernatant was determined by High Performance Liquid Chromatography (HPLC).

The encapsulation efficiency (EE%) was calculated using the following equation:

$$EE\% = \frac{PG_{TOT} - PG_{SURN}}{PG_{TOT}} \times 100 \qquad (1)$$

In the calculation of EE% (Equation (1)), PG_{TOT} corresponds to the total amount of PG used in each sample preparation and PG_{SURN} is the amount of PG in the supernatant after centrifugation. All the measurements were made in triplicate.

PG content was quantified at 254 nm using a Flexar–Perkin Elmer HPLC equipped with a UV detector and a computer-integrating apparatus. The column was a C18 reversed-phase and the mobile phase was a mixture of acetic acid solution (0.5% v/v) and methanol (10:90 v/v and pH = 3.92) at a flow rate of 1.2 mL/min. The retention time was 3.75 min ± 0.01 s. A standard calibration curve was built up by using working standard solutions. Calibration graphs were plotted according to the linear regression analysis, which gave a correlation coefficient value (R^2) of 0.999.

2.6. In Vitro Drug Release Studies

In vitro PG release studies were performed using Franz cells. A dialysis membrane (Spectra/Por® Dialysis Membrane MWCO: 12–14 kD) was previously hydrated with bidistilled water for 24 h and then fixed between the two compartments of Franz cells. The receiving compartment was filled with a water/ethanol solution (40:60 v/v) maintained under constant agitation and at controlled temperature (37 °C). In the donor compartment, 500 µL of the samples (PGNP0.1, PGNP0.5, PGNP0.7, PGNP1) were deposited. At preselected intervals (15, 30, 45, 60, 120, 180, 240, and 300 min), the total content of the receiving compartment (~6.5 mL) was withdrawn, replaced with pre-thermostated, fresh water/ethanol solution, and analyzed by HPLC for PG content. All the analyses were performed in triplicate.

2.7. In Vitro Biocompatibility

The RPMI 2650 human nasal septum carcinoma cell line (Sigma Aldrich, Milan, Italy) was grown as a monolayer in 75 cm^2 flasks, and incubated in 100% humidity and 5% CO_2 at 37 °C, using RPMI1640 supplemented with fetal bovine serum, penicillin/streptomycin, and fungizone as culture medium. For toxicity studies, cells were seeded into 96-well plates (7.5 × 10^3 cells/well) and, after 24 h, were treated for 24 h with PGNP1D-deuterated PG-loaded nanoparticles and related unloaded formulations at different dilutions corresponding to 0.5, 5, 15, and 40 µg/mL of PG. After incubation, cells were washed three times with fresh medium and their viability was determined by the (3(4,5-dimethylthiazolyl-2)-2,5-diphenyltetrazolium bromide) colorimetric assay (MTT), adding 200 µL of MTT reagent (0.5 mg/mL in PBS) to each well. After 2–3 h, the formed formazan crystals were dissolved in DMSO and their concentration was spectrophotometrically quantified at 570 nm with a microplate reader (Synergy 4, Reader BioTek Instruments, AHSI S.P.A, Bernareggio, Monza and Brianza, Italy). All experiments were repeated at least three times. Results are shown as percent of cell viability in comparison with non-treated control cells (100% viability).

2.8. In Vivo Studies

PGNP1D nanoparticle formulation, containing 1 mg/mL of D9-PG (Table 1), was tested on male Sprague–Dawley rats ($n = 16$, weight range 270–300 g). Rats were immobilized in a plexiglass restrainer and exposed to PGNP1D or empty NPs by inhalation via an aerosol apparatus (Nebula M2000, Air Liquide Medical Systems, Bovezzo, Italy).

The rate of flow of the aerosol apparatus was about 0.3 mL/min. The administered dose was approximatively 1 mg/kg per minute or 0.3 mg per animal per minute, since the PG concentration of the PGNP1D nanoparticle formulation is 1 mg/mL. At 15 min, 30 min, 1 h, and 2 h after continuous inhalation, rats were deeply anesthetized and sacrificed by decapitation. Brains and blood were rapidly collected and processed to determine the amount of D9-PG.

All experimental procedures met the guidelines and protocols approved by the European Community (2010/63 UE L 276 20/10/2010) and by the Ethical Commission for Animal Care and Use at the University of Cagliari and Italian Ministry of Health (pr. # 1293/2015-PR, 18/12/2015).

2.9. Progesterone and Deuterated Progesterone (D9-PG) in Plasma and Brain GC-MS Analysis

Quantities of D9-PG in plasma and brain tissue was determined by GC-MS analysis. Plasma samples were initially thawed on ice, and then 200 µL of plasma were withdrawn and extracted with 250 µL of an ice-cold mixture of methanol/water (3:1 v/v). Samples were then loaded on C18 columns (Agilent Technologies, Palo Alto, CA, USA), which were previously activated with 2 mL of methanol and 2 mL of bidistilled water. One mL of methanol was added to each SPE column and recovered. The purified extract was then evaporated to dryness using a gentle nitrogen stream.

Brain samples were initially weighed and thawed on ice. Then, 2 mL of a methanol/acetic acid (99:1 v/v) solution were added to each sample, which was homogenated with a Potter-Elvehjem PTFE pestle and glass tube homogenizer and left overnight. Samples were then centrifugated for 15 min at 4000 rpm and recovered. The pellet was dissolved and extracted again using 0.5 mL of the methanol/acetic acid solution. After centrifugation of the latter obtained solution, the two extracts were combined and evaporated to dryness. Brain and plasma samples were finally derivatized using 100 µL heptafluorobutyric acid (HFBA) and 200 µL acetone. After 30 min at 35 °C, 600 µL hexane were added before GC-MS analysis.

The derivatized samples were analyzed with a Hewlett Packard 6850 Gas Chromatograph, 5973 mass selective detector, and 7683B series injector (Agilent Technologies, Palo Alto, CA, USA), using helium as the carrier gas at 1.0 mL min^{-1} flow. One µL of samples was injected in the split-less mode and resolved on a 30 m × 0.25 mm × 0.25 µm DB-5MS column (Agilent Technologies, Palo Alto, CA, USA). Inlet, interface, and ion source temperatures were 250, 250, and 230 °C, respectively. Oven starting temperature was set to 50 °C, and the final temperature to 230 °C with a heating rate of 5 °C/min for 36 min and then for 2 min at constant temperature. GC-MS mass spectra were recorded in the selected ion monitoring mode (SIM) recording the 510, 495, 425 m/z ions for PG and deuterated PG.

2.10. Statistical Analysis of Data

Results are expressed as the mean ± standard deviation and significance was tested at the 0.01 or 0.05 level of probability (p). For size, zeta potential, drug accumulation, and cytotoxicity, analysis of variance (one way-ANOVA) followed by post-hoc Bonferroni correction were used to substantiate statistical differences between groups using XLSTAT for Excel.

3. Results and Discussion

3.1. TMC Synthesis

In this study PG-loaded hydrogel NPs were prepared by ionotropic gelation technique, using a mixture of TMC/SA and TPP as cross-linker. TMC was synthesized as already reported [21]. The procedure was reproducible and allowed us to obtain TMC with a high degree of quaternization (DQ = 70%), simply extending the reaction time up to seven hours. By means of this procedure, we were able to reduce the methylating agent (CH$_3$I) amount and, as demonstrated by ^{1}H-NMR data, avoid the formation of undesirable side products (such as TMC with a high degree of methoxylation in position 3 and 6 of the glucosamine ring), which decrease the polymer water solubility. Besides, we avoided the use of organic solvents in purification steps.

3.2. Preparation and Characterization of Nanoparticles

The NP composition was selected based on results obtained in an our previous preformulation study in which the effect of both polymers (TMC and SA) and cross-linker (TPP) ratio was deeply investigated [21]. In particular, in this work the volumetric ratio of TMC, SA, and TPP solution was kept constant (6:1:2). Moreover, the amount of TMC was kept higher than that of SA in order to obtain NPs with positive surface charge, useful to promote the interaction with negative sialic residues of the nasal mucosa. Starting from the above reported composition, we prepared five PG NP formulations (PGNP 0, PGNP0.1, PGNP0.5, PGNP0.7, and PGNP1) loaded with different drug concentrations (0, 0.1, 0.5, 0.7, and 1 mg/mL, respectively). Moreover, a D9-PG-loaded NP dispersion was also prepared (PGNP1D, 1 mg/mL). Deuterated drug-loaded NPs have been used for in vivo studies in order to distinguish endogenous and administered PG after the inhalation experiment. Empty (PGNP0) and PG or D9-PG-containing NPs (PGNP0.1, PGNP0.5, PGNP0.7, PGNP1, PGNP1D) were fully characterized by average diameter (nm ± SD), polydispersity index (PDI), ζ potential (ZP), and encapsulation efficiency (EE%) (Table 1). As shown in Table 1, the incorporation of PG or D9-PG led only to a slight variation of the NP mean diameter, PDI, and ζ potential values when compared to the unloaded NP. Indeed, all formulations (unloaded and loaded) showed a mean diameter ranging from 200 nm and 236 nm and a polydispersity index always smaller than 0.23, thus indicating a fairly narrow size distribution.

The zeta potential values, all positive and greater than 28 mV, should ensure NP stability against aggregation phenomena. In general, all loaded formulations showed a high EE%. The amount of PG used for the preparation of the different formulations seems to have only a small influence on the drug encapsulation efficiency (EE%). Indeed, PGNP0.1, prepared with the smallest PG concentration (0.1 mg/mL), showed the highest EE% (95%), but PGNP1, with the highest PG concentration (1 mg/mL) can also incorporate a very high amount of drug (EE% 83).

NP morphology was evaluated via scanning electron microscopy. In Figure 1 an SEM image of freeze-dried PGNP1D nanoparticles is reported. As can be seen, freeze-dried PG-loaded NPs have a regular and rounded shape. Moreover, SEM analyses confirmed the fact that nanoparticles with a mean diameter comparable with that measured by photon correlation spectroscopy are still present in the lyophilized samples.

Table 1. Composition mean diameter (nm), polydispersity index (PDI), and zeta potential (ZP, mV) of freshly prepared progesterone (PG)-loaded nanoparticles. Results are expressed as means of three independent measurements ± standard deviations. EE%: encapsulation efficiency. PGNP0, PGNP0.1, PGNP0.5, PGNP0.7, and PGNP1: PG NP formulations loaded with drug concentrations of 0, 0.1, 0.5, 0.7, and 1 mg/mL, respectively. NP: nanoparticle.

Sample	PG Concentration (mg/mL)	D9-PG Concentration (mg/mL)	Mean Diameter (nm ± SD)	PDI (±SD)	ZP (mV ± SD)	EE%
PGNP0	-	-	208 ± 5	0.19 ± 0.01	+28 ± 2	/
PGNP0.1	0.1	-	222 ± 9	0.23 ± 0.08	+28 ± 1	95 ± 3
PGNP0.5	0.5	-	227 ± 6	0.23 ± 0.04	+30 ± 1	88 ± 5
PGNP0.7	0.7	-	236 ± 6	0.25 ± 0.03	+31 ± 2	85 ± 5
PGNP1	1	-	198 ± 4	0.22 ± 0.02	+29 ± 1	83 ± 2
PGNP1D	-	1	204 ± 5	0.25 ± 0.03	+27 ± 1	80 ± 1

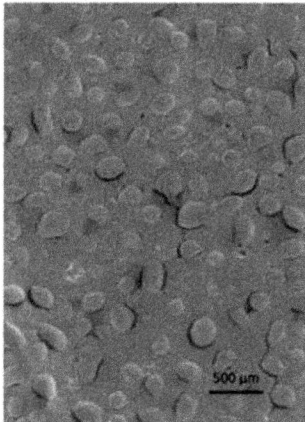

Figure 1. Scanning electron microscopy image of freeze-dried PGNP1D nanoparticles.

3.3. Stability of NPs

Stability studies were performed for 4 weeks, monitoring the variations in size, PDI, and ζ potential of NPs stored at 4 °C (Figures 2 and 3). As shown in Figure 2, the NP mean diameter growth over the studied period was moderate (ranging around 30%). Indeed, all formulations showed a mean diameter of approximately 300 nm after 28 days of storage at 4 °C and, in particular, the smallest size (~290 nm) was measured for PGNP1. Also, polydispersity index values increased after 28 days, thus confirming the fact that NP weak aggregation phenomena occur during storage. Once again, the formulation PGNP1 showed the smallest PDI (nearby 0.30). As expected, zeta potential remains positive for all NP, and almost stable in a narrow range (26–35 mV) over the monitored period (Figure 3).

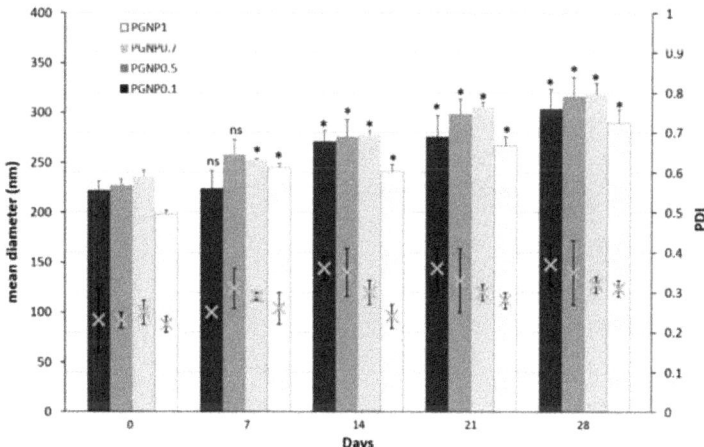

Figure 2. Variation of mean diameter and polydispersity index (PDI) of PG-loaded nanoparticles during 28 days of storage at 4 °C. Results are expressed as means of three independent measurements ± standard deviations. For each formulation, statistical analysis was performed comparing the mean diameter value at each time point with respect to that at time zero. * = different from day 0 ($p \leq 0.05$), ns indicates not significant data ($p > 0.05$).

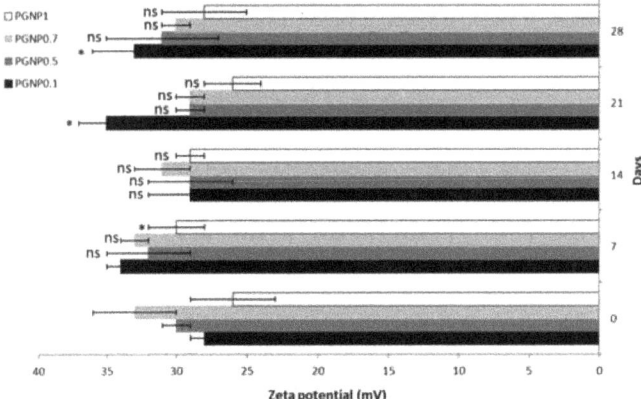

Figure 3. Zeta potential of PG-loaded nanoparticles during 28 days of storage at 4 °C. Results are expressed as means of three independent measurements ± standard deviations. For each formulation, statistical analysis was performed comparing the zeta potential value at each time point with respect to that at time zero. * = different from day 0 ($p \leq 0.05$), ns indicates not significant data ($p > 0.05$).

3.4. PG Release from NPs

The PG release from hydrogel NPs was studied over a period of 5 h in a water/ethanol (40:60 v/v) solution to ensure sink conditions. To this aim, 500 μL of each samples (PGNP0.1, PGNP0.5, PGNP0.7, PGNP1) were deposited in the Franz cell donor compartment while the receiving compartment was filled with a water/ethanol solution (40:60 v/v) maintained at 37 °C and under constant agitation. Results reported in Figure 4 show no burst release for all formulations, thus demonstrating that PG is effectively incorporated into the hydrogel nanoparticles matrix. The PG release profile from formulations PGNP1, PGNP0.7, and PGNP0.5 showed a similar trend, with the release rate directly related to the loaded drug concentration. As for PG release from NPs with the lowest PG concentration, namely PGNP0.1, the rate is significantly the lowest (50.52%). This behavior suggested that the main mechanism by which PG is released from NPs should be a concentration-dependent diffusion process rather than a consequence of matrix hydrogel erosion.

Starting from the release results and taking also into account stability data, we decided to perform the in vivo studies using PGNP1 but loaded with deuterated PG (D9-PG), namely the PGNP1D formulation (Table 1).

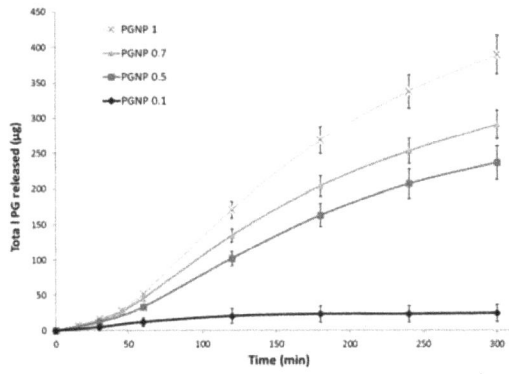

Figure 4. In vitro PG release in water/ethanol (40:60 v/v) solution from PG-loaded nanoparticles.

3.5. In Vitro Biocompatibility

To evaluate the biocompatibility of both PGNP1D-unloaded and deuterated PG-loaded nanoparticles, an in vitro cytotoxicity study was performed using the human nasal septum carcinoma cell line treated with different PG concentrations (0.5, 5, 15, and 40 µg/mL) for 24 h. As can be seen in Figure 5, the unloaded formulation did not induce any toxic effect on RPMI 2650 cells exposed for 24 h up to the highest tested dose. However, the presence of PG reduces the cell viability in an apparently dose-dependent manner. Indeed, at the dose of 40 µg/mL, a 61% cell viability, when compared to non-treated control cells, was observed. These results confirmed data already reported in the literature concerning the apoptosis effect produced by PG at high doses and prolonged exposition times on cells [24].

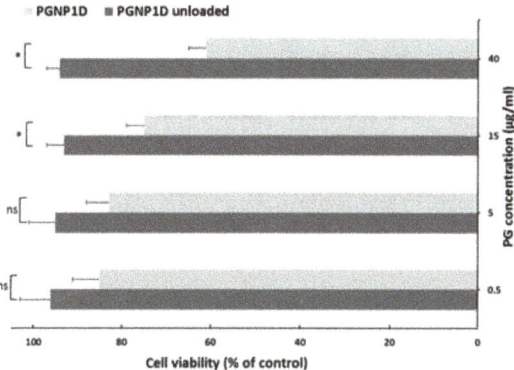

Figure 5. In vitro cytotoxicity studies of PGNP1D and relative unloaded formulations at different dilutions on the human nasal cell line RPMI 2650. The cell viability is recorded as percentage cell viability in comparison with non-treated control cells (100% viability). Results are represented as mean ± SD from three independent experiments. The asterisks indicate statistically significant data (* = $p \leq 0.05$), ns indicates not significant data ($p > 0.05$).

3.6. In Vivo Studies

In vivo studies have been carried out on male rats in order to have an animal model with levels of PG as constant as possible. Indeed, the level of endogenous PG in female rats depends on the estrus phase, and thus it is much more variable than in males [25]. To discriminate endogenous PG from exogenous PG, we administered the PGNP1D or empty nanoparticles via aerosol, and we measured plasma and brain levels of both D-9-progesterone and endogenous progesterone at progressive time points (Figures 6 and 7). Results showed that deuterated PG reached a plasma concentration six-fold higher than endogenous PG as soon as 15 min after nanoparticles inhalation, which lasted for 30 min. Plasma levels of deuterated PG decreased to values close to that of endogenous PG 60 min after inhalation (Figure 6). Analysis of brain tissue showed that deuterated PG increased to a concentration significantly higher than endogenous PG when measured 30 min and 60 min after inhalation, and it returned to endogenous PG level 120 min after inhalation (Figure 7). In Figure 8, the total amount of deuterated PG in plasma and brain tissue at preselected time points up to 120 min is reported. As can be clearly observed from the graph, the maximum amount of D9-PG is detected in plasma after 15 min (~0.5 µg) and it is significantly higher than the maximum detected in brain tissue after 30 min (~0.0083 µg). Therefore, in vivo results demonstrate that the nanoparticles used in the present study efficiently carried PG into the brain, even though we do not have any evidence concerning the pathway by which PG reaches the brain tissue. NPs may allow PG to directly reach the brain parenchyma via the nose-to-brain olfactory pathway, bypassing the BBB. However, obtained results seem also to indicate that PG released from NPs diffuses from the nasal mucosa into the blood stream, from where it may pass the blood–brain barrier according to its lipophilic nature [26].

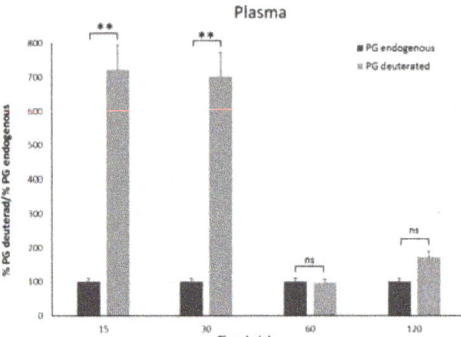

Figure 6. Plasma endogenous and deuterated PG detected on male Sprague–Dawley rats 15 min, 30 min, 1 h, and 2 h after continuous PGNP1D inhalation. The asterisks indicate statistically significant data (** = $p \leq 0.01$), ns indicates not significant data ($p > 0.05$).

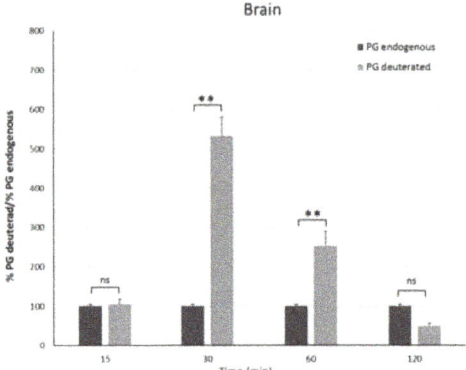

Figure 7. Brain endogenous and deuterated PG detected on male Sprague–Dawley mice 15 min, 30 min, 1 h, and 2 h after continuous PGNP1D inhalation. The asterisks indicate statistically significant data (** = $p \leq 0.01$), ns indicates not significant data ($p > 0.05$).

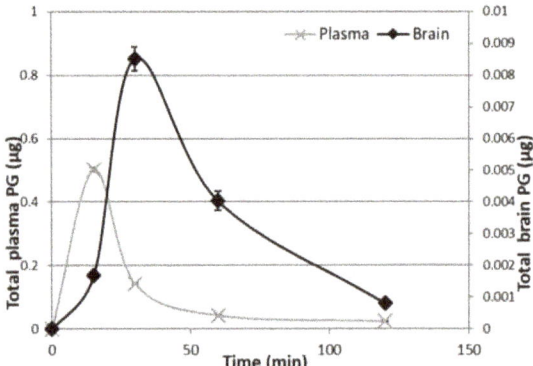

Figure 8. Deuterated PG in plasma and brain 15 min, 30 min, 1 h, and 2 h after continuous PGNP1D inhalation.

4. Conclusions

In this work, NPs loaded with different PG concentrations were obtained from trimethyl chitosan and sodium alginate cross-linked with sodium tripolyphosphate. Among the various prepared NPs, characterization studies allowed us to select the best formulation (PGNP1) in terms of size, stability, and drug release profile. These NPs have been loaded with deuterated PG and tested in vivo on Sprague–Dawley male rats. In vivo results demonstrate that the selected nanoparticles could be an efficient carrier for PG brain delivery useful in the treatment of different neurodegenerative disorders. Further research will be carried out in order to identify the main route involved in PG delivery to the brain tissue.

Author Contributions: Conceptualization, M.C.C., A.R.C., P.C., and C.S.; Data curation, M.C.C., A.M.M., S.E., L.B., and M.C.M.; Formal analysis, M.C.C. and L.B.; Investigation, M.C.C., A.R.C., P.C., A.M.M., S.E., and L.B.; Methodology, P.C. and C.S.; Project administration, A.M.M. and C.S.; Resources, M.C.C. and M.C.M.; Supervision, A.R.C. and C.S.; Validation, S.E. and F.L.; Visualization, M.C.M.; Writing—original draft, M.C.C., A.R.C., P.C., and F.L.; Writing—review and editing, F.L. and C.S.

Funding: This research received no external funding.

Acknowledgments: The author would like to thank Francesca Marongiu for her help.

Conflicts of Interest: The authors declare no conflict of interest.

References

1. Bourque, M.; Morissette, M.; Di Paolo, T. Repurposing sex steroids and related drugs as potential treatment for Parkinson's disease. *Neuropharmacology* **2019**, *147*, 37–54. [CrossRef] [PubMed]
2. Vegeto, E.; Villa, A.; Della Torre, S.; Crippa, V.; Rusmini, P.; Cristofani, R.; Galbiati, M.; Maggi, A.; Poletti, A. The role of sex and sex Hormones in Neurodegenerative Diseases. *Endocr. Rev.* **2019**, in press. [CrossRef] [PubMed]
3. Hirsch, L.; Jette, N.; Frolkis, A.; Steeves, T.; Pringsheim, T. The Incidence of Parkinson's Disease: A Systematic Review and Meta-Analysis. *Neuroepidemiology* **2016**, *46*, 292–300. [CrossRef] [PubMed]
4. Ascherio, A.; Chen, H.; Schwarzschild, M.A.; Zhang, S.M.; Colditz, G.A.; Speizer, F.E. Caffeine, postmenopausal estrogen, and risk of Parkinson's disease. *Neurology* **2003**, *60*, 790–795. [CrossRef] [PubMed]
5. Giatti, S.; Calabrese, D.; Pesaresi, M.; Cermenati, G.; Mitro, N.; Viviani, B.; Garcia-Segura, L.M.; Caruso, D. Levels and actions of progesterone and its metabolites in the nervous system during physiological and pathological conditions. *Prog. Neurobiol.* **2014**, *113*, 56–69.
6. Callier, S.; Morissette, M.; Grandbois, M.; Pélaprat, D.; Di Paolo, T. Neuroprotective properties of 17β-estradiol, progesterone, and raloxifene in MPTP C57Bl/6 mice. *Synapse* **2001**, *41*, 131–138. [CrossRef]
7. Bourque, M.; Morissette, M.; Al Sweidi, S.; Caruso, D.; Melcangi, R.C.; Di Paolo, T. Neuroprotective Effect of Progesterone in MPTP-Treated Male Mice. *Neuroendocrinology* **2016**, *103*, 300–314. [CrossRef]
8. Xiao, G.; Wei, J.; Yan, W.; Wang, W.; Lu, Z. Improved outcomes from the administration of progesterone for patients with acute severe traumatic brain injury: A randomized controlled trial. *Crit. Care* **2008**, *12*, R61. [CrossRef]
9. Wright, D.W.; Kellermann, A.L.; Hertzberg, V.S.; Clark, P.L.; Frankel, M.; Goldstein, F.C.; Salomone, J.P.; Dent, L.L.; Harris, O.A.; Ander, D.S.; et al. ProTECT: A Randomized Clinical Trial of Progesterone for Acute Traumatic Brain Injury. *Ann. Emerg. Med.* **2007**, *49*, 391–402. [CrossRef]
10. Wali, B.; Ishrat, T.; Won, S.; Stein, D.G.; Sayeed, I. Progesterone in experimental permanent stroke: A dose-response and therapeutic time-window study. *Brain* **2014**, *137*, 486–502. [CrossRef]
11. Osmanovic-Barilar, J.; Salkovic-Petrisi, M. Evaluating the Role of Hormone Therapy in Postmenopausal Women with Alzheimer's Disease. *Drugs Aging* **2016**, *33*, 787–808. [CrossRef] [PubMed]
12. Unfer, V.; Casini, M.L.; Marelli, G.; Costabile, L.; Gerli, S.; Di Renzo, G.C. Different routes of progesterone administration and polycystic ovary syndrome: A review of the literature. *Gynecol. Endocrinol.* **2005**, *21*, 119–127. [CrossRef] [PubMed]
13. Tavaniotou, A.; Smitz, J.; Bourgain, C.; Devroey, P. Comparison between different routes of progesterone administration as luteal phase support in infertility treatments. *Hum. Reprod. Update* **2000**, *6*, 139–148. [CrossRef] [PubMed]

14. McAuley, J.W.; Kroboth, F.J.; Kroboth, P.D. Oral administration of micronized progesterone: A review and more experience. *Pharmacotherapy* **1996**, *16*, 453–457.
15. Kozlovskaya, L.; Abou-Kaoud, M.; Stepensky, D. Quantitative analysis of drug delivery to the brain via nasal route. *J. Control. Release* **2014**, *189*, 133–140. [CrossRef]
16. Yuba, E.; Kono, K. Nasal Delivery of Biopharmaceuticals. In *Mucosal Delivery of Biopharmaceuticals*; Springer: Boston, MA, USA, 2014; pp. 197–220.
17. Dhuria, S.V.; Hanson, L.R.; Frey, W.H. Intranasal delivery to the central nervous system: Mechanisms and experimental considerations. *J. Pharm. Sci.* **2010**, *99*, 1654–1673. [CrossRef]
18. Bourganis, V.; Kammona, O.; Alexopoulos, A.; Kiparissides, C. Recent advances in carrier mediated nose-to-brain delivery of pharmaceutics. *Eur. J. Pharm. Biopharm.* **2018**, *128*, 337–362. [CrossRef]
19. Mohammed, M.A.; Syeda, J.T.M.; Wasan, K.M.; Wasan, E.K. An Overview of Chitosan Nanoparticles and Its Application in Non-Parenteral Drug Delivery. *Pharmaceutics* **2017**, *9*, 53. [CrossRef]
20. Warnken, Z.N.; Smyth, H.D.C.; Watts, A.B.; Weitman, S.; Kuhn, J.G.; Williams, R.O. Formulation and device design to increase nose to brain drug delivery. *J. Drug Deliv. Sci. Technol.* **2016**, *35*, 213–222. [CrossRef]
21. Marci, L.; Meloni, M.C.; Maccioni, A.M.; Sinico, C.; Lai, F.; Cardia, M.C. Formulation and characterization studies of trimethyl chitosan / sodium alginate nanoparticles for targeted drug delivery. *ChemistrySelect* **2016**, *1*, 669–674. [CrossRef]
22. Kulkarni, A.D.; Patel, H.M.; Surana, S.J.; Vanjari, Y.H.; Belgamwar, V.S.; Pardeshi, C.V. N,N,N-Trimethyl chitosan: An advanced polymer with myriad of opportunities in nanomedicine. *Carbohydr. Polym.* **2017**, *157*, 875–902. [CrossRef] [PubMed]
23. Mourya, V.K.; Inamdar, N.N. Trimethyl chitosan and its applications in drug delivery. *J. Mater. Sci. Mater. Med.* **2009**, *20*, 1057–1079. [CrossRef] [PubMed]
24. Yu, S.; Lee, M.; Shin, S.; Park, J. Apoptosis induced by progesterone in human ovarian cancer cell line SNU. *J. Cell. Biochem.* **2001**, *82*, 445–451. [CrossRef] [PubMed]
25. Nilsson, M.E.; Vandenput, L.; Tivesten, Å.; Norlén, A.K.; Lagerquist, M.K.; Windahl, S.H.; Börjesson, A.E.; Farman, H.H.; Poutanen, M.; Benrick, A.; et al. Measurement of a Comprehensive Sex Steroid Profile in Rodent Serum by High-Sensitive Gas Chromatography-Tandem Mass Spectrometry. *Endocrinology* **2015**, *156*, 2492–2502. [CrossRef]
26. Ducharme, N.; Banks, W.A.; Morley, J.E.; Robinson, S.M.; Niehoff, M.L.; Mattern, C.; Farr, S.A. Brain distribution and behavioral effects of progesterone and pregnenolone after intranasal or intravenous administration. *Eur. J. Pharmacol.* **2010**, *641*, 128–134. [CrossRef]

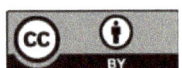

© 2019 by the authors. Licensee MDPI, Basel, Switzerland. This article is an open access article distributed under the terms and conditions of the Creative Commons Attribution (CC BY) license (http://creativecommons.org/licenses/by/4.0/).

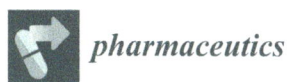

Article

Impact of Different Mucoadhesive Polymeric Nanoparticles Loaded in Thermosensitive Hydrogels on Transcorneal Administration of 5-Fluorouracil

Angela Fabiano [1],*, Anna Maria Piras [1], Lorenzo Guazzelli [1], Barbara Storti [2], Ranieri Bizzarri [2,3] and Ylenia Zambito [1,*]

1. Department of Pharmacy, University of Pisa Via Bonanno, 33, 56126 Pisa, Italy; anna.piras@unipi.it (A.M.P.); lorenzo.guazzelli@unipi.it (L.G.)
2. NEST, Scuola Normale Superiore and Istituto Nanoscienze-CNR, Piazza San Silvestro 12, 56127 Pisa, Italy; barbara.storti@nano.cnr.it (B.S.); ranieri.bizzarri@nano.cnr.it (R.B.)
3. Department of Surgical, Medical and Molecular Pathology, and Critical Care Medicine, University of Pisa, Via Roma 67, 56126 Pisa, Italy
* Correspondence: angela.fabiano@unipi.it (A.F.); ylenia.zambito@unipi.it (Y.Z.); Tel.: +39-050-221-2111 (A.F.); +39-050-221-9657 (Y.Z.)

Received: 30 October 2019; Accepted: 19 November 2019; Published: 21 November 2019

Abstract: In a previous paper a thermosensitive hydrogel formulation based on chitosan or its derivatives (TSOH), containing medicated chitosan nanoparticles (Ch NP) for transcorneal administration of 5-fluorouracil (5-FU) was described. The Ch NP-containing TSOH allowed a time-constant 5-FU concentration in the aqueous for 7 h from instillation. The aim of the present work was to study the impact of the surface characteristics of new NP contained in TSOH on ocular 5-FU bioavailability. The Ch derivatives used to prepare NP were quaternary ammonium-Ch conjugate (QA-Ch), *S*-protected derivative thereof (QA-Ch-*S*-pro), and a sulphobutyl chitosan derivative (SB-Ch). All NP types had 300–400 nm size, 16–18% encapsulation efficiency, and retained the entrapped drug for at least 15 h. Drug release from TSOH containing NP based on QA-Ch or QA-Ch-*S*-pro was virtually equal, whereas with TSOH containing NP based on SB-Ch was significantly slower. Instillation, in rabbit eyes, of NP-containing TSOH based on QA-Ch or SB-Ch led to a plateau in the aqueous concentration vs. time plot in the 1–10 h range with significantly enhanced area under curve (AUC). Negative charges on the NP surface slowed down 5-FU release from TSOH while positive charges increased NP contact with the negatively charged ocular surface. Either results in enhanced ocular bioavailability.

Keywords: thermosensitive hydrogels; mucoadhesive chitosan multifunctional derivatives; mucoadhesive nanoparticles; ocular cancer; microrheology; ocular delivery

1. Introduction

Topical ophthalmic preparations such as eyedrops are the most commonly used ocular drug delivery systems. Unfortunately, the intraocular bioavailability of their active substances is generally less than 5%, due to the anatomical and physiological characteristics of the eyes, including tissue barriers, such as cornea, lens, conjunctiva, and sclera, and various physiological functions, such as lacrimation and consequent dilution, and drug expulsion by tear turnover. As a consequence, to obtain the appropriate intraocular drug concentrations, frequent instillations of eyedrops are needed, which can cause toxic side effects and damage to the ocular tissue [1]. Thus, the traditional ophthalmic preparations and relevant therapeutic protocols cannot provide and maintain effective drug concentrations in the corneal tissue, and this results in a poor ocular bioavailability.

The intraocular bioavailability would improve if the drug transcorneal permeability and precorneal residence were increased [2]. One strategy to improve the corneal permeability is the addition of polymeric penetration enhancers to eyedrop formulations [3–5].

Another interesting approach to ocular drug delivery is the use of hydrogel systems. Among hydrogels the most interesting for the ocular administration of drugs are the thermosensitive hydrogels that can be instilled in the form of drops and become gels once in contact with the eyes [6–8]. In particular, chitosan-based thermosensitive hydrogels have proved to be vehicles of choice for biomedical application because they possess mucoadhesive, antibacterial, biodegradable, and biocompatible properties [7,9].

Another approach aimed at increasing the endo-ocular bioavailability of drugs is the use of nanoparticles (NP) or mucoadhesive vesicles capable of prolonging the contact with eye mucosae and promoting the absorption of entrapped drugs [10,11]. Furthermore, the nanoparticles could be internalized by the corneal cells, and form a reservoir from which the drug could be released over time [12].

Recently, innovative formulations based on thermosensitive hydrogels for the sustained ocular delivery of drugs entrapped in nanosize structures have been proposed [13–15]. In all cases such systems were found to have a greater ability than those based on the simple thermosensitive hydrogels to prolong the drug residence in the precorneal area, promote endoocular bioavailability, and prolong the drug halflife in the aqueous. If nanosystem diffusion in hydrogels is excluded, the above results can be explained by the blinking continuously renewing the hydrogel-cornea contact surface, thus bringing new NP into contact with the cornea.

In our previous work we tried to combine the above strategies by preparing thermosensitive hydrogels (TSOH) based on chitosan and its derivatives containing medicated NP based on unmodified chitosan for transcorneal administration of 5-fluorouracil (5-FU) [13]. Chitosan was chosen because cationic polymers have greater interactivity with the negatively charged ocular surface [16], and also, because chitosan has a lower toxicity than other cationic polymers, such as polyarginine or polyethylenimine [17]. Increased bioavailability of 5-FU in the aqueous with respect to control eyedrops resulted from in vivo experiments with rabbit eyes. The NP-containing hydrogels mediated to a zero-order 5-FU absorption, leading to a time-constant anticancer concentration in the aqueous for up to 7 h from instillation. This was ascribed to the ability of this TSOH to control drug release to a zero order and that of NP to be internalized by corneal cells. In that first study the preparation of thermosensitive hydrogels was studied and developed, while the impact of the surface characteristics of the NP they contained on drug ocular bioavailability was not studied. Such an impact has been investigated in the present study.

Nanoparticles differing in mucoadhesivity and surface charge were prepared for this purpose from chitosan (Ch) derivatives, and NP ability to promote the transcorneal penetration of 5-FU was assessed in vivo. The chitosan derivatives consisted in quaternary ammonium-Ch conjugate (QA-Ch), S-protected derivative thereof (QA-Ch-S-pro), and a sulfobutyl chitosan derivative (SB-Ch). While the properties of quaternary ammonium-Ch conjugate and/or those of the respective S-protected derivatives have widely been described in the literature, the properties of Ch modified by sulfate or sulfonate groups is currently under investigation [18]. The NP were dispersed in TSOH in the sol state and compared on the ground of NP size, surface zeta potential, mucoadhesivity, affinity with the drug, and in vitro drug-release properties, in order to select the systems on which to carry out in vivo pharmacokinetic studies.

2. Materials and Methods

2.1. Materials

Low molecular weight Ch (75–85% deacetylated), 5-FU, β-glycerophosphate (β-GP) disodium salt, sodium tripolyphosphate (TPP), 1,4-butane sulphone, and fluorescein isothiocyanate (FITC),

Type II mucin from porcine stomach, were purchased from Sigma-Aldrich (Milan, Italy). The QA-Ch conjugate was synthesized from Ch according to Zambito et al., 2013 [19], the thiolated S-protected derivative of QA-Ch was synthesized according to Fabiano et al., 2018 [20]. Reduced molecular weight hyaluronic acid (rHA) (viscosimetric molecular weight 470 kDa) was prepared as described by Zambito et al., 2013 [19]. FITC labelling of QA-Ch, QA-Ch-S-pro, and SB-Ch was carried out as previously described [21]. The QA-Ch50 polymer, used to prepare the TSOH, was synthesized according to Zambito et al., 2013 [19]. In the code, 50 means that it was prepared by maintaining the temperature at 50 °C for the entire duration of the reaction. All aqueous solutions/dispersions were prepared with freshly distilled water. QA-Ch was characterized by ^{1}H NMR to determine the degree of substitution with the small side chains containing adjacent quaternary ammonium groups and the length of such chains. Protected thiols present on QA-Ch-S-pro chains were determined by polymer reduction and subsequent quantification of the 6-mercaptonicotinamide protecting group. Only polymers that had the same characteristics as previously obtained [20] were used in this work.

2.2. Synthesis and Characterization of Sulphobutyl Chitosan (SB-Ch)

SB-Ch was synthesized from Ch as previously described [22]. Briefly, 1,4-butane sulphone (3 equivalents per N-acetylglucosamine unit) was added to a Ch solution in acidic water (1% w/w Ch, 2% w/w of acid acetic). The mixture was allowed to react at 60 °C for 6 h. The resulting solution was poured into acetone. The precipitated product was resuspended in demineralized water and purified by dialysis 3 days against water. After dialysis, the polymer solution was lyophilized to obtain the purified SB-Ch (Figure 1). ^{1}H NMR spectrum was recorded in D$_2$O/DCl with a Bruker AC 200 instrument operating at 200.13 MHz (Bruker, Milan, Italy).

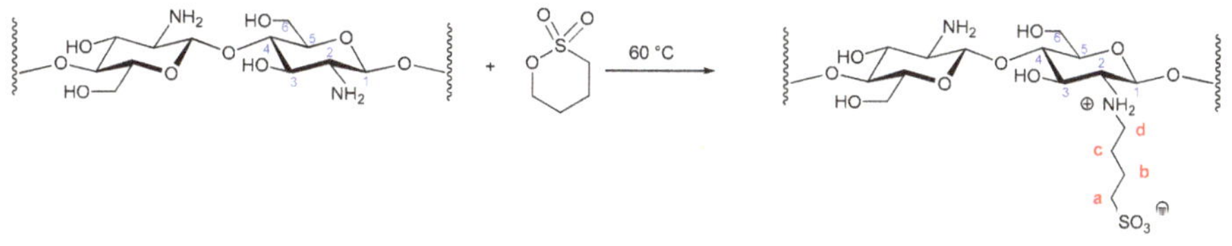

Figure 1. Synthetic route to sulfobutyl chitosan (SB-Ch).

2.3. Preparation of Medicated NP

FITC-labeled or unlabeled NP based on QA-Ch or QA-Ch-S-pro were prepared by self-assembly upon addition of rHA. In detail, a solution of rHA 0.2 mg/mL in phosphate buffer (0.13 M, PB pH 7.4) containing 6.25 mg of 5-FU was added dropwise (500 µL) to 5 mL of 2 mg/mL polymer solution in the same buffer, under stirring at room temperature. Similarly, to prepare FITC-labeled or unlabeled NP based on SB-Ch, a solution of TPP 2 mg/mL in demineralized water containing 6.25 mg of FU was added dropwise (700 µL) to 5 mL of 2 mg/mL SB-Ch in demineralized water, under stirring at room temperature. The final 5-FU concentration in NP systems based on QA-Ch, or QA-Ch-S-pro, or SB-Ch was 1.25 mg/mL, corresponding to the concentration contained in the commercial 5-FU eyedrops. After their preparation, the NP dispersions were checked for particle size and zeta potential (ζ) at a temperature of 25 °C (Zetasizer Nano ZS, Malvern, UK). The ζ values of medicated NP based on QA-Ch, QA-Ch-S-pro, or SB-Ch were determined after NP centrifugation (2000 rpm for 30 min) and their subsequent sediments re-suspended in 1.9 mL of a 0.08 M HCl solution containing 195 µL of NaOH 1 N and 0.8 g/mL of β-GP. Their drug-entrapment efficiency (EE) was evaluated by subjecting the dispersion to centrifugation (20,000 rpm for 30 min at 4 °C) and analyzing the supernatant spectophotometrically at 266 nm. The EE was calculated as follows, using the appropriate calibration curve:

$$EE = (M_t - M_s)/M_t \tag{1}$$

where M_t is the total mass of 5-FU used for the preparation of NP and M_s is the mass found in the supernatant.

2.4. Preparation of Thermosensitive Hydrogels (TSOH) Containing NP Medicated with 5-FU

Thermosensitive ophthalmic hydrogels (TSOH) were prepared according to Fabiano et al. [13]. Briefly, 400 mg of Ch and 100 mg of QA-Ch50 were dissolved in 18 mL of a 0.08 M HCl solution. The resulting solution was kept under magnetic stirring at 4 °C. Then, 5-FU-medicated NP, based on QA-Ch, QA-Ch-S-pro, or SB-Ch, freshly prepared, were added in the sol state under magnetic stirring at 4 °C, before the addition of 450 µl β-GP (0.8 g/mL) solution to obtain TSOH.

2.5. Dynamic Dialysis Studies

To study the reversible drug binding by NP in fluid dispersion we used already reported procedure and theory [23,24]. Briefly, a porous cellulose membrane (cut-off 12.5 kDa) was used to separate the donor compartment of the dialysis cell from the receiving phase (100 mL of PB pH 7.4 for 5-FU-loaded QA-Ch or QA-Ch-S-pro NP or100 mL of demineralized water for 5-FU-loaded SB-Ch NP). The system was thermostated at 35 °C for 5 h, while maintaining sink conditions. At time $t = 0$, 5 mL of freshly prepared 5-FU loaded NP, or plain drug solution (control), or this solution containing 2 mg/mL of QA-Ch or QA-Ch-S-pro dissolved in PB pH 7.4, or 2 mg/mL of SB-Ch in water was introduced in the donor compartment of the cell. In all cases, at the end of experiment, the receiving phase was analyzed spectrophotometrically to determine the drug transport. In the case of NP, the receiving phase was also analyzed for particle size.

2.6. Interrupted-Dialysis Studies

The dynamic dialysis experiment, described in Section 2.5, was stopped after 1, 2, 3, 5, 15, or 24 h, from the start. At each time interval, the donor phase was centrifuged (2000 rpm for 30 min at 4 °C) to determine the drug fraction contained in NP matrix, NP dispersion medium, and acceptor medium, according to reference [25]. The results were plotted as drug fraction in each phase versus time.

2.7. Studies of 5-FU Release from NP-Containing TSOH

5-FU release from TSOH was carried out using a cell and a procedure reported by Fabiano et al. [13]. The gel (0.5 mL) containing medicated NP was introduced in the cylindrical cavity of the cell. A porous cellulose membrane (cut-off 12.5 kDa) was used to separate the gel from the receiving phase (30 mL of PB pH 7.4 for 5-FU-loaded NP based on QA-Ch or QA-Ch-S-pro, or 30 mL of demineralized water for 5-FU-loaded NP based on SB-Ch). At time, $t = 0$, the cell was introduced in a beaker containing the receiving phase thermostated at 35 °C and stirred at 300 rpm. The receiving phase was analyzed spectrophotometrically at 30-min intervals to determine the drug transport kinetics.

2.8. Confocal Microscopy and Image Analysis

To evaluate the possibility of re-dispersing NP into the hydrogel system, the FITC-labelled, 5-FU medicated NP, based on QA-Ch, QA-Ch-S-pro, or SB-Ch were dispersed in the TSOH at room temperature and observed under a confocal laser-scanning microscope (Zeiss LSM 880 with Airyscan, Carl Zeiss, Jena, Germany). The representative fluorescence confocal micrographs of NP were taken in liquid (21 °C) and gel states (4 °C), using a 63x Apochromat NA = 1.4 oil-immersion objective with the pinhole aperture of the confocal system at 1 Airy unit. The excitation wavelength was set at 488 nm (10–20 µW power emission at objective), whereas emission was in the 500–550 nm range. Pixel dwell time was adjusted to 1.52 µs and 512 × 512 pixel images were collected.

Image analysis was carried out by ImageJ v.1.52o (NIH, Bethesda, MD, USA) software. Particle diameters were calculated by tracing an equatorial line over each bead (average of 5–10 beads), collecting the fluorescence profile and fitting it with a Gaussian function. The full width at half maximum (FWHM) of the best-fitting curve was assumed as particle diameter.

2.9. Micro-Rheological Characterization of NP Mucoadhesive Properties

Micro-rheological measurements were carried out using a Zetasizer Nano ZS, Malvern, with a detection angle of 173 °C and a temperature of 25 °C, applying the theory reported by Dodero et al. [26]. The micro-rheological characterization of 5-FU loaded freshly prepared QA-Ch or SB-Ch NP was performed using mucin from porcine stomach, Type II. Ocular mucins are not commercially available, so porcine gastric mucin was used because it has also been applied as a model substance in other studies, investigating ocular mucoadhesion [27]. In order to obtain reliable micro-rheological data, the conditions about the tracer-sample combination were verified as reported by Dodero et al., 2019 [26]. A dispersion of mucin 3 mg/mL in water, was filtered using a cellulose acetate filter (pore size 0.45 μm). A sample was taken from the filtrate and lyophilized to calculate the concentration of dispersed material (1.85 mg/mL). The filtered mucin dispersion was diluted 10 times with a solution of NaCl 0.9%. Then, 5 μL of tracer sample (polystyrene latex particles, diameter 500 nm, Beckman, 5 μl/mL) and 5 μL of NP dispersions prepared as described in Section 2.4 were added to the diluted mucin dispersion. Micro-rheological tests were performed to evaluate viscoelastic properties and assess NP mucoadhesive properties on the basis of the viscosity changes caused by NP addition to a mucin solution.

2.10. In Vivo Studies

For the in vivo studies we used male New Zealand albino rabbits weighing 3–3.5 kg treated as prescribed in the guidelines from the European Community Council Directive 2010/63, approved by the Animal Care Committee of the University of Pisa (D.L. 2014/26, 12 March 2019). Fifty μL (one drop) of the following two types of ophthalmic formulations were instilled in the lower conjunctival sac: (1) a dispersion of QA-Ch-based NP medicated with 1.25 mg/mL of 5-FU in TSOH and (2) a dispersion of SB-Ch-based NP medicated with 1.25 mg/mL 5-FU in TSOH. For the entire duration of the experiments each rabbit eye was checked for signs of conjunctival/cornea edema and/or hyperemia [28]. Before the aspiration of aqueous humor (~60 μL) from the anterior chamber of the eye, the rabbits were anesthetized with one drop of Novesina®. The 5-FU concentration in aqueous humor was determined by high-performance liquid chromatography (HPLC) using the apparatus and the mobile phase described by Fabiano et al. [13]. An Aeris 3.6 μm, PEPTIDE XB-C18 Å, 250 × 4.6 mm column, equilibrated at 30 °C was used and UV detection was set at 266 nm. Standard curves were obtained analyzing six standard drug solutions (concentration range 0.3–1.25 μg/mL) in acetonitrile mixed with aqueous humor (2:1). The resulting mixtures were centrifuged, and the acetonitrile was removed by evaporation at 50 °C. The resulting aqueous product was lyophilized and re-dispersed in a volume of mobile phase corresponding to the initial volume of standard solution. Standard curves were linear ($r^2 > 0.995$, limit of detection 0.2 μg/mL). The retention time was 8.2 min. The concentration of each unknown sample was determined as described above, using a standard curve produced on the same day.

2.11. Data Treatment

Linear plots were obtained by linear regression analysis of data from in vitro experiments. The relevant slope, intercept, and coefficient of determination (r^2) were calculated. The significance of differences was evaluated by Student's t-test ($p < 0.05$). For the in vivo experiments, the linear trapezoidal rule between 0 and 10 h was used to calculate the area under curve (AUC) and the statistical differences were evaluated using the method reported by Schoenwald et al. [29].

3. Results and Discussion

3.1. Synthesis of Sulphobutyl Chitosan (SB-Ch)

^{1}H NMR spectrum (D$_2$O/DCl) of SB-Ch, seen in Figure 2, shows three sets of signals ascribed to the different methylene groups of the sulfobutyl functionalization at 1.32–1.60 ppm (–CH$_{2b}$ and –CH$_{2c}$), 2.62–3.72 ppm (–CH$_{2d}$), and 3.33–3.41 ppm (–CH$_{2a}$ overlapping to protons H-3, H-4, H-5, and H-6 of chitosan). An estimation of the butylsulfonation degree (ca 52%) was possible by comparing the integrals of H-2 of the chitosan backbone, which fell in a quite clean part of the spectrum (2.91–3.20 ppm), and of –CH$_{2d}$ of the sulfobutyl group.

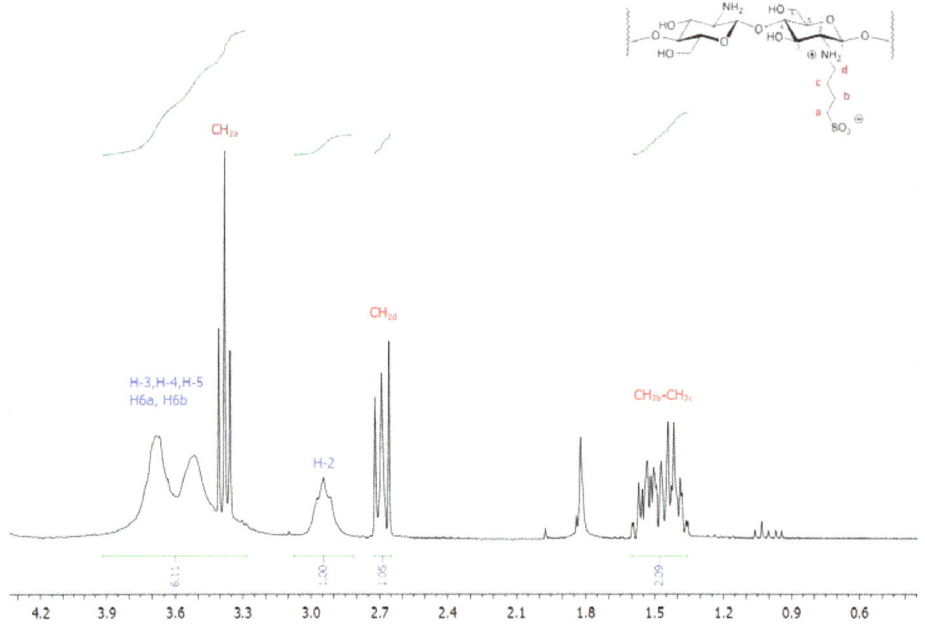

Figure 2. ^{1}H NMR (200.12 MHz, D$_2$O/DCl) spectral region of SB-Ch.

3.2. Characteristics of Medicated NP

The size, polydispersity index, zeta potential (ζ) and encapsulation efficiency (EE) for medicated NP based on QA-Ch, QA-Ch-S-pro, or SB-Ch are found in Table 1. The size and polydispersity index values were not significantly different from each other or from those for NP based on Ch prepared in our preceding paper Fabiano et al. [13] (342.5 ± 15.2). The ζ values for medicated NP based on QA-Ch or QA-Ch-S-pro were positive in agreement with the presence of ammonium quaternary ions on their surface, whereas for medicated NP based on SB-Ch the ζ value was negative in agreement with the presence of superficial sulfonic groups. The EE was in the range 18–15% with no significant difference between the three cases. The prepared NP only differing for their external charge allowed us to evaluate the impact of this property on the system ability to promote the intraocular absorption of 5-FU.

Table 1. Characteristics of medicated nanoparticles (NP) determined immediately after their preparation.

NP Type	Nanoparticle Size, nm (Polydispersity Index)	ζ, mV	EE%
NP quaternary ammonium-Ch conjugate (QA-Ch)	294.3 ± 60.6 (0.4 ± 0.2)	+9.1 ± 0.4	18.4 ± 4.0
NP QA-Ch-S-pro	340.7 ± 100.1 (0.3 ± 0.1)	+9.5 ± 0.1	18.3 ± 0.2
NP SB-Ch	390.6 ± 50.3 (0.2 ± 0.1)	−3.5 ± 0.1	15.6 ± 1.0

3.3. Dynamic Dialysis Studies

Dynamic dialysis data were used to compare reversible drug interactions with the NP in fluid dispersions. According to [23,24], the data obtained were plotted as ln (C_d/C_{d0}) × 100 versus t using the following Equation (2):

$$\ln [(C_d/C_{d0}) \times 100] = 4.605 - K_m F_f t \qquad (2)$$

where C_d is the drug concentration in the donor phase, C_{d0} is the drug concentration in donor phase at $t = 0$, F_f is the non-interacting drug fraction in donor phase, and K_m is the dialysis-rate constant. All plots, reported in Figure 3 were significantly linear (r^2 values, 0.90–0.98) which indicated that in all cases (plain 5-FU, control, NP based on QA-Ch, QA-Ch-S-pro, or SB-Ch) Equation (2) was obeyed and for plain 5-FU (control) the slope of the relative log-linear plot, used to calculate F_f was equal to K_m. The slopes of the straight lines reported in Table 2 indicated a 5-FU binding with all polymers in solution higher than the binding with NP dispersions. From here, it was deduced that the drug fraction reversibly interacting with the polymers in solution was significantly higher than that adsorbed on NP surface. This was probably due to an interaction between the 5-FU and the polycationic polysaccharide Ch. In the case of NP, the positive groups of Ch could be bound to the crosslinker and, hence, less available for 5-FU binding. This, nevertheless, should not impair the NP effectiveness in vivo, in fact, nanoparticles made of mucoahesive polymers are themselves more mucoahesive than the corresponding parent polymers, hence, likely to strongly adhere to the ocular surface [10,20,30].

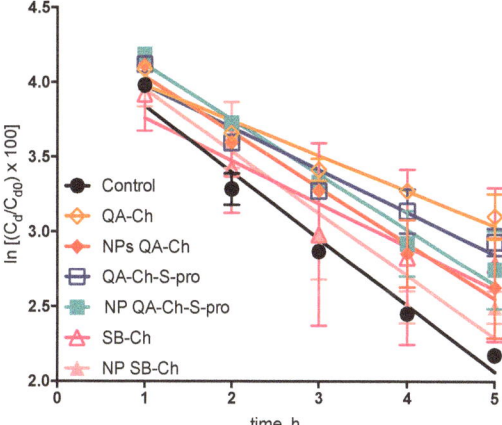

Figure 3. Dynamic dialysis data plotted according to Equation (2). Means ± SD (n = 3–6).

Table 2. Results of dynamic dialysis data plotted in Figure 3 and obtained according to Equation (2).

Formulation	Modulus of Straight-Line Slope ± SD (h^{-1})	r^2	Interaction [a] %
Control	0.44 ± 0.04	0.97	-
QA-Ch	0.23 ± 0.03	0.94	47.7
NP QA-Ch	0.37 ± 0.03	0.98	15.9
QA-Ch-S-pro	0.28 ± 0.04	0.93	36.4
NP QA-Ch-S-pro	0.37 ± 0.03	0.98	15.9
SB-Ch	0.29 ± 0.06	0.90	34.1
NP SB-Ch	0.41 ± 0.06	0.93	6.8

[a] Bound fraction.

3.4. 5-FU Release from NP

The procedure used to study 5-FU release from NP was based on interrupted dialysis, as described in Section 2.6. A dispersion of each freshly prepared NP type, loaded with 5-FU and not separated from the non-entrapped drug was introduced in the donor compartment of the dialysis cell. Hence, not more than 15–18% of the whole 5-FU amount contained in each dispersion was associated with the NP phase, as shown in Table 1. From knowledge of the drug amount used for each NP preparation, the drug amount determined for the NP dispersion medium in donor compartment (DM phase) at each interruption time, the cumulative amount determined for the drug transferred into the receiving medium (RM phase) during each interruption time, and the relevant % 5-FU contained in the NP matrix, i.e., the NPM data reported in Figure 4, could readily be calculated. This data indicated that the 5-FU fraction immobilized in the NP matrix remained virtually constant at the initial value of 15–18% over the first 15 h of experiment, while it seemed to fade after 24 h probably due to some degradation of the NP. Therefore, it is understood that all NP types are able to retain the 5-FU load for a term sufficient for NP to be internalized by corneal cells. It should be noted that the present NP, prepared from Ch derivatives, were able to retain 5-FU for longer than those prepared by Fabiano et al., from Ch (15 vs. 5 h) [13].

3.5. Drug Release from NP-Containing TSOH

Data on drug release from NP-containing TSOH, obtained as described in Section 2.7 and plotted as percentage of drug released versus t or $\sqrt{t}$ are reported in Figure 5a,b, respectively. The release study lasted 5 h since the 5-FU release study for all NP types had shown that the 5-FU % entrapped in the NP was virtually constant for at least 15 h. The drug amount released vs. $\sqrt{t}$ was in all cases linear with comparatively small ordinate intercepts (between −0.99% and 2.88%) and high r^2 values (between 0.96 and 0.99, $n = 3$). This pattern in all cases fitted a well-known model assuming that the release was entirely governed by drug diffusion in the releasing vehicle. The slope of each straight line allowed comparison between the different cases on the basis of drug diffusivity in the hydrogel. The data listed in Table 3 shows that 5-FU release from TSOH containing NP based on QA-Ch or QA-Ch-S-pro was not significantly different from drug release from TSOH containing NP based on Ch, whereas drug release from TSOH containing NP based on SB-Ch was significantly slowed down, with respect to the above, reasonably by the negative charges on the NP surface dispersed in this TSOH. Indeed, TSOH was prepared using a chitosan derivative containing fixed positive charges that could electrostatically interact with the negative charges of SB-Ch, and this interaction could slow down the 5-FU release from TSOH.

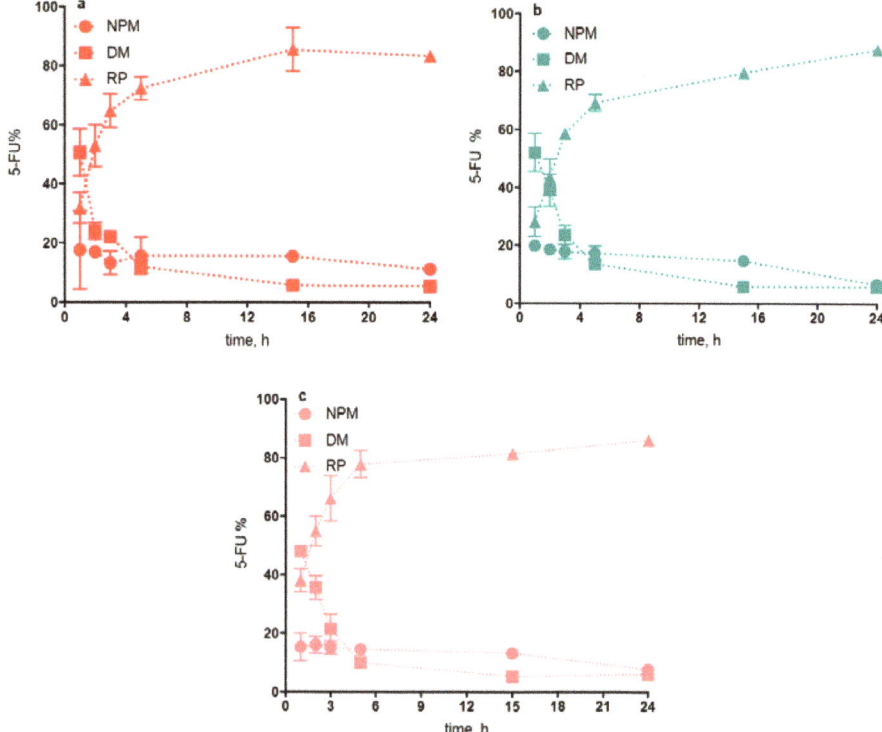

Figure 4. Interrupted dialysis studies: kinetic analysis of dialysis phases for 5-fluorouracil (5-FU)-loaded QA-Ch NP (**a**), QA-Ch-S-pro NP (**b**), and SB-Ch NP (**c**). Percent 5-FU in: NP matrix (NPM); NP dispersion medium (DM); and receiving phase (RP). Means ± SD ($n = 3$).

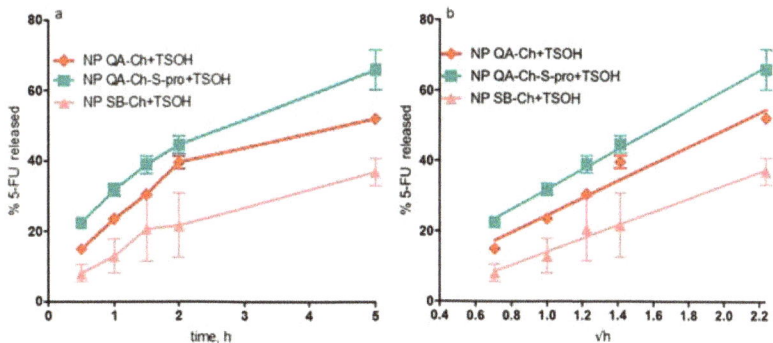

Figure 5. 5-FU released (%) from NP-containing thermosensitive hydrogels (TSOH) vs. time (hours) (**a**) or vs. $\sqrt{t}$ (**b**).

Table 3. Characteristics of 5-FU release from NP-containing TSOH.

Formulation	Slope of √t Plot (%/√h)	Cumulative Release at 5 h (%)
Ch NP+TSOH [a]	3.34 ± 0.32	59.50 ± 0.90
QA-Ch NP+TSOH	3.14 ± 0.39	52.23 ± 1.07
QA-Ch-S-pro NP+TSOH	3.64 ± 3.12	65.93 ± 5.70
SB-Ch NP+TSOH	2.43 ± 0.21 *	37.00 ± 3.82 *

[a] Data taken from Fabiano et al., 2017 [13]. * Significantly different from all the others ($p < 0.05$).

3.6. Confocal Microscopy and Image Analysis

Particle fluorescence allowed their visualization in both the sol and gel states by means of fluorescence confocal microscopy [13]. From particle images, their size could be inferred (Table 4, Figure 6) affording interesting information on the role of gelification on their aggregation status. Gelation did not affect the size of SB-Ch NP (Table 4, entries 1,2; Figure 6a,b) which remained close to the optical diffraction limit of the microscopy apparatus (~0.2 µm). Conversely, QA-Ch NP in the gel phase showed the presence of two main particle populations: one, with a size comparable to that of SB-Ch NP, the other twice as large (Table 4, entry 3; Figure 6c). A bimodal pattern was observed also with QA-Ch-S-pro NP, although in this case the smaller peak was about 0.6 µm and the larger was, on the average, more than 4 µm with a rather large dispersion as indicated by the relevant standard error (SE) values (Table 4, entry 4; Figure 6d). These findings strongly suggest a moderate aggregation of QA-Ch NP, each aggregate possibly consisting of two particles sticking together, in the sol state, and a much larger aggregate state for QA-Ch-S-pro NP in the gel state. These data encouraged us to continue the study only with NP based on QA-Ch and SB-Ch.

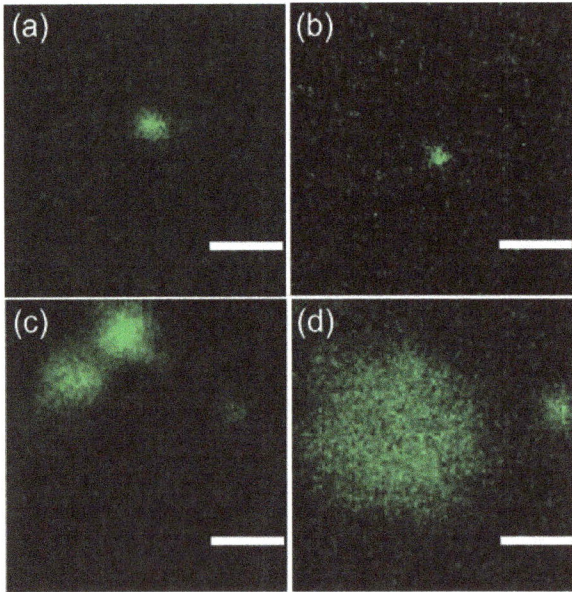

Figure 6. Representative fluorescence confocal micrographs of NP. For all images, the same field of view and pixel size was adopted, to allow a direct visual comparison of NP size. (**a**) SB-Ch NP (sol state), (**b**) SB-Ch NP (gel state), (**c**) QA-Ch NP (gel state), and (**d**) QA-Ch-S-pro NP (gel state). Scale bar: 1 µm.

Table 4. Size of the particles as determined by confocal fluorescence microscopy. Each entry refers to one experiment where the size was calculated as the average of five full width at half maximum (FWHM) measurements (see Materials and Methods section).

Entry	Particle (Status)	Mean Size ± SE (µm)
1	SB-Ch NP (sol)	0.27 ± 0.02
2	SB-Ch NP (gel)	0.33 ± 0.02
3	QA-Ch NP (gel)	0.70 ± 0.07; 0.29 ± 0.01
4	QA-Ch-S-pro NP (gel)	4.26 ± 1.67; 0.61 ± 0.15

3.7. Micro-Rheological Characterization of NP Mucoadhesive Properties

The elastic (or storage) modulus, G′, the viscous (or loss) modulus, G″, and the complex viscosity, η*, are reported in Figure 7. As can be seen, there was an increase in η* of mucin dispersion in the presence of NP based on either QA-Ch or SB-Ch, compared to plain mucin dispersion. The increase of η* was reflected in the increase of both G′ and G″ moduli. In particular, the increase in G′ is indicative of the development of an inter-connected microstructure between mucin macromolecules and NP based on QA-Ch, resulting in a stronger mucoadhesivity of these NP with respect to the NP based on SB-Ch. However, G′ for NP based on SB-Ch was higher than G′ for mucin, due to the intrinsic mucoadhesivity of Ch, i.e., the pristine material used to prepare SB-Ch. These data demonstrate that the sign of the NP surface charge can actually influence their mucoadhesivity. Moreover, it is known that the mucus glycoproteins bear negatively charged sialic moieties that are capable of forming ionic bonds with oppositely charged chemical species [31].

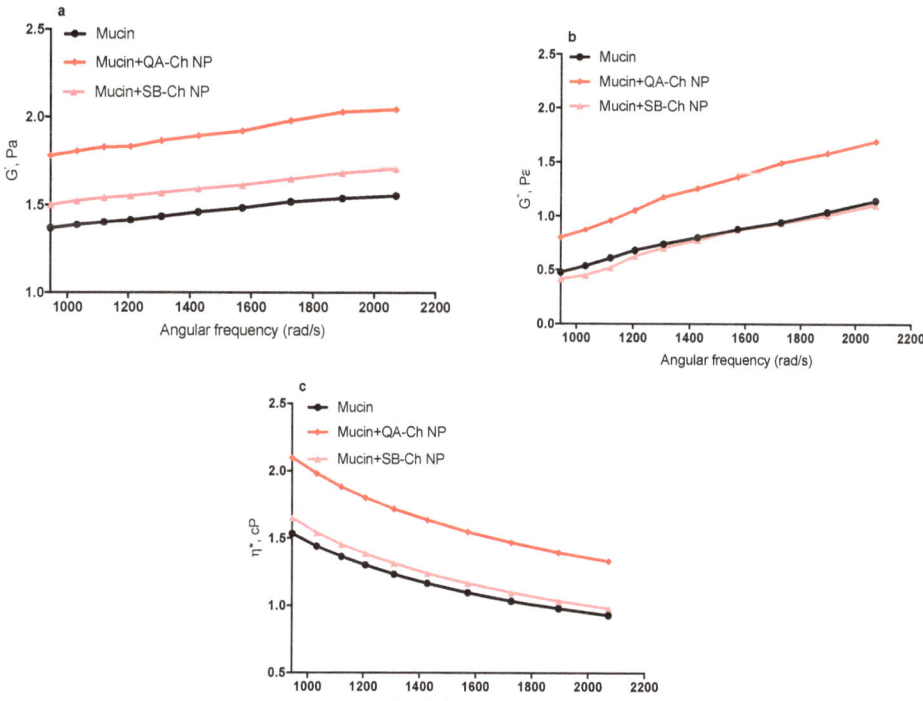

Figure 7. Elastic modulus, G′ (**a**), viscous modulus, G″ (**b**), and complex viscosity, η* (**c**), of QA-Ch and SB-Ch NP with respect to mucin dispersion.

3.8. In Vivo Tests

During each experiment, we observed that all the ophthalmic drops instilled in rabbit eyes caused no conjunctival/corneal edema and/or hyperemia. The pharmacokinetic profiles in the aqueous and the relative AUC values are reported in Figure 8 and Table 5, respectively. The results of the in vivo tests shown in Figure 8 demonstrate the ability of the TSOH containing NP based on QA-Ch or SB-Ch to increase the 5-FU bioavailability with respect to the control, TSOH, and Ch NP-containing TSOH [13]. Indeed, the AUC values relative to QA-Ch NP+TSOH and SB-Ch NP+TSOH listed in Table 5, are significantly higher than those relative to the control, TSOH, and Ch NP+TSOH, with a concentration plateau in the range 1–10 h. These results demonstrate that the QA-Ch NP+TSOH and SB-Ch NP+TSOH systems have much more ability to prolong the drug precorneal residence time than the control, TSOH, or Ch NP-containing TSOH. In view of the ability of NP to retain the drug for longer, the plateau in the 1–10 h range is in-keeping with the hypothesis of an intraocular drug absorption controlled by gel erosion in pre-corneal area accompanied by release of drug-loaded NP that are then internalized in corneal cells.

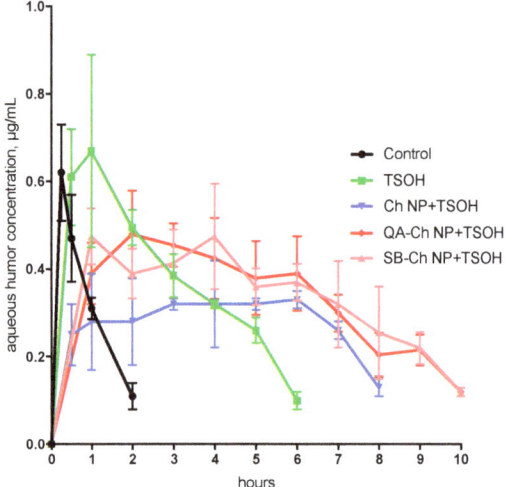

Figure 8. Pharmacokinetics in the aqueous following instillation of ophthalmic drops. Means ± SD (n = 6). Control, TSOH, and Ch NP+TSOH profiles are taken from Fabiano et al. [13].

Table 5. AUC data obtained in vivo in rabbit eyes.

Formulation	AUC_{0-10}, µg h/mL	AUC_{rel}
Control [a]	0.62 ± 0.1	-
TSOH [a]	2.32 ± 0.26 *	3.7
Ch NP+TSOH [a]	2.23 ± 0.39 *	3.6
QA-Ch NP+TSOH	3.30 ± 0.52 *,**	5.3
SB-Ch NP+TSOH	3.34 ± 0.53 *,**	5.4

[a] Data taken from Fabiano et al., 2017 [13]; * $p < 0.05$ versus control, ** $p < 0.05$ versus TSOH, and Ch NP+TSOH.

It is interesting to note that no differences were seen, in Figure 8, in the concentration in the aqueous vs. time profiles between any of the three NP-containing TSOH formulations. This can be ascribed to the presence in all formulations of a significant 5-FU dose fraction not entrapped in NP, but free to permeate across the cornea by passive diffusion. Such a drug fraction is unaffected by the different NP ability to be internalized in corneal cells, which can indeed be influenced by the NP surface characteristics.

The data altogether demonstrate the importance of NP mucoadhesion properties and of their ability to interact with the vehicle. In fact, QA-Ch NP-containing TSOH showed an AUC value higher than that for TSOH or Ch NP+ TSOH probably thanks to their fixed positive charges that prolong the drug retention time and increase the drug contact with the anterior surface of the eyes and thereby, enhance ocular absorption via paracellular transport through the tight junctions of corneal epithelia [16]. On the other hand, SB-Ch NP+TSOH showed an AUC value similar to that of QA-Ch NP+TSOH probably due to its ability to slow down the 5-FU release from the vehicle, as demonstrated in Section 3.5.

These present results are in agreement with those shown in a preceding paper where it was found that the more effective NP were able to concurrently adhere to the ocular surface and strongly interact with the drug molecules in solution [10]. After all, although less mucoadhesive than QA-Ch NP, the SB-Ch NP also showed some mucoadhesivity due to the intrinsic mucoadhesivity of the Ch backbone.

4. Conclusions

These results indicate that the present SB-Ch NP-containing thermosensitive hydrogels are able to prolong 5-FU ocular residence thanks to the synergistic effect of negative charges on NP surface and positive charges present in the TSOH. Furthermore, in the case of QA-Ch NP-containing thermosensitive hydrogels the presence of positive charges on NP surface prolongs their contact with corneal and conjunctival surfaces that are negatively charged. As a result, both NP-containing QA-Ch-based and SB-Ch-based TSOH were able to increase the ocular 5-FU bioavailability. NP-containing thermosensitive hydrogels could be administered as conventional eyedrops and still represent an alternative, more effective formulation than the commercial 5-FU eyedrops, with reduced 5-FU applied dose and instillation frequency. However stability studies of the formulations must be carried out in the future to understand if they can really be commercialized.

Author Contributions: Conceptualization, A.F. and Y.Z.; methodology, A.F., A.M.P., R.B. and Y.Z.; validation, A.F., A.M.P., and Y.Z..; formal analysis, A.F., A.M.P., L.G., B.S. and R.B., data curation, A.F., A.M.P., R.B. and Y.Z.; writing—original draft preparation, A.F. and Y.Z.; writing—review and editing, all authors; supervision, Y.Z.

Funding: This research was funded by University of Pisa grant numbers PRA 2018_18.

Conflicts of Interest: The authors declare no conflict of interest.

References

1. Gaudana, R.; Ananthula, H.K.; Parenky, A.; Mitra, A.K. Ocular drug delivery. *AAPS J.* **2010**, *12*, 348–360. [CrossRef] [PubMed]
2. Üstündağ-Okur, N.; Gökçe, E.H.; Bozbıyık, D.I.; Eğrilmez, S.; Özer, Ö.; Ertan, G. Preparation and in vitro–in vivo evaluation of ofloxacin loaded ophthalmic nano structured lipid carriers modified with chitosan oligosaccharide lactate for the treatment of bacterial keratitis. *Eur. J. Pharm. Sci.* **2014**, *63*, 204–215. [CrossRef] [PubMed]
3. Di Colo, G.; Zambito, Y.; Zaino, C. Polymeric enhancers of mucosal epithelia permeability: Synthesis, transepithelial penetration-enhancing properties, mechanism of action, safety issues. *J. Pharm. Sci.* **2008**, *97*, 1652–1680. [CrossRef] [PubMed]
4. Zambito, Y.; Di Colo, G. Chitosan and its derivatives as intraocular penetration enhancers. *J. Drug Deliv. Sci. Technol.* **2010**, *20*, 45–52. [CrossRef]
5. Zambito, Y.; Di Colo, G. Thiolated quaternary ammonium–chitosan conjugates for enhanced precorneal retention, transcorneal permeation and intraocular absorption of dexamethasone. *Eur. J. Pharm. Biopharm.* **2010**, *75*, 194–199. [CrossRef] [PubMed]
6. Berger, J.; Reist, M.; Chenite, A.; Felt-Baeyens, O.; Mayer, J.M.; Gurny, R. Pseudo-thermosetting chitosan hydrogels for biomedical application. *Int. J. Pharm.* **2005**, *288*, 197–206. [CrossRef]
7. Chenite, A.; Chaput, C.; Wang, D.; Combes, C.; Buschmann, M.D.; Hoemann, C.D.; Selmani, A. Novel injectable neutral solutions of chitosan form biodegradable gels in situ. *Biomaterials* **2000**, *21*, 2155–2161. [CrossRef]

8. Wang, Q.; Zuo, Z.; Cheung CK, C.; Leung, S.S.Y. Updates on thermosensitive hydrogel for nasal, ocular and cutaneous delivery. *Int. J. Pharm.* **2019**, *559*, 86–101. [CrossRef]
9. Ruel-Gariepy, E.; Leroux, J.C. In situ-forming hydrogels—review of temperature-sensitive systems. *Eur. J. Pharm. Biopharm.* **2004**, *58*, 409–426. [CrossRef]
10. Fabiano, A.; Chetoni, P.; Zambito, Y. Mucoadhesive nano-sized supramolecular assemblies for improved pre-corneal drug residence time. *Drug Dev. Ind. Pharm.* **2015**, *41*, 2069–2076. [CrossRef]
11. Bonferoni, M.C.; Sandri, G.; Dellera, E.; Rossi, S.; Ferrari, F.; Zambito, Y.; Caramella, C. Palmitoyl glycol chitosan micelles for corneal delivery of cyclosporine. *J. Biomed. Nanotechnol.* **2016**, *12*, 231–240. [CrossRef] [PubMed]
12. Diebold, Y.; Jarrín, M.; Saez, V.; Carvalho, E.L.; Orea, M.; Calonge, M.; Alonso, M.J. Ocular drug delivery by liposome–chitosan nanoparticle complexes (LCS-NP). *Biomaterials* **2007**, *28*, 1553–1564. [CrossRef] [PubMed]
13. Fabiano, A.; Bizzarri, R.; Zambito, Y. Thermosensitive hydrogel based on chitosan and its derivatives containing medicated nanoparticles for transcorneal administration of 5-fluorouracil. *Int. J. Nanomed.* **2017**, *12*, 633. [CrossRef] [PubMed]
14. Morsi, N.; Ghorab, D.; Refai, H.; Teba, H. Ketoroloac trometamine loaded nanodispersion incorporated into thermosensitive in situgel for prolonged ocular delivery. *Int. J. Pharm.* **2016**, *506*, 57–67. [CrossRef] [PubMed]
15. Mo, Z.; Ban, J.; Zhang, Y.; Du, Y.; Wen, Y.; Huang, X.; Xie, Q.; Shen, L.; Zhang, S.; Deng, H.; et al. Nanostructured lipid carriers-based thermosensitive eye drops for enhanced, sustained delivery of dexamethasone. *Nanomedicine* **2018**, *13*, 1239–1253. [CrossRef]
16. Nagarwal, R.C.; Kumar, R.; Pandit, J.K. Chitosan coated sodium alginate–chitosan nanoparticles loaded with 5-FU for ocular delivery: In vitro characterization and in vivo study in rabbit eye. *Eur. J. Pharm. Sci.* **2012**, *47*, 678–685. [CrossRef]
17. Bernkop-Schnürch, A.; Dünnhaupt, S. Chitosan-Based Drug Delivery Systems. *Eur. J. Pharm. Biopharm.* **2012**, *81*, 463–469. [CrossRef]
18. Dimassi, S.; Tabary, N.; Chai, F.; Blanchemain, N.; Martel, B. Sulfonated and sulfated chitosan derivatives for biomedical applications: A review. *Carbohydr. Polym.* **2018**, *202*, 382–396. [CrossRef]
19. Zambito, Y.; Felice, F.; Fabiano, A.; Di Stefano, R.; Di Colo, G. Mucoadhesive nanoparticles made of thiolated quaternary chitosan crosslinked with hyaluronan. *Carbohydr. Polym.* **2013**, *92*, 33–39. [CrossRef] [PubMed]
20. Fabiano, A.; Piras, A.M.; Uccello-Barretta, G.; Balzano, F.; Cesari, A.; Testai, L.; Zambito, Y. Impact of mucoadhesive polymeric nanoparticulate systems on oral bioavailability of a macromolecular model drug. *Eur. J. Pharm. Biopharm.* **2018**, *130*, 281–289. [CrossRef]
21. Felice, F.; Zambito, Y.; Belardinelli, E.; D'Onofrio, C.; Fabiano, A.; Balbarini, A.; Di Stefano, R. Delivery of natural polyphenols by polymeric nanoparticles improves the resistance of endothelial progenitor cells to oxidative stress. *Eur. J. Pharm. Sci.* **2013**, *50*, 393–399. [CrossRef] [PubMed]
22. Tsai, H.S.; Wang, Y.Z.; Lin, J.J.; Lien, W.F. Preparation and properties of sulfopropyl chitosan derivatives with various sulfonation degree. *J. Appl. Polym.* **2010**, *116*, 1686–1693. [CrossRef]
23. Di Colo, G.; Zambito, Y.; Zaino, C.; Sansò, M. Selected polysaccharides at comparison for their mucoadhesiveness and effect on precorneal residence of different drugs in the rabbit model. *Drug Dev. Ind. Pharm.* **2009**, *35*, 941–949. [CrossRef] [PubMed]
24. Uccello-Barretta, G.; Nazzi, S.; Balzano, F.; Di Colo, G.; Zambito, Y.; Zaino, C.; Benvenuti, M. Enhanced affinity of ketotifen toward tamarind seed polysaccharide in comparison with hydroxyethylcellulose and hyaluronic acid: A nuclear magnetic resonance investigation. *Bioorg. Med. Chem.* **2008**, *16*, 7371–7376. [CrossRef]
25. Zambito, Y.; Pedreschi, E.; Di Colo, G. Is dialysis a reliable method for studying drug release from nanoparticulate systems?—A case study. *Int. J. Pharm.* **2012**, *434*, 28–34. [CrossRef]
26. Dodero, A.; Williams, R.; Gagliardi, S.; Vicini, S.; Alloisio, M.; Castellano, M. A micro-rheological and rheological study of biopolymers solutions: Hyaluronic acid. *Carbohydr. Polym.* **2019**, *203*, 349–355. [CrossRef]
27. Ceulemans, J.; Vermeire, A.; Adriaens, E.; Remon, J.P.; Ludwig, A. Evaluation of a mucoadhesive tablet for ocular use. *J. Control. Release* **2001**, *77*, 333–344. [CrossRef]
28. Lallemand, F.; Furrer, P.; Felt-Baeyens, O.; Gex-Fabry, M.; Dumont, J.M.; Besseghir, K.; Gurny, R. A novel water-soluble cyclosporine a prodrug: Ocular tolerance and in vivo kinetics. *Int. J. Pharm.* **2005**, *295*, 7–14. [CrossRef]

29. Schoenwald, R.D.; Harris, R.G.; Turner, D.; Knowles, W.; Chien, D.S. Ophthalmic bioequivalence of steroid/antibiotic combination formulations. *Biopharm. Drug Dispos.* **1987**, *8*, 527–548. [CrossRef]
30. Fabiano, A.; Zambito, Y.; Bernkop-Schnürch, A. About the impact of water movement on the permeation behaviour of nanoparticles in mucus. *Int. J. Pharm.* **2017**, *517*, 279–285. [CrossRef]
31. Bansil, R.; Turner, B.S. The biology of mucus: Composition, synthesis and organization. *Adv. Drug Deliv. Rev.* **2018**, *124*, 3–15. [CrossRef] [PubMed]

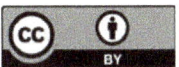

© 2019 by the authors. Licensee MDPI, Basel, Switzerland. This article is an open access article distributed under the terms and conditions of the Creative Commons Attribution (CC BY) license (http://creativecommons.org/licenses/by/4.0/).

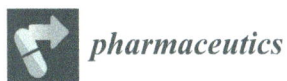

Article

A Mixed Thermosensitive Hydrogel System for Sustained Delivery of Tacrolimus for Immunosuppressive Therapy

Hsiu-Chao Lin [1,†], Madonna Rica Anggelia [2,3,†], Chih-Chi Cheng [1], Kuan-Lin Ku [1], Hui-Yun Cheng [2], Chih-Jen Wen [2], Aline Yen Ling Wang [2], Cheng-Hung Lin [2,3,*] and I-Ming Chu [1,*]

[1] Department of Chemical Engineering, National Tsing Hua University, Hsinchu 300, Taiwan
[2] Center for Vascularized Composite Allotransplantation, Department of Plastic and Reconstructive Surgery, Chang Gung Memorial Hospital, Chang Gung Medical College and Chang Gung University, Taoyuan 333, Taiwan
[3] Graduate Institute of Biomedical Sciences, College of Medicine, Chang Gung University, Taoyuan 333, Taiwan
* Correspondence: lukechlin@gmail.com (C.-H.L.); imchu@che.nthu.edu.tw (I.-M.C.); Tel.: +886-3-3281200 (C.-H.L.); +886-3-5713704 (I.-M.C.); Fax: +886-3-3289582 (C.-H.L.); +886-3-5715408 (I.-M.C.)
† These authors contributed equally to this work.

Received: 11 July 2019; Accepted: 12 August 2019; Published: 14 August 2019

Abstract: Tacrolimus is an immunosuppressive agent for acute rejection after allotransplantation. However, the low aqueous solubility of tacrolimus poses difficulties in formulating an injection dosage. Polypeptide thermosensitive hydrogels can maintain a sustained release depot to deliver tacrolimus. The copolymers, which consist of poloxamer and poly(L-alanine) with L-lysine segments at both ends (P–Lys–Ala–PLX), are able to carry tacrolimus in an in situ gelled form with acceptable biocompatibility, biodegradability, and low gelling concentrations from 3 to 7 wt %. By adding Pluronic F-127 to formulate a mixed hydrogel system, the drug release rate can be adjusted to maintain suitable drug levels in animals with transplants. Under this formulation, the in vitro release of tacrolimus was stable for more than 100 days, while in vivo release of tacrolimus in mouse model showed that rejection from skin allotransplantation was prevented for at least three weeks with one single administration. Using these mixed hydrogel systems for sustaining delivery of tacrolimus demonstrates advancement in immunosuppressive therapy.

Keywords: allotransplantation; hydrogels; sustained delivery; tacrolimus

1. Introduction

Hydrogels are composed of crosslinked polymeric networks that can form highly hydrated semisolid materials. Because their diverse capacity to carry therapeutic agents in a depot-like form allows sustained release, hydrogels have been utilized in many applications, including drug delivery, cell therapy, and tissue engineering [1–4].

Among various types of hydrogels, thermosensitive poly(ethylene glycol)-co-poly(amino acids) hydrogels are capable of in situ gelling upon injection to appropriate sites in the body. They can deliver drugs or cells to specific sites with minimum invasiveness while serving as a depot for extended delivery [5–9]. These polymers belong to LCST-type materials; thus, when above a certain temperature, their aqueous solution undergoes a phase transition to the gel state, depending on the concentration. The gelling process involves a reduced hydrogen bond interaction between the hydrophilic segments of polymers and water as the temperature rises [10,11]. Different types of hydrophilic polymers are used in this gelling process, including various hydrogels, poly(ethylene glycol) (PEG) [12], methoxy poly(ethylene glycol) (mPEG) [13], and PEO–PPO–PEO copolymers (mainly the Pluronic® or poloxamer (PLX) series) [14]. Several types of polypeptides have been used in the hydrophobic portion of the polymer [12,15,16]. The fact that peptides have secondary interactions between or within themselves complicates the gelling process of these amino acid-based hydrogels, creating different types of self-assembled morphology [17–20]. Additionally, because peptide bonds possess low hydrolytic rates, compared with ester bonds, for example, hydrogels degrade at extremely slow rates. Therefore, side effects caused by long-term foreign body reactions may be a concern, or the release rates of some drugs might be too slow for intended applications.

In this study, a suitable formulation of a hydrogel carrier was sought for tacrolimus, an immunosuppressive, antirejection drug. Tacrolimus is a hydrophobic substance with low aqueous solubility. Controlled delivery of tacrolimus would avoid the low bioavailability problem and improve patient compliance statistics by reducing the administration frequency. Several delivery systems for tacrolimus have been reported, including mPEG-poly(lactic acid) nanoparticles [21], poly(lactide-co-glycolide) microspheres [22], and triglycerol monostearate hydrogels [23]. The in situ gelation property of the system studied here has several advantages over particulate systems or conventional hydrogel systems, including longer release time, higher encapsulation efficiency, easy administration, and applicability to various types of drugs. In particular, by combining two types of hydrogel components, the possibility of increasing the flexibility of carriers to suit distinct pharmaceutical entities and modifying release rates for better clinical outcomes is explored.

2. Materials and Methods

2.1. Materials

O,O′-Bis(2-aminopropyl) polypropylene glycol-block-polyethylene glycol-block-polypropylene glycol (Poloxamer, PLX, PPG–PEG–PPG, Mn = 900), L-alanine, hydrogen bromide (HBr/acetic acid), and a LIVE/DEAD staining kit were purchased from Sigma-Aldrich (St. Louis, MO, USA). Tacrolimus (FK506) was obtained from LC Labs (Woburn, MA, USA). Trifluoroacetic acid-d (TFA-d) and trifluoroacetic acid (TFA) were purchased from Alfa Aesar (Wall Hill, MA, USA). L-lysine-(Z) was commercially obtained from ACROS (Morris Plains, NJ, USA). Diethyl ether, hexane, and ethanol (95%) were purchased from Echo Chemicals (Toufen, Miaoli, Taiwan). Dimethyl sulfoxide (DMSO) was obtained from J.T. Baker. Dulbecco's modified eagle's medium (DMEM), fetal bovine serum (FBS), and antimycotics–antibiotics were purchased from Gibco (Grand Island, NY, USA). Toluene and tetrahydrofuran (THF) were obtained from TEDIA (Fairfield, OH, USA), and chloroform, dichloromethane (DCM), and N,N-dimethylformaide (DMF) were purchased from AVANTOR (Center Valley, PA, USA). All solvents were dried over CaH_2 before used.

2.2. Synthesis of L-alanine N-Carboxyanhydride (Ala-NCA), L-Lysine-(Z) N-Carboxyanhydride (Lys-(Z)-NCA), and P–Lys–Ala–PLX Block Copolymer

The copolymer synthesis was similar to that in our previous study conducted in 2016 [14] in which L-alanine (5.0 g and 56.1 mmol) and triphosgene (16.65 g, 56.3 mmol) were dissolved in anhydrous THF (150 mL) and gently stirred at 45 °C under nitrogen flux. After the reaction period of approximately 12 h, the mixture turned clear and the solution was condensed to a final volume of 15 mL through rotary evaporation. The product was precipitated in excess n-hexane. A similar preparation method was employed in this study: L-lysine-(Z) (5.0 g, 17.8 mmol) using 3.2 g of triphosgene (10.7 mmol) was dissolved in 60 mL of anhydrous THF. The reaction was completed within 4 h, and the mixture was then condensed and finally precipitated.

The block copolymer P–Lys–Ala–PLX was prepared through a two-step ring-opening polymerization of Ala–NCA and Lys–(Z)–NCA with PLX as the macroinitiator. Briefly, PLX (4.0 g, 5 mmol) was dissolved in 15 mL of toluene and azeotropically distilled to a final volume of approximately

5 mL to remove residual water. Ala-NCA (5.198 g) was added to the reaction flask and dissolved in 20-fold of anhydrous chloroform/DMF (2:1). The mixture was stirred at 40 °C for 24 h until the reaction was complete and then precipitated with diethyl ether. Next, pre-weighed Lys–(Z)–NCA (3.063 g) was added into the reaction flask, and the reaction was carried out at 40 °C for 24 h again. The final product was precipitated with diethyl ether.

The copolymer (Z)–Lys–Ala–PLX–Ala–Lys–(Z) was dissolved in TFA (1 g/10 mL), and a solution of 33 wt % HBr/acetic acid (0.3 mL/mol L-lysine) was added and stirred at 0 °C for 1 h. After precipitation with diethyl ether, the product was dialyzed (MWCO 1000) using a spectrum dialysis bag, lyophilized, and stored in a vacuum atmosphere for future use.

2.3. ^1H Nuclear Magnetic Resonanc (NMR) Spectroscopy

A ^1H NMR spectrum of the 0.5 wt % copolymer solution in TFA-d was obtained using a Varian UNITY INOVA 500 MHz spectrometer (Palo Alto, CA, USA) to verify the chemical structure of the product.

2.4. Fourier-Transformed Infrared Spectroscopy (FT-IR)

Fourier-transformed infrared spectroscopy (FT-IR) was performed using an FTIR spectrometer (Nicolet™ iS50, Thermo Fisher Scientific, Waltham, MA, USA) equipped with an attenuated total reflectance (ATR) module. The copolymer solution prepared at 5 wt % in deionized water was injected into the test chamber. Spectra were collected at a temperature ranging from 10 to 50 °C at increments of 10 °C. The sample was equilibrated for 20 min at each temperature. The amide I band region of 1600–1700 cm^{-1} was used to collect information on secondary structures and conducted for chemical structure verification.

2.5. Sol-to-gel Phase Transition

The sol-to-gel transition behavior of copolymers prepared at various concentrations was investigated using the test tube inversion method. Samples were prepared in test tubes at 3 to 7 wt % in deionized water and placed in a tube rotator overnight at 4 °C until the solutes were completely dissolved. The inverted test tube test was performed at a temperature range of 10–50 °C, at increments of 1 °C. At each temperature, the sample was allowed to equilibrate for 10 min. The gelation point was designated when the solution stopped flowing while inverted and gently agitated.

2.6. Scanning Electron Microscope (SEM)

The copolymer mixed gel solution was prepared at 5 wt % in P–Lys–Ala–PLX and 1 wt % in Pluronic F-127 that allowed full equilibration at 4 °C overnight for future use. The hydrogel microstructure was examined using a JEOL JSM-7001F SEM system (Peabody, MA, USA). Briefly, hydrogels were gelled at 37 °C and then submerged in liquid nitrogen prior to lyophilization. To investigate the cross section, lyophilized hydrogels were carefully cut open using a scalpel blade.

2.7. Degradation Test

The in vitro degradation of hydrogels (100 μL) in phosphate-buffered saline (PBS) and PBS containing elastase (5 U/mL) was analyzed. Briefly, copolymer solutions were gelled in 1.5 mL tubes at 37 °C for 30 min prior to adding 1 mL of the respective degradation mediums. The medium was replaced at each time point, and the residual was weighted after washing and lyophilization.

2.8. Biocompatibility

The cell compatibility of the prepared mixed hydrogel was assessed. Briefly, human embryonic kidney cells (293T) were loaded onto a 24-well transwell plate at 6 × 10^3 cells per well and grown in DMEM media, supplemented with 10% FBS and 1% antimycotics–antibiotics. Exactly 100 μL of the copolymer solution was gelled at 37 °C in the transwell insert overlaid with 1 mL of culture media. LIVE/DEAD staining with fluorescence microscopy observation was performed on the third and seventh days to quantitate the viability of the cells, and a 3-(4,5-dimethylthiazol-2-yl)-2,5-diphenyltetrazolium bromide (MTT) assay was simultaneously performed to detect cell proliferation. Briefly, cells were treated with 3-(4,5-dimethylthiazol-2-yl)-2,5-diphenyltetrazolium bromide (10% v/v in medium) in each well for 3 hours before 200 μL of DMSO was added. The solution was collected and analyzed.

2.9. Drug Release In Vitro

The hydrogels P–Lys–Ala–PLX 5 wt % and Pluronic F-127 1 wt % were combined, solubilized in deionized water, and then mixed with tacrolimus in tubes to afford 1 mL solutions of the final drug concentration with 10 or 20 mg/mL. A negative control of the mixed hydrogel without tacrolimus was used. 100 μL copolymer solutions were loaded into a 1.5 mL tube and kept at 37 °C for 10 min before adding 1 mL of PBS with 2% tween 20 as the conditional medium. At each time point, aliquots were collected using HPLC analysis to ascertain the tacrolimus concentration. A linear calibration curve over the concentration range of 1000 μg/mL to 1 μg/mL was constructed, and the tacrolimus concentration was interpolated accordingly.

2.10. Drug Release In Vivo

Male Lewis (LEW) rats, weighing 300 to 350 g, were obtained from the National Laboratory Animal Center and were housed under pathogen-free conditions at the Animal Center of Linkou Chang Gung Memorial Hospital according to protocols approved by Institutional Animal Care and Use Committee of Chang Gung Memorial Hospital (IACUC No. 2017121807, approved date, 14 May 2018). Those rats ($n = 3$) were injected subcutaneously with 1 mL mixed hydrogels loaded with tacrolimus at 10 mg/mL. To analyze the in vivo release rate of tacrolimus, whole blood was drawn from the tail vein of those rats on days 7, 14, and 28 and put into the VACUETTE® EDTA tubes. Whole blood concentration of tacrolimus was quantitated by liquid chromatography-tandem mass spectrometry (LC-MS/MS) (Waters, Milford, MA, USA) at the Department of Laboratory Medicine, Linkou Chang Gung Memorial Hospital. The performance characteristics and assay method has been described previously. [24] The method for tacrolimus assay showed linearity over the calibrator range, $r > 0.999$, with the range measurement: 1.1–38.5 ng/mL and accuracy 108%. For intra-day and inter-day precision, the CV was <6.6%. This method showed no carryover or ion suppressant. The calibration solution (6PLUS1® RMultilevel Calibrator Immunosuppressants in Whole Blood) was purchased from Chromsystems (Munich, Germany) and contained tacrolimus and a blank calibration fluid (blank calibrator)). Further, 100 μL of calibration solution, quality control solution, and sample were loaded into a 1.5 mL centrifuge tube, and 300 μL of 0.1 M zinc sulfate containing internal standards (FK-506) were added. The mixtures were then vigorously vortexed for 30 s then centrifuged at 12,000 rpm for 15 min to completely precipitate the protein. The 300 μL supernatant was removed, placed in a 96-well collection tray, and put into the autosampler.

3. Results and Discussion

3.1. The Synthesis and Characterization of P–Lys–Ala–PLX and Pluronic F-127

Thermosensitive hydrogels composed of amphiphilic block copolymers were used in this study, specifically PLX-poly(L-alanine-lysine) (P–Lys–Ala–PLX). The ^{1}H-NMR spectra of the triblock copolymer are illustrated in Figure 1A, where peaks corresponding to copolymers are observed and successful synthesis of copolymers is confirmed. The molecular weights, as measured by Gel Permeation Chromatography (GPC) and ^{1}H NMR, are displayed in Table 1. Briefly, the molar mass polydispersity of the triblock copolymer is 1.51, and the weight average molecular weight (Mw) is 3817 Da.

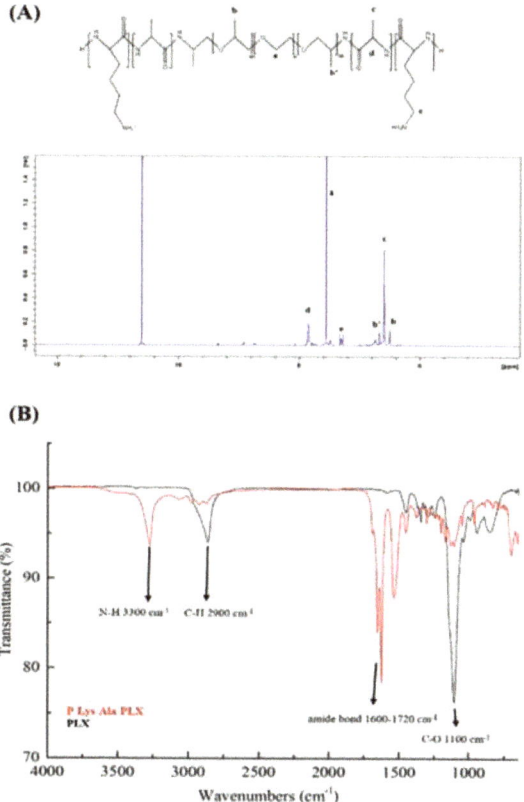

Figure 1. (**A**) ^{1}H-NMR of poloxamer (PLX)-poly(L-alanine-lysine) (P–Lys–Ala–PLX) copolymer in trifluoroacetic acid-d (TFA-d). (**B**) FT-IR spectra of P–Lys–Ala–PLX (red line) and PLX (black line) samples obtained via an attenuated total reflectance (ATR) module (2900 cm^{-1}, alkane of Pluronic F-127; 3345 cm^{-1}, amide of poly(L-alanine) and poly(L-lysine); 1637 cm^{-1} and 1540 cm^{-1}, amide I and II of poly(L-alanine) and poly(L-lysine); 1100 cm^{-1}, carbon-oxygen bond of PLX.

Table 1. The molecular weight and polydispersity as determined by GPC and ^{1}H NMR.

	Ala	Lys	Mn [a]	Mw [b]	PDI [b]
P–Lys–Ala–PLX	19.4	1.8	2528	3817	1.51

[a]. Determined by ^{1}H NMR. [b]. Determined by GPC.

ATR-FTIR was used to verify the synthesis of the copolymer P–Lys–Ala–PLX and compared with that of O,O'-Bis(2-aminopropyl) polypropylene glycol-block-polyethylene glycol-block-polypropylene glycol (Poloxamer, PLX), which has the same characteristic peaks as the PLX segment of P–Lys–Ala–PLX. As in Figure 1B, peaks at 3300 cm^{-1} (N–H bond) and 1600–1720 cm^{-1} (amide bond) are from polypeptides, while those found at 2900 cm^{-1} (C–H) and 1100 cm^{-1} (C–O) are from the PLX segment. The characterization and structure of the triblock copolymer P–Lys–Ala–PLX is explained in our 2016 study [14].

The sol–gel transition phase diagram is represented in Figure 2. In the room to body temperature range, P–Lys–Ala–PLX underwent a sol-to-gel transition in the concentration range from 3% to 7%. The gelation temperature decreased as the concentration of copolymers increased. For solutions with a copolymer concentration lower than 3 wt %, hydrogels were unable to form stable gels under the inverted test tube test despite significant increases in viscosity at higher temperatures. Consequently, copolymer concentrations of 4 to 5 wt % were chosen for further formulation studies.

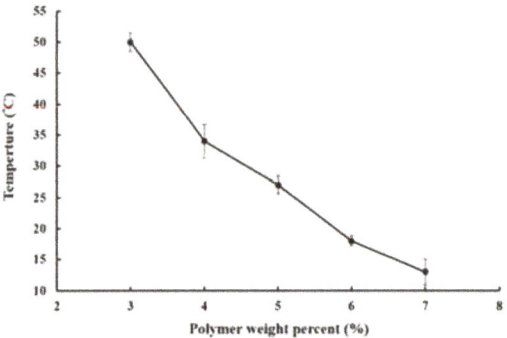

Figure 2. Sol–gel transition profile of aqueous solutions of P–Lys–Ala–PLX.

The internal structure of the P–Lys–Ala–PLX hydrogel was examined through scanning electronic microscopy, as portrayed in Figure 3. A plate-like structure was dominant with some fibrous features within. This type of morphology is typical for PLX-poly(alanine) hydrogels.

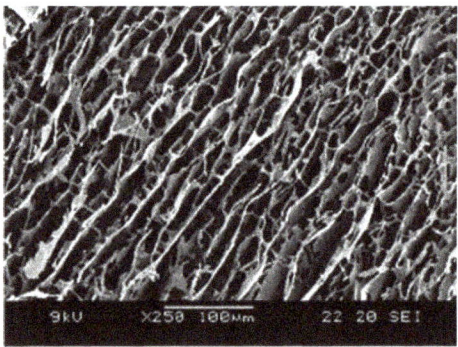

Figure 3. SEM image of P–Lys–Ala–PLX hydrogels.

3.2. Development of Mixed Hydrogel Formulation

After the preliminary in vivo drug release tests with the P–Lys–Ala–PLX hydrogel, extremely slow tacrolimus release rates and a considerably low plasma concentration of tacrolimus were observed. Unexpected transplant rejection resulted from these tests (data not shown) because drug concentrations were low. The slow in vivo release rate of the drug may be caused by the slow degradation rate of the hydrogel in vivo. Therefore, the hydrogel formulation should be modified to accelerate drug release at effective concentrations and sustain the release for more than 30 days. Pluronic F-127 has been mentioned to modulate the drug release rate [25]. The addition of Pluronic F-127, an approved fast-degrading hydrogel, to the P–Lys–Ala–PLX hydrogel system may provide a solution to accelerate the release rate.

A series of hydrogel formulations of 1 to 3 wt % Pluronic F-127 powder mixed into 4 or 5 wt % P–Lys–Ala–PLX were studied, as shown in Table 2. Sol-to-gel transition properties, cytotoxicity, drug encapsulation efficiency, and the release rate were measured. The formulation of 5 wt % P–Lys–Ala–PLX with 1 wt % Pluronic F-127 (sample 5:1) had a lower transition temperature than the other three groups, as demonstrated in Figure 4A. Additionally, the sample 5:1 had the highest drug encapsulation efficiency (Figure 4B). Consequently, the formulation of the sample 5:1 was chosen for further studies.

Table 2. The series formulation test group of the mixed hydrogels.

Group	P–Lys–Ala–PLX	Pluronic F-127
1	4 wt %	2 wt %
2	5 wt %	1 wt %
3	5 wt %	2 wt %
4	5 wt %	3 wt %

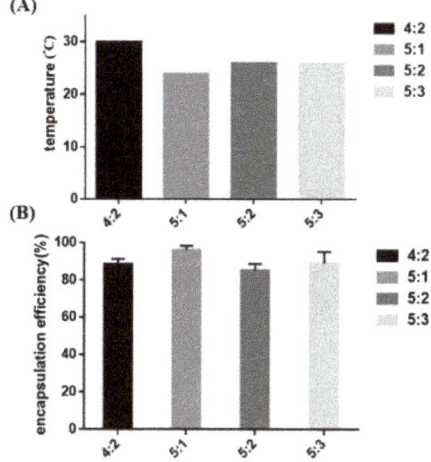

Figure 4. (A) The sol-to-gel transition temperature of mixed hydrogels without tacrolimus; (B) the encapsulation efficiency of tacrolimus in mixed hydrogels.

3.3. Biodegradability

Degradation behavior of hydrogels in a buffer solution with and without the enzyme elastase at 37 °C was observed. P–Lys–Ala–PLX gels (5 wt %) incubated with elastase (5 U/mL) resulted in a mass loss of 40% after 14 days, as displayed in Figure 5, whereas gels incubated with the buffer solution lost only 10% of the original mass. The sample 5:1 incubated with elastase had a mass loss of 50% after 14 days, whereas those without the enzyme lost only 15% of the original mass. The mass loss of mixed hydrogels was higher than that of the P–Lys–Ala–PLX hydrogel because Pluronic F-127 was more prone to dissolve back to an aqueous solution. In short, hydrogels were stable when proteinases were absent, and Pluronic F-127 accelerated degradation rates.

SEM micrographs of lyophilized P–Lys–Ala–PLX and a sample 5:1 mixed hydrogel are shown in Figure 6. The mixed hydrogels exhibited more porous structures and space resulting from the incorporation of Pluronic F-127. After the 14-day degradation, samples of mixed hydrogels revealed larger pores and looser structure resulting from the faster dissolution or disintegration of Pluronic F-127.

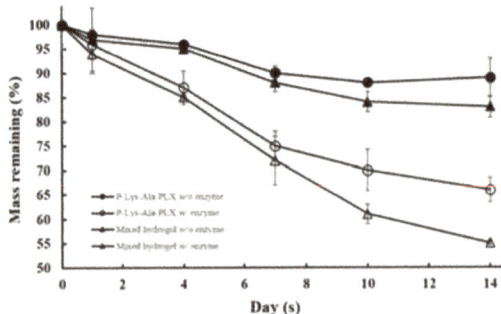

Figure 5. Degradation profiles of P–Lys–Ala–PLX and sample 5:1 mixed hydrogel in phosphate-buffered saline (PBS) with or without 5 U/mL elastase ($n = 6$).

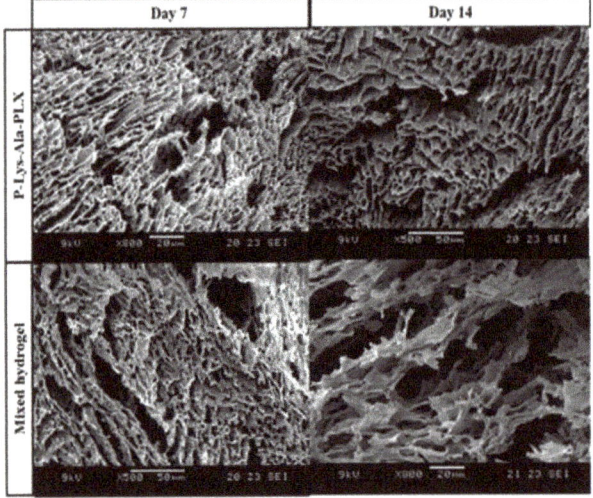

Figure 6. SEM microphotographs of P–Lys–Ala–PLX hydrogel and sample 5:1 mixed hydrogel after degradation in PBS with 5 U/mL elastase at 37 °C for 7 and 14 days.

3.4. Biocompatibility

The dispersion of insoluble tacrolimus particles in the hydrogel solution was rather challenging [21,22]. Certain solvents must be used to dissolve tacrolimus during the encapsulation process to assure an even distribution of the drug. Acceptable solvents should be nontoxic to cells and not interfere in the sol–gel transition of the polymeric system.

Several solvents that can dissolve tacrolimus were chosen, including DMSO, ethanol, and transcutol P. Ethanol had the least toxicity and highest dissolving power when water was present (data not shown). To reduce the toxicity of ethanol to the cells, tacrolimus was dissolved in ethanol as 100 mg/mL or 200 mg/mL stock solutions, which were then used to prepare the 10 mg/mL and 20 mg/mL drug-carrying hydrogels, respectively. Tacrolimus encapsulated in the gel gradually precipitated out as small evenly dispersed solid particles when ethanol diffused into the surrounding aqueous environment. When the gel pellet was placed in a 10-time volume of medium and the residual ethanol concentration was below 1 wt %, its conditioned medium exerted little effect on the cells in the in vitro toxicity test (see Figure 7).

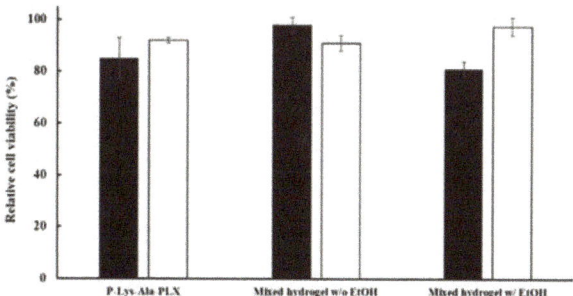

Figure 7. Cytotoxicity of conditioned mediums of various formulations by the MTT assay. Mixed hydrogels: 5:1 P–Lys–Ala–PLX to Pluronic F-127. Ethanol was added to the gel as in the 10 mg/mL formulation but without the drug. The black bar was on day 3 (black) and the white bar was on day 7.

Cellular compatibility under encapsulation of prepared hydrogels was evaluated using LIVE/DEAD staining, in which live cells stained green and dead cells were red. To evaluate the cytotoxicity of materials, in the medium, cells were cultivated in contact with hydrogels in transwells. The cells showed acceptable viability in culture for 3 to 7 days with both P–Lys–Ala–PLX and mixed hydrogels, as related in Figure 8.

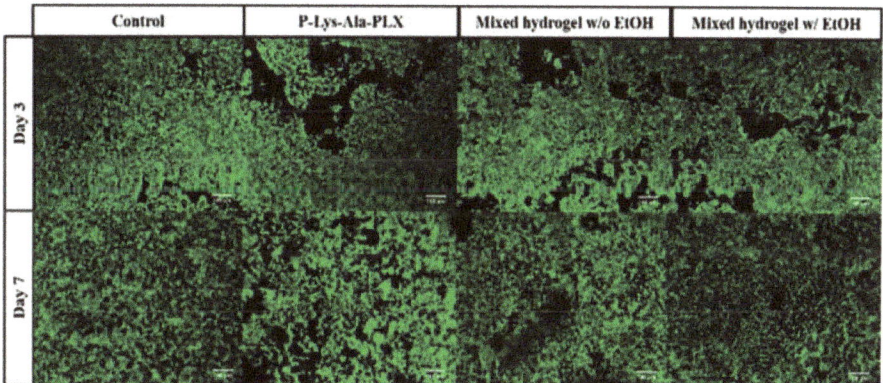

Figure 8. The LIVE/DEAD staining of 293T cells was co-cultured with various hydrogels without the drug.

3.5. Tacrolimus Encapsulation and Release

The feasibility of hydrogels as an efficient local drug delivery system for tacrolimus was studied first under in vitro conditions. The encapsulation efficiency and release of tacrolimus in mixed hydrogel were measured. The values of encapsulation efficiency (EE) of the sample 5:1 mixed hydrogel were measured at two levels of drug content, where EE = (experimental drug loading)/(theoretical drug loading) × 100%. The results are presented in Table 3. The data indicated the hydrogel encapsulated tacrolimus rather well, with the EE at approximately 96%–98% in triplicate samples. Drug release rates in P–Lys–Ala–PLX or the sample 5:1 mixed hydrogel was measured for a one-month period. The release rates were stable and higher in the mixed hydrogel at both drug content levels, as illustrated in Figure 9. No burst release was observed, and the sustained release of tacrolimus was achieved. Release rates correlated with hydrogel degradation (e.g., see Figure 5) and thereby suggest that the enhanced disintegration of mixed hydrogels was responsible for higher drug release rates in mixed hydrogels. These results demonstrate the ability to modify the release rate by using mixed hydrogels.

Table 3. The encapsulation efficiency of 5:1 mixed hydrogel for tacrolimus.

Group	Encapsulation Efficiency (%)
10 mg/mL	96.13 ± 1.56
20 mg/mL	98.5 ± 0.97

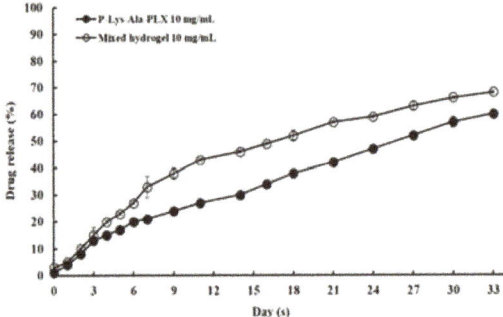

Figure 9. In vitro tacrolimus release as a fraction of total encapsulated drug.

For the mixed hydrogel with 10 mg/mL tacrolimus group, preliminary in vivo drug release tests were conducted. The aim was to establish a correlation between our in vitro release data and the corresponding data in a plasma concentration when 1 mL of the formulation was injected subcutaneously in a mouse. More comprehensive pharmacokinetic work, together with allotransplantation animal study, is currently underway, and results will be presented in a separate paper. As exhibited in Table 4, plasma concentrations of tacrolimus during a 28-day period after administration were stable at approximately 10 ng/mL, a level generally considered clinically relevant [23,26]. Therefore, the linear in vitro release rates reflected consistent in vivo plasma concentrations.

Table 4. Whole blood concentrations of tacrolimus: In vivo drug release results from mixed hydrogels containing 10 mg/mL tacrolimus.

Tacrolimus (ng/mL)	Time (Days)		
	7 (n = 3)	14 (n = 3)	28 (n = 3)
	8.5 ± 1.5	12.2 ± 2.1	10.1 ± 1.6

4. Conclusions

Tacrolimus is a potent immunosuppressive age that can be used for patients who receive allotransplantation. The current daily or twice-daily oral dosage forms may encounter patient compliance problems. Encapsulation of tacrolimus by in situ gelling hydrogels is a feasible way to deliver this drug. Using the mixed hydrogel system developed in this study, steady and extended delivery was achieved. The use of toxic solvents was avoided and the formulation exhibited high biocompatibility with 293T cells in vitro with high encapsulation efficiency of drug and good gelling properties. Preliminary in vivo data also confirm a stable plasma concentration of the drug for an extended period of time. In summary, the newly designed formulation of mixed hydrogels is a promising delivery system for tacrolimus and, perhaps, other highly hydrophobic compounds.

Author Contributions: Conceptualization, I.-M.C. and C.-H.L.; methodology, A.Y.L.W.; software, C.-J.W.; validation, C.-C.C., H.-C.L. and M.R.A.; formal analysis, K.-L.K. and H.-Y.C.; investigation, C.-C.C.; writing—original draft preparation, H.-C.L. and M.R.A.; writing—review and editing, I.-M.C.; supervision, I.-M.C. and C.-H.L.; project administration, I.-M.C. and C.-H.L.; funding acquisition, I.-M.C. and C.-H.L.

Funding: This research was funded by grants from the Ministry of Science and Technology, Taiwan (107-2314B007004 and 108-2314B007001) and Chang Gung Medical Foundation (CMRPG3B0261 and CMRPG3C1531-3).

Conflicts of Interest: The authors declare no conflict of interest.

References

1. Hoare, T.R.; Kohane, D.S. Hydrogels in drug delivery: Progress and challenges. *Polymer* **2008**, *49*, 1993–2007. [CrossRef]
2. Wichterle, O.; Lim, D. Hydrophilic Gels for Biological Use. *Nature* **1960**, *185*, 117. [CrossRef]
3. Drury, J.L.; Mooney, D.J. Hydrogels for tissue engineering: Scaffold design variables and applications. *Biomaterials* **2003**, *24*, 4337–4351. [CrossRef]
4. Kopeček, J. Hydrogel biomaterials: A smart future? *Biomaterials* **2007**, *28*, 5185–5192. [CrossRef] [PubMed]
5. Ko, D.Y.; Shinde, U.; Yeon, B.; Jeong, B. Recent progress of in situ formed gels for biomedical applications. *Prog. Polym. Sci.* **2013**, *38*, 672–701. [CrossRef]
6. Jeong, Y.; Joo, M.K.; Bahk, K.H.; Choi, Y.Y.; Kim, H.T.; Kim, W.K.; Lee, H.J.; Sohn, Y.S.; Jeong, B. Enzymatically degradable temperature-sensitive polypeptide as a new in-situ gelling biomaterial. *J. Control. Release* **2009**, *137*, 25–30. [CrossRef] [PubMed]
7. Boustta, M.; Colombo, P.-E.; Lenglet, S.; Poujol, S.; Vert, M. Versatile UCST-based thermoresponsive hydrogels for loco-regional sustained drug delivery. *J. Control. Release* **2014**, *174*, 1–6. [CrossRef] [PubMed]
8. Klouda, L. Thermoresponsive hydrogels in biomedical applications: A seven-year update. *Eur. J. Pharm. Biopharm.* **2015**, *97*, 338–349. [CrossRef]
9. Yu, L.; Ding, J. Injectable hydrogels as unique biomedical materials. *Chem. Soc. Rev.* **2008**, *37*, 1473–1481. [CrossRef]
10. Nguyen, M.K.; Lee, D.S. Injectable Biodegradable Hydrogels. *Macromol. Biosci.* **2010**, *10*, 563–579. [CrossRef]
11. Yu, L.; Chang, G.; Zhang, H.; Ding, J. Temperature-induced spontaneous sol–gel transitions of poly (D,L-lactic acid-co-glycolic acid) *b* poly (ethylene glycol)-*b*-poly (D,L-lactic acid-co-glycolic acid) triblock copolymers and their end-capped derivatives in water. *J. Polym. Sci. Part A Polym. Chem.* **2007**, *45*, 1122–1133. [CrossRef]
12. Yeon, B.; Park, M.H.; Moon, H.J.; Kim, S.J.; Cheon, Y.W.; Jeong, B. 3D culture of adipose-tissue-derived stem cells mainly leads to chondrogenesis in poly (ethylene glycol)-poly (L-alanine) diblock copolymer thermogel. *Biomacromolecules* **2013**, *14*, 3256–3266. [CrossRef] [PubMed]
13. Peng, S.; Lai, Z.T.; Hong, D.W.; Chu, I.M.; Lai, P.L. Controlled release of strontium through neutralization reaction within a methoxy (polyethylene glycol)-polyester hydrogel. *J. Appl. Biomater. Funct. Mater.* **2017**, *15*, e162–e169. [CrossRef] [PubMed]
14. Lin, J.-Y.; Lai, P.-L.; Lin, Y.-K.; Peng, S.; Lee, L.-Y.; Chen, C.-N.; Chu, I.M. A poloxamer-polypeptide thermosensitive hydrogel as a cell scaffold and sustained release depot. *Polym. Chem.* **2016**, *7*, 2976–2985. [CrossRef]
15. Yun, E.J.; Yon, B.; Joo, M.K.; Jeong, B. Cell therapy for skin wound using fibroblast encapsulated poly (ethylene glycol)-poly (L-alanine) thermogel. *Biomacromolecules* **2012**, *13*, 1106–1111. [CrossRef] [PubMed]
16. Chiang, P.R.; Lin, T.Y.; Tsai, H.C.; Chen, H.L.; Liu, S.Y.; Chen, F.R.; Hwang, Y.S.; Chu, I.M. Thermosensitive hydrogel from oligopeptide-containing amphiphilic block copolymer: Effect of peptide functional group on self-assembly and gelation behavior. *Langmuir* **2013**, *29*, 15981–15991. [CrossRef] [PubMed]
17. Cui, H.; Zhuang, X.; He, C.; Wei, Y.; Chen, X. High performance and reversible ionic polypeptide hydrogel based on charge-driven assembly for biomedical applications. *Acta Biomater.* **2015**, *11*, 183–190. [CrossRef] [PubMed]
18. Cheng, Y.; He, C.; Xiao, C.; Ding, J.; Zhuang, X.; Huang, Y.; Chen, X. Decisive role of hydrophobic side groups of polypeptides in thermosensitive gelation. *Biomacromolecules* **2012**, *13*, 2053–2059. [CrossRef] [PubMed]
19. Oh, H.J.; Joo, M.K.; Sohn, Y.S.; Jeong, B. Secondary Structure Effect of Polypeptide on Reverse Thermal Gelation and Degradation of l/dl-Poly (alanine)–Poloxamer–l/dl-Poly (alanine) Copolymers. *Macromolecules* **2008**, *41*, 8204–8209. [CrossRef]

20. Choi, Y.Y.; Jang, J.H.; Park, M.H.; Choi, B.G.; Chi, B.; Jeong, B. Block length affects secondary structure, nanoassembly and thermosensitivity of poly (ethylene glycol)-poly (L-alanine) block copolymers. *J. Mater. Chem.* **2010**, *20*, 3416–3421. [CrossRef]
21. Xu, W.; Ling, P.; Zhang, T. Toward immunosuppressive effects on liver transplantation in rat model: Tacrolimus loaded poly (ethylene glycol)-poly (D,L-lactide) nanoparticle with longer survival time. *Int. J. Pharm.* **2014**, *460*, 173–180. [CrossRef] [PubMed]
22. Tajdaran, K.; Shoichet, M.S.; Gordon, T.; Borschel, G.H. A novel polymeric drug delivery system for localized and sustained release of tacrolimus (FK506). *Biotechnol. Bioeng.* **2015**, *112*, 1948–1953. [CrossRef] [PubMed]
23. Gajanayake, T.; Olariu, R.; Leclere, F.M.; Dhayani, A.; Yang, Z.; Bongoni, A.K.; Banz, Y.; Constantinescu, M.A.; Karp, J.M.; Vemula, P.K.; et al. A single localized dose of enzyme-responsive hydrogel improves long-term survival of a vascularized composite allograft. *Sci. Transl. Med.* **2014**, *6*, 249ra110. [CrossRef] [PubMed]
24. Huang, Y.F.; Lai, P.C.; Huang, Y.C.; Chiang, Y.S.; You, H.L.; Lin, C.N.; Ning, H.C. Development of an ultra-performance liquid chromatography tandem mass spectrometric method for simultaneous quantitating four immunosuppressant drugs. *J. Biomed. Lab. Sci.* **2015**, *27*, 61–68.
25. Kojarunchitt, T.; Hook, S.; Rizwan, S.; Rades, T.; Baldursdottir, S. Development and characterisation of modified poloxamer 407 thermoresponsive depot systems containing cubosomes. *Int. J. Pharm.* **2011**, *408*, 20–26. [CrossRef] [PubMed]
26. Kojima, R.; Yoshida, T.; Tasaki, H.; Umejima, H.; Maeda, M.; Higashi, Y.; Watanabe, S.; Oku, N. Release mechanisms of tacrolimus-loaded PLGA and PLA microspheres and immunosuppressive effects of the microspheres in a rat heart transplantation model. *Int. J. Pharm.* **2015**, *492*, 20–27. [CrossRef] [PubMed]

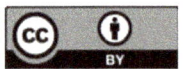

© 2019 by the authors. Licensee MDPI, Basel, Switzerland. This article is an open access article distributed under the terms and conditions of the Creative Commons Attribution (CC BY) license (http://creativecommons.org/licenses/by/4.0/).

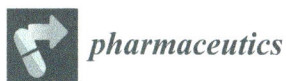

Article

Development of Functionalized Carbon Nano-Onions Reinforced Zein Protein Hydrogel Interfaces for Controlled Drug Release

Narsimha Mamidi [1,*], Aldo González-Ortiz [1], Irasema Lopez Romo [2] and Enrique V. Barrera [3,4]

1. Tecnologico de Monterrey, Department of Chemistry and Nanotechnology, School of Engineering and Science, Monterrey 64849, Nuevo Leon, Mexico
2. Tecnologico de Monterrey, Department of Biotechnology, School of Engineering and Science, Monterrey 64849, Nuevo Leon, Mexico
3. Department of Materials Science and NanoEngineering, Rice University, Houston, TX 77005, USA
4. Department of Chemistry, Rice University, Houston, TX 77005, USA
* Correspondence: nmamidi@tec.mx; Tel.: +81-83582000-4593

Received: 30 September 2019; Accepted: 11 November 2019; Published: 20 November 2019

Abstract: In the current study, poly 4-mercaptophenyl methacrylate-carbon nano-onions (PMPMA-CNOs = f-CNOs) reinforced natural protein (zein) composites (zein/f-CNOs) are fabricated using the acoustic cavitation technique. The influence of f-CNOs inclusion on the microstructural properties, morphology, mechanical, cytocompatibility, in-vitro degradation, and swelling behavior of the hydrogels are studied. The tensile results showed that zein/f-CNOs hydrogels fabricated by the acoustic cavitation system exhibited good tensile strength (90.18 MPa), compared with the hydrogels fabricated by the traditional method and only microwave radiation method. It reveals the magnitude of physisorption and degree of colloidal stability of f-CNOs within the zein matrix under acoustic cavitation conditions. The swelling behaviors of hydrogels were also tested and improved results were noticed. The cytotoxicity of hydrogels was tested with osteoblast cells. The results showed good cell viability and cell growth. To explore the efficacy of hydrogels as drug transporters, 5-fluorouracil (5-FU) release was measured under gastric and intestinal pH environment. The results showed pH-responsive sustained drug release over 15 days of study, and pH 7.4 showed a more rapid drug release than pH 2.0 and 4.5. Nonetheless, all the results suggest that zein/f-CNOs hydrogel could be a potential pH-responsive drug transporter for a colon-selective delivery system.

Keywords: zein/poly 4-mercaptophenyl methacrylate-carbon nano-onions hydrogels; acoustic cavitation method; pH-responsive drug release; cytocompatibility

1. Introduction

Hydrogels are incipient three-dimensional (3D) networking structures that are able to swell in aqueous or non-aqueous fluids without dissolving. The hydrogels have been used in tissue engineering, drug release, material separation, and artificial organs, due to their excellent flexibility, high moisture content, and outstanding viscoelasticity [1]. Various hydrogels have been fabricated from synthetic and/or natural polymers with an emphasis on regenerative medicine, drug delivery, and tissue adhesives [2]. Such developed hydrogels are able to mimic the native extracellular matrix (ECM) and support cellular growth and tissue regeneration [3]. Besides, hydrogels are used in cell-matrix, 3D culturing cell-cell interactions, cellular proliferation, differentiation, and migration [4,5]. In this regard, naturally occurring biopolymers comprising hydrogels have potential advantages over synthetic polymers, including low cost, good cytocompatibility, less immunogenicity, degradability in physiological conditions, and wide availability [6]. Thus, several hydrogels developed from alginate, chitosan, hyaluronic acid, fibrinogen, collagen, and zein have been reported [7–12]. Consequently, it is vital to fabricate plant protein-derived hydrogels for biomedical applications. Zein is a natural plant protein and extracted from corn. Zein is hydrophobic and water-insoluble due to lack of prolamin [13–16]. Zein protein has been used in drug delivery, food packaging, and coatings [15,17]. However, there are some issues, such as shrinkage in water, low mechanical strength, and rapid degradation that impede the biomedical applications of pure zein. Therefore, several chemical modification and physical treatments have been developed to improve the mechanical strength, water-resistance, and plasticity of zein protein [18–22]. Moreover, zein was covalently functionalized with gold nanoparticles, polycaprolactone (PCL), and 3-glycidoxypropyltrimethoxysilane to improve mechanical and degradability, respectively [23–25]. In order to improve the above properties of zein, poly 4-mercaptophenyl methacrylate-carbon nano-onions were incorporated within zein protein to fabricate zein/f-CNOs composite hydrogels.

Carbon-nano-onions (CNOs) are a class of carbon nanomaterials that contain concentric graphitic shells and are described by Ugarte in 1992 [26]. CNOs have been widely used in catalysis, supercapacitors, lithium-ion batteries, cell imaging, and diagnostic, therapeutic, and other biomedical applications because of their good physicochemical properties [27–32]. Among different carbon nanomaterials, CNOs are the most promising carbon material for biomedical applications because of their tolerance to transport in the circulatory systems with negligible toxicity and good cytocompatibility [31]. Moreover, several studies demonstrated that CNOs are highly biocompatible compared to MWCNTs, and CNOs showed less inflammation than CNTs [32]. Pristine CNOs, oxidized CNOs, and PEGylated CNOs are nontoxic and presented more than 85% of cell viability with fibroblasts [33]. Recently, ultra-high molecular weight polyethylene/4-mercaptophenyl methacrylate functionalized carbon nano-onions (UHMWPE/f-CNOs) nanocomposites were developed [34]. The mechanical, cytocompatibile, and thermal properties of the UHMWPE were significantly enhanced in the presence of 0.1 wt% of functionalized CNOs [34]. These outstanding results of f-CNOs motivated us to design and fabricate f-CNOs incorporated zein/f-CNOs hydrogels. Thus, it is of great interest to explore the application of CNOs as a second phase reinforcement in the fabrication of novel hydrogels.

The proper synthetic route of nanomaterials is essential in biomedical application, where the sonochemical method offers an easy path of synthesis. Sonochemistry is an emerging synthetic method to fabricate nanomaterials. Sonochemistry is a simple, facile, and short-time physicochemical method liable to the high-intensity ultrasound and acoustic cavitation phenomenon [35,36]. A sonochemical method has been used to develop several nanomaterials with an emphasis on controlled drug delivery [37,38]. Nonetheless, to the best of our knowledge, the fabrication of plant protein (zein)/f-CNOs composite hydrogels have not yet been established, until now, for controlled drug release. Thus, it is hypothesized that f-CNOs can uniformly disperse and reinforce within the zein matrix by sonochemical method. The homogeneous dispersion of CNOs not only improves the mechanical properties of zein/f-CNOs composite hydrogels but also enhances biodegradability, swelling, drug release, and cytocompatibility.

The aim of the current study is to fabricate poly 4-mercaptophenyl methacrylated CNOs loaded zein protein hydrogels using acoustic cavitation technique. Besides, we will investigate the physicochemical properties, mechanical properties, drug release under physiological conditions, and cytocompatibility of hydrogels.

2. Experimental Section

2.1. Materials and Methods

All the reagents and organic solvents were purchased from commercial suppliers and used without further purification. Zein protein, methacryloyl chloride (MA), *N*-hydroxysuccinimide (NHS), 1-ethyl-3-(3-dimethylaminopropyl) carbodiimide (EDC), 5-Fluorouracil (5-FU), glutaraldehyde (GA), and 2,2′-Azobis(2-methylpropionitrile) (AIBN) were procured from Sigma Aldrich (St. Louis, MO,

USA.). Osteoblast cells were obtained from the American Type Culture Collection (ATCC, Manassas, VA, USA.). Dulbecco's modified Eagle's medium/F12 without phenol red (DMEM/F12), phosphate buffered saline (PBS) pH 7.4, fetal bovine serum (FBS), penicillin/streptomycin, and trypsin were acquired from Gibco Invitrogen (Camarillo, CA, USA.). CellTiter96®AQueous One Solution Cell Proliferation Assay was bought from Promega, (Fitchburg, WI, USA.). LIVE/DEAD Cell Imaging Kit was purchased from Molecular Probes, Life Technologies Corp. (Carlsbad, CA, U.S.A.).

2.2. Synthesis

2.2.1. Preparation of Composite Hydrogels

The synthesis of poly 4-mercaptophenyl methacrylated-CNOs was accomplished according to the previous report [34].

Synthesis of CNOs-MP

Briefly, 100 mg of pristine carbon nano-onions were dispersed in 50 mL of anhydrous DMF for 30 min using an ultrasonic bath. Then, 350 mg of *N*-hydroxysuccinimide (NHS) and 350 mg 4-dimethylaminopyridine (DMAP) were added to the dispersion solution and further sonicated for 30 min. After that, 1-ethyl-3-(3-dimethylaminopropyl) carbodiimide (EDC, 570 mg) was added and sonicated for 30 min. Next, 100 mg of 4-mercaptophenol (MP) was added and stirring was continued for 48 h at 60 °C under N_2. After the completion of the reaction (monitored thin layer chromatography), the stirring was stopped and the reaction mixture was cooled to ambient temperature. Next, the supernatant was discarded using centrifugation. The resulting black solid was thoroughly washed with DMF, methanol, DMF/triethylamine (9.9: 01), and ethyl acetate to obtain 4-mercaptophenylated CNOs (CNOs-MP).

Synthesis of CNOs-PMPMA

The mixture of 50 mg of CNOs-MP and 1.0 mL of diisopropylethylamine was dispersed in 50 mL of anhydrous tetrahydrofuran (THF) for 30 min using an ultrasonic bath. Then, 1.0 mL of methacryloyl chloride (MA) was added to the above mixture and stirred at room temperature for 24 h. Subsequently, the supernatant was discarded using centrifugation to attain a black solid. The resulted black solid was washed thoroughly with THF, dichloromethane, and HCl (0.01 M aqueous) to provide monomer CNOs-MPMA as a black solid. Then, 50 mg of CNOs-MPMA and azobisisobutyronitrile (AIBN, 1 wt%) were dissolved in 20 mL of anhydrous THF and sonicated for 30 min. Next, the reaction mixture was stirred at 70 °C for 48 h. Subsequently, the reaction mixture was cooled to ambient temperature and the supernatant was removed by centrifugation to attain CNOs-PMPMA as a black solid. The solid was washed with dichloromethane and diethyl ether and vacuum dried and stored in a desiccator until further use. The functionalized CNOs-PMPMA (f-CNOs) were characterized using ^{1}H-NMR, Raman, TGA, and GPC analysis.

In order to prepare zein/f-CNOs hydrogels, initially, 2 mg/mL of f-CNOs was ultrasonicated for 30 min in water/1,4-dioxane (1:1) to obtain the homogenous dispersion. Then, 1.0 g of zein protein (in 10 mL of water/1,4-dioxane; 1:1) was added into the f-CNOs solution. The resulting reaction mixture was treated with GA (1%, *w/w*) as a crosslinking agent under three different reaction conditions as showed in the Table 1.

To prepare the drug-loaded hydrogels, 10 mg/mL of 5-FU was added to the above solutions before the addition of crosslinker to incorporate the drug within the polymer matrix. This could prevent the surface drug loading, burst release, and aid the sustained release.

Table 1. Reaction conditions and fabrication methods of hydrogels.

Entry	Method	Zein/f-CNOs	Cross-Linker (GA)	Time (min.)	Hydrogel [d]
1.	Conventional	(1.0 g/2.0 mg)	(1%, w/w)	180 [a]	CZCNOs
2.	Microwave	(1.0 g/2.0 mg)	(1%, w/w)	40 [b]	MZCNOs
3.	Acoustic cavitation (ultra-sonic)	(1.0 g/2.0 mg)	(1%, w/w)	30 [c]	UZCNOs

[a] The reaction mixture was stirred at 65 °C for 180 min; [b] 500 W of power was applied for 40 min; [c] The reaction mixture was ultra-sonicated for 30 min; [d] The homogeneous reaction mixture was poured into a glass petri dish and left to stand overnight for gel formation.

2.3. Characterizations of Composite Hydrogels

Scanning electron microscopy (SEM, ZEISS EVO®MA 25, Ostalbkreis, Baden-Württemberg, Germany) was used to study the surface morphological properties of composite hydrogels. For this, all the hydrogel samples were flash-frozen in liquid nitrogen and then fractured. Prior to the SEM analysis, the cross-sections of the freeze-dried hydrogel specimens were gold coated. Tensile strength and elongation at break testing were measured to evaluate the mechanical properties of composite hydrogels samples. A tensile testing machine (Instron 3365, Instron, and Norwood, MA, USA.) was used to measure the tensile properties of specimens. The size of the hydrogel sample was 33.0 mm × 6.0 mm × 2.0 mm, and the crosshead speed was 50 mm/min.

To get the information about the functional groups presented in the hydrogel structure, the Fourier transform infrared (FTIR) spectroscopy (Perkin Elmer Universal ATR Sampling Accessory Frontier, Waltham, MA, USA) was used to scrutinize the zein/f-CNOs composite hydrogel specimens in the wavenumber range of 400–4000 cm^{-1} at room temperature.

2.3.1. Dynamic Light Scattering (DLS) and Zeta-Potential Experiments

DLS measurements were recorded using the Malvern Nano-ZS instrument and the data analyzed by Zetasizer software (version 7.12), Malvern Instruments Ltd., Worcestershire, WR14 1XZ, United Kingdom. 500 µg/mL of f-CNOs were probe sonicated in water and DMEM cell medium for 60 min. Then, the final concentration (500 µg/mL) of f-CNOs was diluted into 50, 25, 5, and 1 µg/mL in water and DMEM cell medium to measure the size of the particles. The dispensable zeta potential cuvettes were used to record the Zeta potential measurements. All the zeta measurements were run in triplicate per each sample and averaged to attain the final results.

2.3.2. Swelling of Hydrogels

Swelling ratio measurements of hydrogels were recorded by gravimetrically on a definite amount of dried hydrogel samples. Initially, the freeze-dried and pre-weighed hydrogel samples were immersed in DMEM (pH 7.4) at predetermined time intervals.

The swollen hydrogels were drawn from DMEM and the non-adsorbed medium was soaked mildly with filter paper and weighed with a microbalance. The swelling ratio (SR) was measured using the following equation:

$$SR = \frac{(Ws - Wd)}{Wd} \times 100 \tag{1}$$

where W_s is the weight of hydrogels at equilibrium state and W_d is the weight of the hydrogels at the dry state. The swelling rate of the composite hydrogels was calculated according to the following equation

$$v = \frac{(Wt2 - Wt1)}{Wd(t2 - t1)} \tag{2}$$

where $t1$ and $t2$ were the mean of the swelling time, and W_{t1} and W_{t2} were the weight of the sample at $t1$ and $t2$, and W_d was the weight of dried hydrogels.

2.3.3. In Vitro Degradation of Hydrogels

In vitro degradation of hydrogels was measured with respect to weight loss. For this, initially weighed hydrogel specimens (W_0) were immersed in DMEM (pH 7.4) medium and incubated at 37 °C for 25 days. Then, the samples were taken out from the medium at predetermined time intervals, washed and dried in the desiccator for 12 h and weighed (W_t). The weight loss ratio calculated as $100 \times \frac{W_0 - W_t}{W_0}$. The weight remaining ratio was calculated as $1 - \left[100 \times \frac{W_0 - W_t}{W_0}\right]$.

2.3.4. In Vitro Drug Release from Hydrogels

UV-spectrophotometer (Agilent Technologies, 89090A) was used to measure the 5-FU release from the hydrogel specimens. For this, 30 mg of 5-FU-loaded hydrogel samples were immersed in 10 mL of DMEM (pH 2.0, 4.5, 7.4, and 9.0) and gently incubated at 37 °C. At predetermined time intervals, 2 mL of 5-FU released medium was collected and replaced with 2 mL of fresh DMEM medium to maintain the solution volume constant. The drug release was determined at λ_{max} = 265 nm to attain 5-FU concentration. The 5-FU release from hydrogel samples against time intervals was established. The pH-values (pH 2.0, 4.5, 7.4, and 9.0) of DMEM medium was adjusted with 1 M HCl or 1 M NaOH. Triplicate measurements were carried out. The drug release (%) was calculated from the following formula:

$$\text{drug release (\%)} = \frac{\text{Mass of drug loaded Gel} - \text{Mass of drug released}}{\text{Mass of drug released}}$$

2.3.5. Cytotoxicity Evaluation of Composite Hydrogels

The human osteoblasts (bone-forming cells) were used to evaluate in vitro cytocompatibility of hydrogels. For this, osteoblast cells were cultured on the surface of the hydrogel samples. Cell viability and morphology were also studied.

Cell Viability of Hydrogels

Cell viability was measured using CellTiter96®AQueous One Solution Cell Proliferation Assay. Initially, disk-shaped (~6.3 mm in diameter) hydrogels were prepared and then cut into thin sections and these hydrogel specimens were sterilized by ethanol (70% v/v) followed by UV irradiation. After that, the sterilized hydrogel specimens were decorated on a 96-well plate and then, human fetal osteoblastic cells (hFOB 1.19) at a density of 1×10^4 cells per well (~3.12×10^4 cells/cm^{-2}) were seeded over the hydrogels. The non-adherent cells were removed on the next day. The cell number was calculated after 1, 2, and 3 days post-seeding, using CellTiter96®. Furthermore, the LIVE/DEAD Cell Staining Kit was used to measure the cell viability of hydrogels and the images were recorded using fluorescence microscopy. The tissue culture plate was used as a control in 96-well plates. The experiments were run in triplicate.

Morphological Evaluations of Osteoblasts on Hydrogels

Prior to cell seeding on 24-well plates, hydrogels were cut into a disk shape. After that, human fetal osteoblastic cells (hFOB 1.19) at a density of 1×10^4 cells/mL were seeded on the surface of hydrogels in DMEM/F12 medium supplemented with 0.3 mg/mL of G418 disulfate salt, 2.5 mM of L-glutamine, 1% of penicillin/streptomycin and 10% of fetal bovine serum. The cells were incubated for 24 h in a humidified atmosphere at 5% CO_2. Then, the medium was transferred from the well plates and washed several times with phosphate buffer solution. After 3 days of incubation, cell images were recorded by an optical microscope (Model IN200A-5M, Amscope, Chino, CA, USA).

2.4. Statistical Analysis

All the experiments were carried out in triplicate and quantitative data were presented as mean ± standard deviation (SD) with n = 3. Statistical analysis was determined by one-way analysis of variance (ANOVA) and Tukey's post hoc tests using Minitab17 (Minitab, State College, PA, USA). $p < 0.05$ was considered statistically significant.

3. Results

3.1. Synthesis

Recently, we synthesized poly 4-mercaptophenyl methacrylated CNOs (f-CNOs) starting from the thioester coupling of 4-mercaptophenol with COOH-CNOs followed by methacrylatation and polymerization [34]. Then, UHMWPE/f-CNOs nanocomposites were developed through reinforcing f-CNOs with long-chain UHMWPE. A small quantity of f-CNOs improved the mechanical and cytocompatibility of UHMWPE. The uniform dispersion of f-CNOs particles throughout the hydrogel matrix is necessary to achieve good physicochemical properties of zein/f-CNOs hydrogels. Therefore, f-CNOs were synthesized and zein/f-CNOs (UZCNOs) hydrogels were fabricated by reinforcing f-CNOs within the zein matrix through acoustic cavitation method (Figure 1a). The acoustic cavitation promoted 5-FU loaded UZCNOs hydrogels were crosslinked with GA. The UZCNOs hydrogels were pH sensitive, pH-responsive, and pH 7.4 and pH 9.0 exhibited quicker drug release than pH 2.0 and pH 4.5 medium (Figure 1b). Moreover, the synthesized f-CNOs were dispersed in physiological buffer (DMEM) or aqueous environment and stabilized uniform colloidal dispersion was observed over 12 months (Figure 1c). The digital photo of zein/f-CNOs hydrogel composite is presented in Figure 1d and the inverted image unveils the evidence of the gelation.

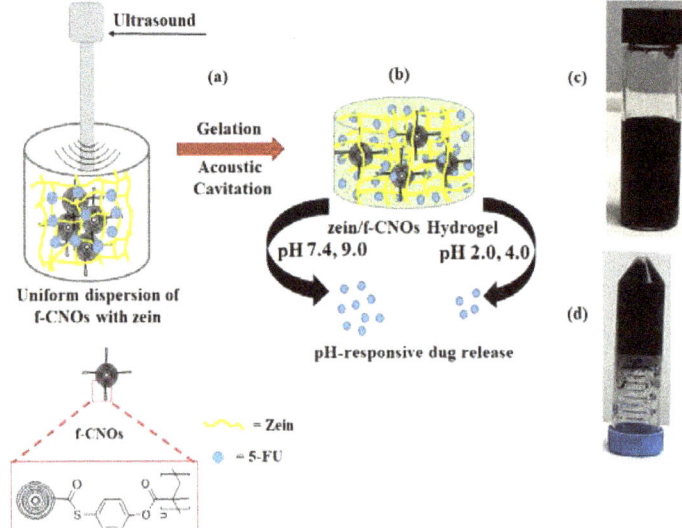

Figure 1. Synthetic illustration of (**a**) hydrogel preparation via acoustic cavitation, (**b**) cartoon diagram of hydrogel, (**c**) digital photograph of uniformly dispersed f-CNOs in DMEM after 1 year, and (**d**) digital photographs of fabricated UZCNOs hydrogel composite. f-CNOs indicates functionalized CNOs.

3.2. Dynamic Light Scattering (DLS) and Zeta-Potential Measurements

The dispersion and stability of pure COOH-CNOs and f-CNOs were scrutinized under physiological environment by DLS measurements. The dispersion of pristine COOH-CNOs particles showed approximately 110 nm, whereas f-CNOs particles exhibited around 147 nm in DMEM (Figure 2a). The particle size of pristine CNOs and f-CNOs was not changed with the concentration and time, indicating a stabilized colloidal dispersion even at relatively high concentrations. Besides, zeta potential measurements of pristine CNOs and f-CNOs were measured in DMEM and water.

The pristine CNOs exhibited ξ-potential values around −35 and −27 mV in DMEM and water, respectively, suggesting that they form uniform dispersions and that the COOH group has a substantial effect on the charge capacity of pristine CNOs (Figure 2b). Accordingly, positive (+ 30 and + 23 mV) ξ-potential values were observed in DMEM, and water, respectively (Figure 2b), indicating the chemical conjugation of the MPMA group on the surface of COOH-CNOs.

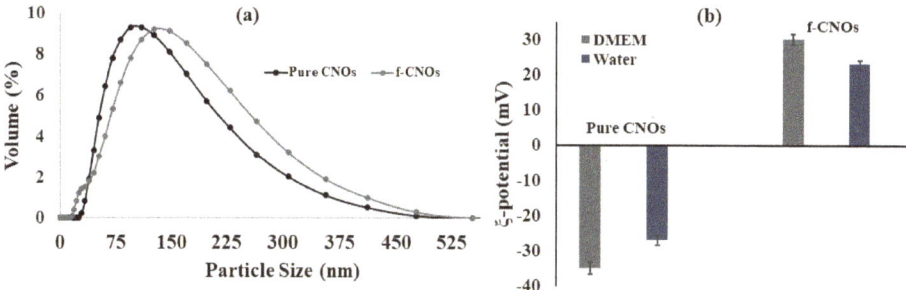

Figure 2. (a) Illustration of DLS particle size distribution, and (b) ξ-potential measurement of pristine CNOs and f-CNOs dispersions in DMEM.

3.3. SEM Analysis

The SEM analysis was performed to obtain microstructure morphologies of composite hydrogels and the resulting SEM images are illustrated in Figure 3. As shown in the SEM images, CZCNOs, MZCNOs, and UZCNOs hydrogel composites exhibited a porous and continuous structure. However, the porosity and internal morphology of hydrogels were reliant on the fabrication method. Particularly, the conventional thermal method provided CZCNOs showed constrained structure with low porosity (Figure 3a,d). On the other hand, MZCNOs hydrogel provided by microwave radiation showed a somewhat improved porosity (Figure 3b), and the porosity can be observed in the high magnification image of MZCNOs hydrogel (Figure 3e). Whereas UZCNOs hydrogel fabricated by acoustic cavitation exhibited sponge-like structure with good porosity, this porous morphology can restore the water uptake properties of the UZCNOs hydrogel (Figure 3c,f).

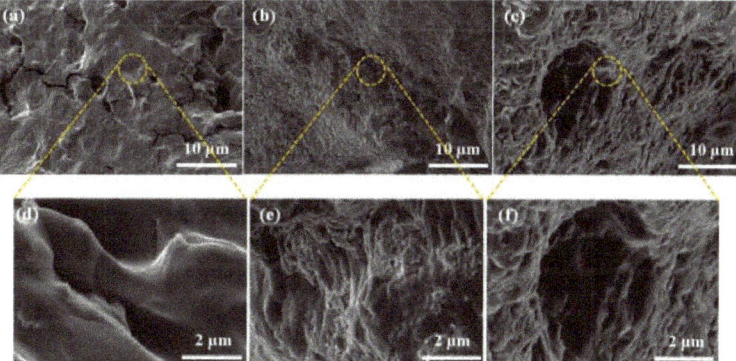

Figure 3. SEM image of composite hydrogel after freeze-drying (a,d) CZCNOs, (b,e) MZCNOs, and (c,f) UZCNOs, respectively. (d–f) Indicates the high magnification SEM images of CZCNOs, MZCNOs, and UZCNOs hydrogels, respectively.

3.4. FTIR and Tensile Measurements

FTIR analysis was utilized to understand the possible interactions between zein and f-CNOs (Figure 4a). PMPMA chemically conjugated CNOs exhibited a major absorption band at 1745 cm^{-1} for C=O stretching and 1560–1418 cm^{-1} for vibrational starching of the phenyl ring. Besides, 1263–1003 cm^{-1} bands were absorbed for C–O–C stretching and 2960 cm^{-1} for aliphatic C–H stretching of PMPMA moiety. The f-CNOs also showed a sharp peak at 685 cm^{-1} for the C–H bending vibration (out of plane) of phenyl moiety. On the other hand, pristine zein showed a broad absorption band in the frequency range of 3524–3133 cm^{-1} for amide A (N–H stretching vibration) and 2964–2923 cm^{-1} for C–H stretching vibrations of aliphatic functional groups. In addition, the zein protein exhibited a band at 1648 cm^{-1} for amide-I and stretching vibration of C=O bond, and at 1551 cm^{-1} for amide-II and C–N bond, respectively [26]. Several absorption peaks of the N–H bending and C–N stretching of zein protein were detected at 1521–1374, 1241, and 1080 cm^{-1}, respectively. As shown in Figure 4a, UZCNOs composite hydrogel showed a broad absorption band in the range of 3530–3137 cm^{-1}, and 2967–2930 cm^{-1} for amide A (N–H stretching vibration), and C–H stretching vibrations of aliphatic functional groups, respectively. UZCNOs sample also showed the absorption peak at 1665 cm^{-1} for amide-I, and C=O stretching, respectively. The C–N bond and amide-II of UZCNOs hydrogels were detected in the frequency range of 1525–1380 cm^{-1}. Furthermore, UZCNOs hydrogel showed the absorption bands at higher a frequency range for C–N stretching, and N–H bending, respectively. Notably, C–H bending (out of plane) of phenyl moiety (f-CNOs) was absorbed at 690 cm^{-1}.

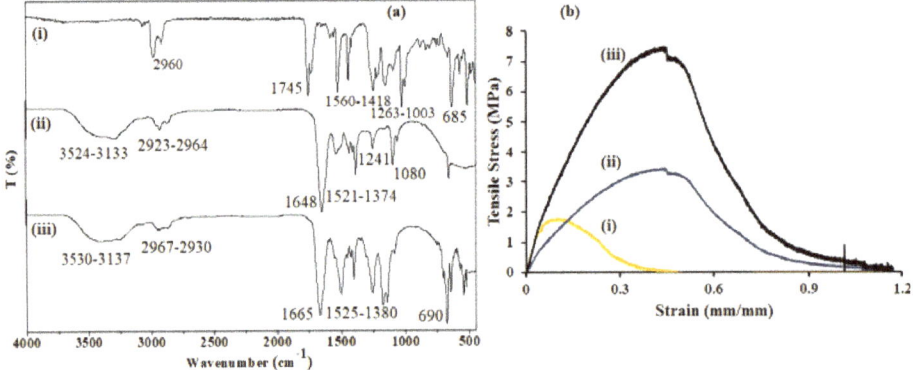

Figure 4. (a) FTIR spectra of (i) pure f-CNOs, (ii) pristine zein, and (iii) UZCNOs. (b) Tensile graph of (i) CZCNOs, (ii) MZCNOs, and (iii) UZCNOs hydrogels, respectively.

The tolerance of high loads and sustained deformation of the hydrogel are important characteristics in drug delivery applications. Consequently, the mechanical properties of UZCNOs hydrogel composite were recorded and non-linear stress/strain curves are illustrated in Figure 4b. The mechanical properties of UZCNOs hydrogels were significantly ($p < 0.05$) enhanced with the addition of f-CNOs. Specifically, UZCNOs hydrogel composite showed 7.7 ± 0.25 MPa of tensile strength, whereas MZCNOs hydrogel composite exhibited 4.2 ± 1.12 MPa of tensile strength (Figure 4b). These results revealed that UZCNOs hydrogel composite displayed higher tensile strength and lower strain than MZCNOs hydrogel. This could be due to the crosslinking density, electrostatic interactions or hydrogen bonding between f-CNOs and zein protein under acoustic cavitation environment. In addition, the tensile strength of CZCNOs hydrogel was measured (0.98 ± 1.25 MPa) and compared with UZCNOs hydrogel.

3.5. Swelling and Degradation Measurements

Usually, the water absorption of the hydrogel can be influenced by the aggregate structure and chemical structure. Thus, the swelling ratio and swelling rate of the fabricated hydrogels with different methods were measured using the gravimetric method and the results were presented in Figure 5a,b, respectively. From Figure 5a, it can be seen that the percentage swelling of the composite hydrogels was more than 150%. Particularly, UZCNOs hydrogel synthesized by acoustic cavitation and MZCNOs synthesized by microwave radiation showed the higher mass swelling ratio (>255%), this indicates that f-CNOs have a detrimental effect on the swelling ratio. Besides, the swelling rate of hydrogels was measured and is illustrated in Figure 5b. According to Figure 5, the swelling rates of the all the composite hydrogels were gradually decreased and reached equilibrium values, which indicates that the swelling behavior of hydrogels could be controlled with a short period for zein/f-CNOs hydrogels. Subsequently, this can be a rapid absorbent.

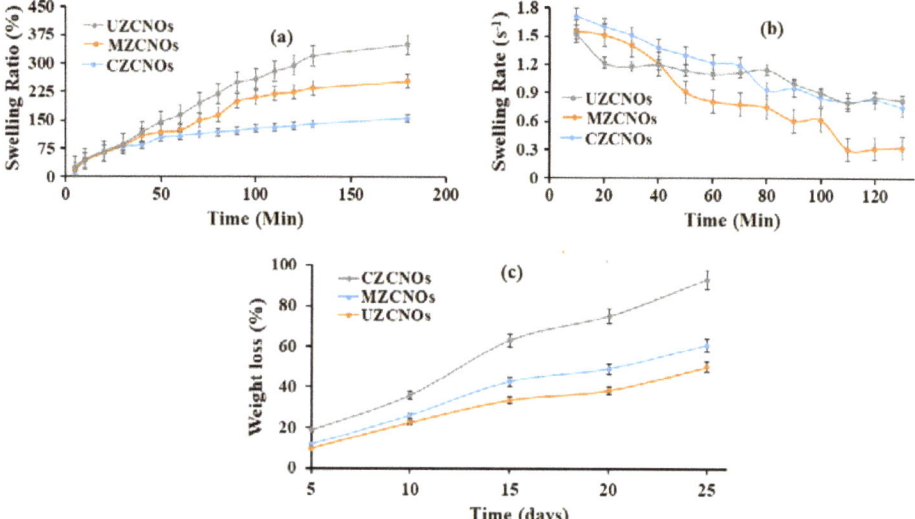

Figure 5. (a) Swelling ratio, (b) swelling rate, and (c) degradation curves of (i) CZCNO, MZCNOs, and UZCNOs hydrogels, respectively, in DMEM (pH 7.4) at room temperature.

The biodegradation characteristics of composite hydrogels display an important role in drug delivery and tissue engineering. Consequently, the degradation of hydrogels was measured in DMEM (pH 7.4) at 37 °C and the results are illustrated in Figure 5c. The CZCNOs hydrogel showed approximately 93% of degradation in 25 days of incubation. This could be due to the existence of weak electrostatic interactions and a difference in crosslinking density under the conventional method. On the other hand, MZCNOs and UZCNOs hydrogels showed sustained weight loss up to 25 days of incubation (Figure 5c). The UZCNOs hydrogel exhibited a lower degradation rate than MZCNOs hydrogels. Specifically, UZCNOs hydrogel showed around 50% of degradation in 25 days of study. This could be due to the strong electrostatic interactions and higher crosslinking density under acoustic cavitation. Whereas MZCNOs hydrogel exhibited approximately 61% of degradation in 25 days of study.

3.6. PH-Responsive Drug Release

In vitro release of 5-FU from composite hydrogels was performed by immersing the 5-FU loaded hydrogels in DMEM at pH 2.0, 4.5, 7.4, and 9.0. The drug release curves are presented in Figure 6. Initially, the 5-FU release from CZCNOs, MZCNOs, and UZCNOs hydrogels was measured at pH 2.0 over 15 days (Figure 6a). Under these conditions, composite hydrogels showed prolonged drug release. Particularly, the CZCNOs sample exhibited approximately 52% and the MZCNOs sample showed 69%

of drug release over 15 days of study (Figure 6a). On the other hand, the UZCNOs sample showed 85% of drug release over 15 days at pH 2.0.

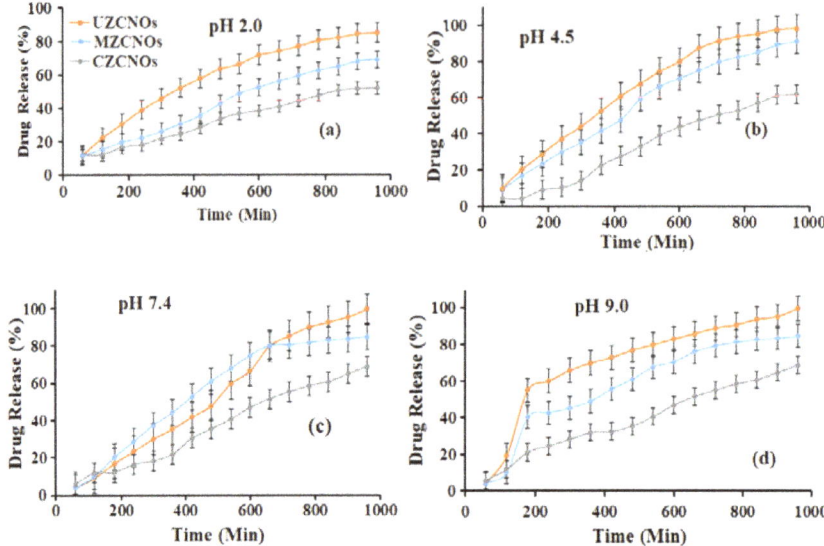

Figure 6. The graph illustrating the cumulative release of 5-FU from CZCNOs, MZCNOs, and UZCNOs composite hydrogels in DMEM at (**a**) pH 2.0, (**b**) pH 4.5, (**c**) pH 7.4, and (**d**) pH 9.0 at 37 °C, respectively.

To improve the drug release profile, pH 4.5 was used and measured the 5-FU release from composite hydrogel specimens (Figure 6b). As expected, CZCNOs hydrogel specimen exhibited around 62% of drug release over 15 days of study, which improved 8% of drug release at pH 4.5 (Figure 6b). The MZCNOs hydrogels sample showed around 91% of 5-FU release after 15 days of study and 20% of drug release was improved by changing pH 2.0 to pH 4.5., whereas the UZCNOs hydrogel sample synthesized by acoustic cavitation method exhibited approximately 94% of drug release at pH 4.5 over 15 days of incubation and reached plateau (Figure 6b).

In addition, 5-FU release was carried out in DMEM at pH 7.4 at room temperature (Figure 6c). This pH environment is defensible to the normal cells and reduces drug loss during drug transportation. Besides, pH 7.4 can control drug release behavior of hydrogel specimens while they present at the cytoplasm of normal cells or intracellular environment. The CZCNOs hydrogel showed around 67% of sustained drug release over 15 days of study. The MZCNOs hydrogel exhibited 85% of sustained drug release, whereas UZCNOs hydrogel samples displayed approximately 97% of sustained drug release over 15 days of study and reached a plateau.

Furthermore, 5-FU release was measured at pH 9.0 and the results are illustrated in Figure 6d. The UZCNOs hydrogel specimen showed approximately 52% of burst release on the third day of study. After that, around 99.9% of the drug was released in 15 days of study and reached a plateau (Figure 6d). On the other hand, MZCNOs hydrogels showed around 40% of burst release on the third day, followed by 85% of sustained drug release over 15 days of study, which is very similar to the pH 7.4 study (Figure 6d). Finally, CZCNOs hydrogels showed approximately 70% of sustained drug release over 15 days of incubation (Figure 6d).

3.7. In Vitro Cytocompatibility Measurements

The CellTiter96® AQueous One Solution was used to measure the cell viability of composite hydrogels and the results are depicted in Figure 7. The osteoblast cells were cultured on the pre-sterilized hydrogels specimens. On the first day of incubation, very similar cell viability was observed in CZCNOs, MZCNOs, and UZCNOs composite hydrogels. On the second day of study, MZCNOs, and UZCNOs hydrogel samples showed slightly improved cell viability, whereas CZCNOs hydrogel sample exhibited comparable viability on the same day of study (Figure 7). However, on the third day of incubation, the UZCNOs hydrogel specimen exhibited a better cell viability than the MZCNOs and CZCNOs hydrogel specimens.

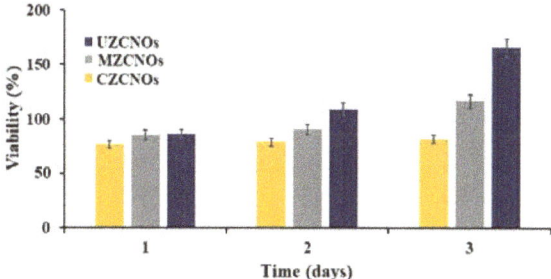

Figure 7. Cell viability of CZCNOs, MZCNOs, and UZCNOs composite hydrogels. Data represent mean ± SD ($n = 3$). Statistically significant difference ($p < 0.05$) was observed between the cell viability parameters of CZCNOs, MZCNOs, and UZCNOs samples.

The LIVE/DEAD kit was also utilized to evaluate the cytotoxicity of f-CNOs in zein/f-CNOs composite hydrogels and the resulting optical images are depicted in Figure 8. The cell culture plate was used as a controller and it exhibited some DEAD cells after three days of study (Figure 8a). The CZCNOs hydrogel sample showed a decent percentage (77 ± 1.30%) of LIVE cells along with some of the DEAD cells (Figure 8b). The MZCNOs hydrogel sample displayed approximately 93 ± 0.81% of LIVE cells along with a small number of DEAD cells (Figure 8c). Interestingly, UZCNOs sample exhibited more than 97 ± 0.41% of LIVE cells (Figure 8d).

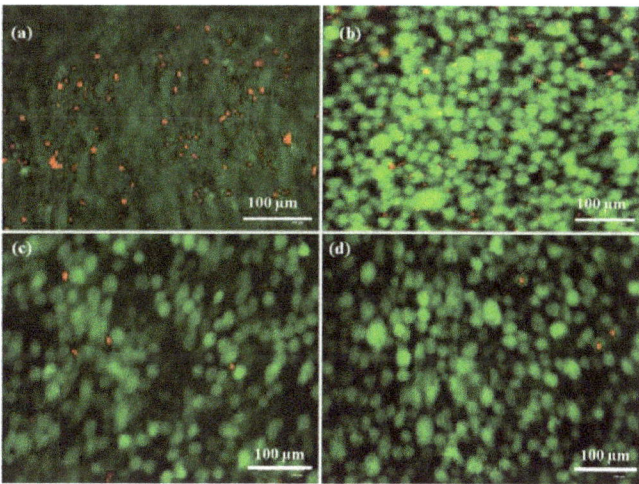

Figure 8. Optical images of osteoblast cells on the surface of zein/f-CNOs composite hydrogels after 3 days of study: (**a**) The control (tissue culture plate), (**b**) CZCNOs, (**c**) MZCNOs, and (**d**) UZCNOs; green indicates LIVE cells, and red indicates DEAD, respectively. Scale bar = 100 μm.

4. Discussion

The homogeneous colloidal dispersion measurements suggested that the functionalized CNOs could stabilize in the aqueous environment. The acoustic cavitation wave or acoustic cavitation is the superlative stringent source of exfoliation of 2D nanomaterials. The fluctuation of pressure in the liquid environment generates the acoustic cavitation that creates bubble growth followed by bubble collapse and finally internal turbulence. This ultrasound energy renovates into high temperature and pressure. Ultrasound waves transfer through carbon nanoparticles (CNOs) which are held by weak interactions, including the Van der Waals forces and/or π–π stacking. Thus, acoustic cavitation is a good choice to achieve the uniform dispersion and stability of CNOs in the aqueous environment. Colloidal stable CNOs produced by acoustic cavitation are effective to enhance the electrical, tensile, and biocompatible assets of the nanocomposites. Consequently, uniformly dispersed and colloidal stabilized f-CNOs were reinforced with zein and fabricated zein/f-CNOs hydrogel composite through the acoustic cavitation method. Thus, the positive and negative ξ-potential values described the proton exchange phenomenon between the polar groups present on the surface of CNOs and the solvent system. When COOH-CNOs were dispersed in DMEM and water, CNOs groups were able to donate protons to the medium, exhibiting the negative ξ-potential values. On the other hand, chemically conjugated CNOs (f-CNOs) were unable to offer protons to the medium, switching the ξ-potential to positive values. The SEM analysis of UZCNOs hydrogel exhibited a sponge-like structure with porous morphology.

All these absorption bands of pristine zein were altered in the FTIR spectrum of UZCNOs hydrogel composite, suggesting that there were hydrophobic interactions or π-π stacking between the zein protein and f-CNOs. Thus, UZCNOs hydrogel composite showed a peak at 1665 cm^{-1} for C=O stretching vibration and amide-I, whereas, 1525 cm^{-1} for amide II and the C–N bond, respectively. Likewise, the N–H bending and C–N stretching peaks of UZCNOs hydrogel were shifted to a higher frequency range, which reveals that f-CNOs were completely blended within the hydrogel matrix. Thus, FTIR spectra show physicochemical interactions between zein protein and f-CNOs. The tensile results suggest that the UZCNOs hydrogel produced by acoustic cavitation has exhibited approximately seven times higher tensile strength than CZCNOs hydrogel produced by a conventional stirring method. Accordingly, the mechanical measurements reveal that the hydrogel fabrication method could be critical to obtaining enhanced tensile properties.

The percentage of the swelling ratio of the CZCNOs hydrogel synthesized by the traditional stirring method was significantly lower than UZCNOs and MZCNOs (Figure 5a). This could be due to the difference in crosslinking density. By comparing the swelling results from Figure 5a, it can be revealed that the swelling ratio of CZCNOs hydrogel was remarkably lower than MZCNOs and UZCNOs hydrogels, which indicates that the crosslinking density was higher for hydrogels fabricated by radiation and acoustic cavitation. The UZCNOs hydrogels showed the lowest degradation in 25 days of incubation. This could be due to the existence of moderate electrostatic interactions and the difference in crosslinking density under the microwave method. Overall, the fabrication method had a considerable impact on the degradation measurements.

The UZCNOs hydrogels exhibited higher drug release than MZCNOs and CZCNOs hydrogels at pH 2.0 and 4.5. This could be due to the π-π stacking and Van der Waal forces between hydrogels and 5-FU. These characteristics might have slowed the diffusion rate of 5-FU from the composite hydrogels. Besides, it is hypothesized that the solubility and diffusion of 5-FU dawdled in the presence of f-CNOs. Moreover, the fabrication method, lower swelling ratio, and mobility of f-CNOs played a key role in the drug release measurements. In addition, UZCNOs hydrogel showed improved drug release (97%) at pH 7.4. We relate this to the high swelling ratio of the hydrogels at pH 7.4. Furthermore, the 5-FU release rate is significantly proportional to the swelling behavior of the hydrogel network. Whereas at pH 9.0 we did not see a significant improvement in the drug release of MZCNOs and CZCNOs specimens by increasing from pH 7.4 to pH 9.0, however, the UZCNOs hydrogel sample exhibited burst release followed by sustained drug release up to 15 days of study. It could be due to the hydrophilic nature of 5-FU within the gel matrix, which led to faster diffusion from the hydrogel into the medium.

The drug release results at pH 7.4 and 9.0 are attributed to π–π stacking of 5-FU molecules on the surface of composite hydrogels. 5-FU is a chemotherapeutic agent and is used clinically for colorectal carcinoma and there is a great need for colon-specific controlled delivery systems to treat directly at a disease site in the colon [39]. The results of in vitro 5-FU release from zein/f-CNOs suggest that the UZCNOs could be a prospective pH-sensitive transporter for colon-specific drug delivery. It is well known that the natural pH environment of the gastrointestinal tract differs from acidic (stomach) to slightly basic (intestinal). Particularly, the gastrointestinal tract increases its pH environment from the stomach (pH 1.4–3.0) to the terminal ileum (pH 7.5 ± 0.5). Such pH environment decreases to 6.4 ± 0.6 at the beginning of the colon, which slightly rises to pH 6.6 ± 0.8 in the middle of the colon and reaches 7.0 ± 0.7 in the left colon [40]. Therefore, it is important to consider the pH environment of the gastrointestinal tract while designing peroral dosage forms. The pH-responsive release of 5-FU from the UZCNOs hydrogels could indicate that zein/f-CNOs composite has an admirable protective effect for the oral delivery system of peptides and other drugs, which are easily ruined by gastric acid. Thus, the loaded drug can be released in a lesser amount from the hydrogel as it travels through the stomach. After reaching the colon, a significant amount of drug retained in the gel matrix could be released from the hydrogel.

Besides, UZCNOs hydrogels displayed higher cell viability ($p < 0.05$) than MZCNOs and CZCNOs hydrogels. This could be due to the enhanced tensile strength, lower degradation, higher hydrophobicity, and crosslinking density of UZCNOs hydrogel synthesized by acoustic cavitation method. The cell viability results revealed that the percentage of cell viability was dependent on the fabrication method of hydrogels. Moreover, cell viability suggests that UZCNOs composite hydrogels would useful as potential drug transporters with good cytocompatibility.

The LIVE/DEAD results suggest that the cell growth was considerably enhanced with f-CNOs inclusion and cells were extensively attached on the surface of the composite hydrogels. This could be due to the excellent cytocompatibility behavior and less degradability of f-CNOs. Overall, UZCNOs hydrogels exhibited better cell growth than a controller, MZCNOs, and CZCNOs samples. The LIVE/DEAD measurements also suggest a positive effect of f-CNOs on the osteoblast cells. Moreover, spherical cellular morphology was also observed on the surface of the hydrogels due to a contact angle with the cell medium, surface morphology, and surface chemical interactions of cells with hydrogels. In addition, it is also posited that the homogeneous colloidal dispersion of f-CNOs within the hydrogel matrix and wrapping with zein produced strengthened zein/f-CNOs hydrogels with amenable cytocompatibility. Nonetheless, improved mechanical strength, admiral cytocompatibility, the pH-responsive sustained drug release, and good pH-sensitivity of UZCNOs hydrogels can be useful as potential drug transporters for oral colon delivery systems and cartilage tissue engineering.

Author Contributions: Conceptualization, N.M.; methodology, A.G.-O.; formal analysis, I.L.R.; investigation, N.M., A.G.-O., I.L.R., and E.V.B.; resources, data curation, writing—original draft preparation, project administration, and funding acquisition, N.M.; writing—review and editing, E.V.B.

Funding: This research received no external funding.

Acknowledgments: We gratefully acknowledge Consejo Nacional de Ciencia y Tecnología de México (CONACYT) for the materials and Tecnologico de Monterrey for the infrastructure facilities.

Conflicts of Interest: The authors declare no conflict of interest.

References

1. Sangeetha, K.; Thamizhavel, A.; Girija, E.K. Effect of gelatin on the in situ formation of Alginate/Hydroxyapatite nanocomposite. *Mater. Lett.* **2013**, *91*, 27–30. [CrossRef]
2. Annabi, N.; Tamayol, A.; Uquillas, J.A.; Akbari, M.; Bertassoni, L.E.; Cha, C.; Camci-Unal, G.; Dokmeci, M.R.; Peppas, N.A.; Khademhosseini, A. 25th anniversary article: Rational design and applications of hydrogels in regenerative medicine. *Adv. Mater.* **2014**, *26*, 85–124. [CrossRef] [PubMed]

3. Alge, D.L.; Anseth, K.S. Bioactive hydrogels: Lighting the way. *Nat. Mater.* **2013**, *12*, 950–952. [CrossRef]
4. Yue, K.; Trujillo-de Santiago, G.; Alvarez, M.M.; Tamayol, A.; Annabi, N.; Khademhosseini, A. Synthesis, properties, and biomedical applications of gelatin methacryloyl (GelMA) hydrogels. *Biomaterials* **2015**, *73*, 254–271. [CrossRef] [PubMed]
5. West, J.L. Protein-patterned hydrogels: Customized cell microenvironments. *Nat. Mater.* **2011**, *10*, 727–729. [CrossRef] [PubMed]
6. Silva, R.; Fabry, B. Boccaccini, A.R. Fibrous protein-based hydrogels for cell encapsulation. *Biomaterials* **2014**, *35*, 6727–6738. [CrossRef] [PubMed]
7. Zhang, Z.; Zhang, R.; Zou, L.; McClements, D.J. Protein encapsulation in alginate hydrogel beads: Effect of pH on microgel stability, protein retention and protein release. *Food Hydrocoll.* **2016**, *58*, 308–315. [CrossRef]
8. Hamid, H.; Sara, M.; Samuel, M.H.; Alan, E.T. Chitosan based hydrogels and their applications for drug delivery in wound dressings: A review. *Carbohydr. Polym.* **2018**, *199*, 445–460. [CrossRef] [PubMed]
9. Dorsey, S.M.; McGarvey, J.R.; Wang, H.; Nikou, A.; Arama, L.; Koomalsingh, K.J.; Kondo, N.; Gorman, J.H.; Pilla, J.J.; Gorman, R.C.; et al. MRI evaluation of injectable hyaluronic acid-based hydrogel therapy to limit ventricular remodeling after myocardial infarction. *Biomaterials* **2015**, *69*, 65–75. [CrossRef] [PubMed]
10. Thanavel, R.; Seong, S.A.A. Fibrinogen and fibrin based micro and nano scaffolds incorporated with drugs, proteins, cells and genes for therapeutic biomedical applications. *Int. J. Nanomed.* **2013**, *8*, 3641–3662.
11. Ravichandran, R.; Islam, M.M.; Alarcon, E.I.; Samanta, A.; Wang, S.; Lundstrom, P.; Hilborn, J.; Griffith, M.; Phopase, J. Functionalised type-I collagen as a hydrogel building block for bio-orthogonal tissue engineering applications. *J. Mater. Chem. B.* **2016**, *4*, 318–326. [CrossRef]
12. Labib, G. Overview on zein protein: A promising pharmaceutical excipient in drug delivery systems and tissue engineering. *Expert Opin. Drug Deliv.* **2018**, *15*, 65–75. [CrossRef] [PubMed]
13. Apoorva, G.; Mandeep, S.B. Ag Nanometallic Surfaces for Self-Assembled Ordered Morphologies of Zein. *ACS Omega.* **2018**, *3*, 10851–10857. [CrossRef]
14. De Folter, J.W.J.; Van Ruijven, M.W.M.; Velikov, K.P. Oil-in-water Pickering emulsions stabilized by colloidal particles from the water-insoluble protein zein. *Soft Matter.* **2012**, *8*, 6807–6815. [CrossRef]
15. Paliwal, R.; Palakurthi, S. Zein in controlled drug delivery and tissue engineering. *J. Control. Release* **2014**, *189*, 108–122. [CrossRef] [PubMed]
16. Zhang, Y.; Cui, L.; Che, X.; Zhang, H.; Shi, N.; Li, C.; Chen, Y.; Kong, W. Zein-based films and their usage for controlled delivery: Origin, classes and current landscape. *J. Control. Release* **2015**, *206*, 206–219. [CrossRef]
17. Lin, J.; Li, C.; Zhao, Y.; Hu, J.; Zhang, L.M. Co-electrospun nanofibrous membranes of collagen and zein for wound healing. *ACS Appl. Mater. Interfaces* **2012**, *4*, 1050–1057. [CrossRef]
18. Wang, Y.; Padua, G.W. Nanoscale characterization of zein self-assembly. *Langmuir* **2012**, *28*, 2429–2435. [CrossRef]
19. Chen, Y.; Ye, R.; Xu, H. Physicochemical Properties of Zein-Based Films by Electrophoretic Deposition Using Indium Tin Oxide Electrodes: Vertical and Horizontal Electric Fields. *Int. J. Food Prop.* **2016**, *19*, 945–957. [CrossRef]
20. Dong, F.; Zhang, M.; Tang, W.W.; Wang, Y. Formation and mechanism of superhydrophobic/hydrophobic surfaces made from amphiphiles through droplet-mediated evaporation-induced self-assembly. *J. Phys. Chem. B* **2015**, *119*, 5321–5327. [CrossRef]
21. Hao, L.; Lin, G.; Chen, C.; Zhou, H.; Chen, H.; Zhou, X. Phosphorylated Zein as Biodegradable and Aqueous Nanocarriers for Pesticides with Sustained-Release and anti-UV Properties. *J. Agric. Food Chem.* **2019**, *67*, 9989–9999. [CrossRef] [PubMed]
22. Mamidi, N.; Romo, I.L.; Leija Gutiérrez, H.M.; Barrera, E.V.; Elías-Zúñiga, A. Development of forcespun fiber-aligned scaffolds from gelatin-zein composites for potential use in tissue engineering and drug release. *MRS Commun.* **2018**, *8*, 885–892. [CrossRef]
23. Verdolotti, L.; Lavorgna, M.; Oliviero, M.; Sorrentino, A.; Iozzino, V.; Buonocore, G.; Iannace, S. Functional zein-siloxane biohybrids. *ACS Sustain. Chem. Eng.* **2014**, *2*, 254–263. [CrossRef]
24. Yoosaf, M.A.P.; Jayaprakash, A.; Ghosh, S.; Jaswal, V.S.; Singh, K.; Mandal, S.; Shahid, M.; Yadav, M.; Das, S.; Kumar., P. Zein film functionalized with gold nanoparticles and the factors affecting its mechanical properties. *RSC Adv.* **2019**, *9*, 25184–25188. [CrossRef]
25. Wu, Q.; Yoshino, T.; Sakabe, H.; Zhang, H.; Isobe, S. Chemical modification of zein by bifunctional polycaprolactone (PCL). *Polymer* **2003**, *44*, 3909–3919. [CrossRef]

26. Ugarte, D. Curling and closure of graphitic networks under electron-beam irradiation. *Nature* **1992**, *359*, 710–713. [CrossRef]
27. Han, F.D.; Yao, B.; Bai, Y.J. Preparation of carbon nano-onions and their application as anode materials for rechargeable lithium-ion batteries. *J. Phys. Chem. C.* **2011**, *115*, 8923–8927. [CrossRef]
28. Pech, D.; Brunet, M.; Durou, H.; Huang, P.H.; Mochalin, V.; Gogotsi, Y.; Taberna, P.L.; Simon, P. Ultrahigh-power micrometre-sized supercapacitors based on onion-like carbon. *Nat. Nanotechnol.* **2010**, *5*, 651–654. [CrossRef]
29. Mykhailiv, O.; Zubyk, H.; Plonska-Brzezinska, M.E. Carbon nano-onions: Unique carbon nanostructures with fascinating properties and their potential applications. *Inorg. Chim. Acta* **2017**, *468*, 49–66. [CrossRef]
30. Frasconi, M.; Marotta, R.; Markey, L.; Flavin, K.; Spampinato, V.; Ceccone, G.; Echegoyen, L.; Scanlan, E.M.; Giordani, S. Multi-Functionalized Carbon Nano-onions as Imaging Probes for Cancer Cells. *Chem A Eur. J.* **2015**, *21*, 19071–19080. [CrossRef]
31. Camisasca, A.; Giordani, S. Carbon nano-onions in biomedical applications: Promising theranostic agents. *Inorg. Chim. Acta* **2017**, *468*, 67–76. [CrossRef]
32. Yang, M.; Flavin, K.; Kopf, I.; Radics, G.; Hearnden, C.H.A.; McManus, G.J.; Moran, B.; Villalta-Cerdas, A.; Echegoyen, L.A.; Giordani, S.; et al. Functionalization of carbon nanoparticles modulates inflammatory cell recruitment and NLRP3 inflammasome activation. *Small* **2013**, *9*, 4194–4206. [CrossRef] [PubMed]
33. Luszczyn, J.; Plonska-Brzezinska, M.E.; Palkar, A.; Dubis, A.T.; Simionescu, A.; Simionescu, D.T.; KalskaSzostko, B.; Winkler, K.; Echegoyen, L. Small noncytotoxic carbon nano-onions: First covalent functionalization with biomolecules. *Chem - A Eur. J.* **2010**, *16*, 4870–4880. [CrossRef] [PubMed]
34. Mamidi, N.; Gamero, M.R.M.; Castrejón, J.V.; Zúñiga, A.E. Development of ultra-high molecular weight polyethylene-functionalized carbon nano-onions composites for biomedical applications. *Diam. Relat. Mater.* **2019**, *97*, 107435. [CrossRef]
35. Rooze, J.; Rebrov, E.V.; Schouten, J.C.; Keurentjes, J.T.F. Dissolved gas and ultrasonic cavitation—A review. *Ultrason. Sonochem.* **2013**, *20*, 1–11. [CrossRef]
36. Wu, J.; Zhu, Y.J.; Cao, S.W.; Chen, F. Hierachically nanostructured mesoporous spheres of calcium silicate hydrate: Surfactant-free sonochemical synthesis and drug-delivery system with ultrahigh drug-loading capacity. *Adv. Mater.* **2010**, *22*, 749–753. [CrossRef]
37. Li, Z.F.; Yang, T.; Lin, C.M.; Li, Q.S.; Liu, S.F.; Xu, F.Z.; Wang, H.Y.; Cui, X.J. Sonochemical Synthesis of Hydrophilic Drug Loaded Multifunctional Bovine Serum Albumin Nanocapsules. *ACS Appl. Mater. Interfaces* **2015**, *7*, 19390–19397. [CrossRef]
38. Li, Z.; Du, X.; Cui, X.; Wang, Z. Ultrasonic-assisted fabrication and release kinetics of two model redox-responsive magnetic microcapsules for hydrophobic drug delivery. *Ultrason Sonochem.* **2019**, *57*, 223–232. [CrossRef]
39. Krishnaiah, Y.S.R.; Khan, M.A. Strategies of targeting oral drug delivery systems to the colon and their potential use for the treatment of colorectal cancer. *Pharm. Dev. Technol.* **2012**, *17*, 521–540. [CrossRef]
40. Amidon, S.; Brown, J.E.; Dave, V.S. Colon-Targeted Oral Drug Delivery Systems: Design Trends and Approaches. *AAPS PharmSciTech* **2015**, *16*, 731–741. [CrossRef]

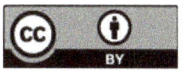

© 2019 by the authors. Licensee MDPI, Basel, Switzerland. This article is an open access article distributed under the terms and conditions of the Creative Commons Attribution (CC BY) license (http://creativecommons.org/licenses/by/4.0/).

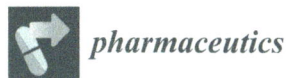

Article

Carbamazepine Gel Formulation as a Sustained Release Epilepsy Medication for Pediatric Use

Saeid Mezail Mawazi [1,2], Sinan Mohammed Abdullah Al-Mahmood [3], Bappaditya Chatterjee [1,4], Hazrina AB. Hadi [1] and Abd Almonem Doolaanea [1,5,*]

1. Department of Pharmaceutical Technology, Kulliyyah of Pharmacy, International Islamic University Malaysia, Kuantan 25200, Malaysia; saeidmezail@yahoo.com (S.M.M.); bdpharmaju@gmail.com (B.C.); hazrina.hadi@gmail.com (H.A.H.)
2. School of Pharmacy, PICOMS International University College, Batu Muda, Batu caves, Kuala Lumpur 68100, Malaysia
3. Pharmacy College, Al-Kitab University, Kirkuk 36010, Iraq; sinan.almawla@gmail.com
4. Department of Pharmaceutics, SPPSPTM, SVKM's NMIMS (Deemed to be University), Mumbai 400056, India
5. IKOP Sdn Bhd, Kulliyyah of Pharmacy, International Islamic University Malaysia, Kuantan 25200, Malaysia
* Correspondence: abdalmonemdoolaanea@yahoo.com; Tel.: +60-136-238-628

Received: 24 July 2019; Accepted: 10 September 2019; Published: 20 September 2019

Abstract: This study aimed to develop a carbamazepine (CBZ) sustained release formulation suitable for pediatric use with a lower risk of precipitation. The CBZ was first prepared as sustained release microparticles, and then the microparticles were embedded in alginate beads, and finally, the beads were suspended in a gel vehicle. The microparticles were prepared by a solvent evaporation method utilizing ethyl cellulose as a sustained release polymer and were evaluated for particle size, encapsulation efficiency, and release profile. The beads were fabricated by the dropwise addition of sodium alginate in calcium chloride solution and characterized for size, shape, and release properties. The gel was prepared using iota carrageenan as the gelling agent and evaluated for appearance, syneresis, drug content uniformity, rheology, release profile, and stability. The microparticles exhibited a particle size of 135.01 ± 0.61 µm with a monodisperse distribution and an encapsulation efficiency of $83.89 \pm 3.98\%$. The beads were monodispersed with an average size of 1.4 ± 0.05 mm and a sphericity factor of less than 0.05. The gel was prepared using a 1:1 ratio (gel vehicle to beads) and exhibited no syneresis, good homogeneity, and good shear-thinning properties. The release profile from the beads and from the gel was not significantly affected, maintaining similarity to the tablet form. The gel properties were maintained for one month real time stability, but the accelerated stability showed reduced viscosity and pH with time. In conclusion, CBZ in a gel sustained release dosage form combines the advantages of the suspension form in terms of dosing flexibility, and the advantages of the tablet form in regards to the sustained release profile. This dosage form should be further investigated in vivo in animal models before being considered in clinical trials.

Keywords: gel; sustained release; carbamazepine; epilepsy; pediatric

---

1. Introduction

Carbamazepine (CBZ) is an epilepsy treatment used by patients of different age groups, including pediatrics and especially children below six years old. However, the sustained release dosage is only available as a solid oral dosage form (tablet or capsule). Children below six years old usually have difficulty swallowing solid oral dosage forms [1–3]. The United States Food and Drug Administration (FDA) and European Medical Agency (EMA) have encouraged developers to make sustained release formulations for pediatric use [4–6]. CBZ can be given as a suspension for children in 2–4 doses per day, but several side effects have been reported due to precipitation of the suspension [7–9]. This highlights the need for a new formulation that can provide a sustained release and avoid precipitation of CBZ. This study aimed to achieve these goals. Making a sustained release formulation suitable for children with swallowing difficulties (below six years old) is challenging. Based on EMA guidelines, currently only solution and suspension formulations are suitable for this age group [4–6]. While a sustained release form is difficult to develop, the suspension dosage form was considered.

Carbamazepine (CBZ) is an anticonvulsant drug used for the treatment of neuralgia, trigeminal, epilepsy, and bipolar disorder. CBZ is a white-yellowish, bitter tasting powder that is insoluble in water [10,11]. The FDA approved carbamazepine formulations include chewable tablets (Tegretol®), a suspension (Tegretol®), sustained release capsules (Carbatrol®), and sustained release tablets (Tegretol®-XR) [7]. Following a twice a day dosage regimen, the suspension provides higher peak levels and lower trough levels than those obtained from conventional tablets for the same dosage regimen. On the other hand, following a thrice daily dosage regimen, the CBZ suspension affords steady-state plasma levels comparable to CBZ tablets given twice a day when administered at the same total mg daily dose [7]. Following a twice daily dosage regimen, CBZ extended-release tablets afford steady-state plasma levels comparable to conventional CBZ tablets given four times a day, when administered at the same total mg daily dose [7]. CBZ is prescribed for children under 6 years of age at a dose of 10 to 20 mg/kg/day twice a day or three times a day. The dose is increased weekly to achieve an optimal clinical response, and administration may be increased to three times a day or four times a day. As such, the suspension dosage form allows dosing flexibility. However, it lacks the property of sustained release. This is available only in the solid oral dosage forms, like tablets and capsules. There is still a need for a sustained release CBZ formulation to be developed that provides both the required release profile and dosing flexibility.

The International Conference on Harmonisation of Technical Requirements for Registration of Pharmaceuticals for Human Use (ICH) has classified five different age groups: preterm new-borns infants, new-born infants (0–27 days), infants and toddlers (28 days–23 months), children (2–11 years), and adolescents (12 to 16–18 years, depending on the region) [12,13]. Due to the anatomy of their buccal cavity development, this young population is usually unable to swallow capsules or tablets. However, children may be able to swallow small tablets but not larger tablets. According to the Guideline on Development of Medicines for Paediatric Use, the acceptability of the tablets depends on their age and the size of the tablets [5,6]. For children from 2 to 5 years old (pre-school), the preferred dosage forms are solutions and suspensions, with the ability to swallow tablets smaller than 5 mm [5]. However, overdose caused by suspension sedimentation is one of the common reported issues with CBZ suspensions.

Most of the CBZ sustained release formulations have been developed as tablets. Only a few formulations have been attempted for paediatric use. Among them, nanoparticles and microparticles are the most reported, despite the authors not claiming their suitability for the paediatric population [14–20]. However, as multiparticulate systems with a size that can be swallowed by children younger than six years old, those dosage forms might be useful [21].

There are several types of polymers or coating materials, such as celluloses (like ethyl cellulose, methyl cellulose, carboxymethyl cellulose), gums (like gum Arabic), carrageenans (kappa carrageenan, iota carrageenan, and lambda carrageenan), and alginates (sodium alginate). Ethyl cellulose (EC) is the most stable polymer among the cellulose derivatives. It can resist alkalis in both concentrated and diluted solutions. It only adsorbs a very small amount of water from the moist air or from aqueous solutions during immersion [22]. There are three types of carrageenan—kappa carrageenan, iota carrageenan, and lambda carrageenan. Iota carrageenan is the only type that shows no syneresis [23]. Sodium alginate is a natural polysaccharide polymer that is soluble in cold and hot water. It is biocompatible, non-toxic, and widely used in pharmaceutical beads, microparticles, nano-particles, and sustained release preparations [24]. Beads of alginate are easily prepared by crosslinking with divalent cations, such as calcium.

Oral gel is a fundamental solution for dysphagic patients and is frequently prescribed for geriatrics [25,26]. The gel has the advantage of preventing precipitation due high viscosity. In addition, when the gel is shear-thinned, it allows flexible dosing because it flows easily upon application of suitable stress, like withdrawal by syringe. Gel formulations have been developed for some drugs already, such as paracetamol [27]. Gel formulations can be designed for immediate release or sustained release [28]. One study described a CBZ oral gel and performed a comparison study between different gelling agents and a stability study for those gelling agents, but the release was almost completed in 1 h (immediate release dosage form) [25,26]. There is no existing report on a sustained release gel formulation for CBZ.

In this study, a CBZ sustained release formulation suitable for pediatric use, especially for children below six years old, was developed based on multiparticulate systems (microparticles and beads). These particles were embedded in a gel as the final dosage form. The in vitro release properties were compared with those of commercial CBZ sustained release tablets.

2. Materials and Methods

2.1. Materials

Carbamazepine (CBZ) was purchased from Anuja Healthcare Limited (Punjab, India). Ethyl cellulose (EC) was bought from DOW chemicals (Louisiana, Greensburg, PA, USA). Polyvinyl alcohol (PVA), dichloromethane, and other chemicals were procured from Merck (Hohenbrunn, Germany). Sodium alginate was purchased from FMC (Philadelphia, PA, USA). Calcium chloride was obtained from Merck (Darmstadt, Germany). Iota carrageenan and honey powder were sourced from the Modernist Pantry (Portsmouth, NH, US). Propyl paraben was bought from Parchem (New Rochelle, NY, USA).

2.2. Preparation and Characterization of CBZ-Loaded Microparticles

CBZ was encapsulated in ethyl cellulose microspheres using the solvent evaporation technique. Briefly, 200 mg of CBZ and 200 mg of EC were dissolved in 10 mL dichloromethane to create the oil phase. The aqueous phase was prepared by dissolving PVA in water at 1% w/v concentration. Ten mL of the oil phase was added to 30 mL of the aqueous phase (ratio of 1:3) and mixed at 6000 rpm using a homogenizer for 180 s. The mixture was added to 120 mL of the dispersion medium of distilled water (ratio 1:3 emulsion to dispersion medium) and stirred for 3 h at room temperature to evaporate the organic solvent. Microparticles were collected by filtration then washed three times with distilled water [29,30].

The particle size of the CBZ-loaded microparticles was evaluated by suspending the microparticles in distilled water, followed by the measurement using a laser diffraction particle sizer (BT-9300H, Liaoning, China). Polydispersity of the microparticles was evaluated by calculating the span value (Equation (1)).

$$\text{Span value} = (D90 - D10)/D50, \quad (1)$$

where D10: 10% of the particles are smaller than this diameter; D50: 50% of the particles are smaller than this diameter; D90: 90% of the particles are smaller than this diameter [31].

The particle morphology was observed under a light stereomicroscope (Nikon SMZ745, Tokyo, Japan) attached to a Nikon special lens (Nikon DS-Fi2, Tokyo, Japan).

The presence of CBZ in the microparticles was confirmed by attenuated total reflectance Fourier transform infrared (ATR-FTIR) spectroscopy. Ethyl cellulose, CBZ, and CBZ microparticles were scanned in the range 4000–400 cm^{-1} using a Perkin-Elmer FTIR spectrometer (Perkin Elmer Corp., Norwalk, CT, USA).

The amount of CBZ encapsulated in the microparticles was determined by adding 10 mg of microparticles into 100 mL phosphate buffer at pH 6.8 and stirring at 200 rpm using an incubator shaker (INNOVA 4000, GMI, Ramsey, MN, USA) at 37 ± 0.05 °C for 4 h. Then, the sample was filtered (Whatman filter paper grade 1) and analyzed ($n = 3$) at 286 nm using a UV-spectrophotometer (SHIMADZU UV-1800, Kyoto, Japan). Encapsulation efficiency was calculated by dividing the actual amount of CBZ in the microparticles by the theoretical amount.

2.3. Encapsulation of CBZ-Loaded Microparticles in Alginate Beads

A quantity of the microparticles equivalent to 200 mg of CBZ was suspended in 5 mL of 2% w/v sodium alginate solution using a magnetic stirrer. The electrospray apparatus was assembled using a high voltage power supply from Genvolt (Shropshire, UK) and a syringe pump from Shenchen Pump (Baoding, China), and a stainless-steel needle. The microparticle-in-alginate suspension was extruded into 1% w/v calcium chloride solution using the electrospray at a 1 mL/min flow rate, with a 10 cm distance between the needle head and calcium chloride solution, and 4000 kV. Alginate beads were formed instantly by means of crosslinking between the alginate and calcium ions. The beads were collected using a metal mesh and washed using distilled water.

The particle size of 10 beads was determined using a digital microscope, U500 Shenzhen (Guangdong, China). The sphericity factor (SF) was used as an indication of the shape of the beads and calculated using Equation (2).

$$\text{Sphericity factor (SF)} = (D_{max} - D_{min})/(D_{max} + D_{min}), \qquad (2)$$

where D_{max} is the longest diameter and D_{min} is the shortest diameter of the same bead.

The EE of the CBZ in the alginate beads was measured to ensure the loading of CBZ-loaded microparticles inside the beads. An indirect method was utilized by measuring the un-encapsulated amount of CBZ. Un-encapsulated CBZ leaks into calcium chloride solution either as soluble CBZ or as microparticles. Soluble CBZ was quantified using a spectrophotometer at a 286 nm wavelength. Meanwhile, measurement at 600 nm was also conducted and used to measure the turbidity in the calcium chloride solution resulting from the presence of microparticles that have not been embedded in the beads.

2.4. Loading of CBZ Alginate Beads in a Gel Vehicle

The gel vehicle was prepared by heating 40 mL of distilled water up to 90 °C, followed by addition of the gelling agent under continuous stirring. After complete dissolving and cooling, propyl paraben sodium was added as preservative then the solution was made up to 50 mL with distilled water. Two types of carrageenan (iota or kappa) at two concentrations (1 and 2.5% w/v) were used as gelling agents. CBZ alginate beads containing 2000 mg CBZ (about 50 mL as volume) were added into the gel vehicle at 40 °C, then left to cool down at room temperature to produce the gel formulation. The final gel formulation was prepared in two ratios—1 to 1 and 1 to 2 volume ratios of beads to iota carrageenan jelly. Therefore, the volume fraction of the alginate beads in the final gel was 1/2 (for the 1 to 1 ratio) and 1/3 (for the 1 to 2 ratio).

2.5. Characterization of CBZ Oral Gel

2.5.1. Physical Appearance and Syneresis

Visual observation of the fabricated CBZ-oral gels was undertaken to assess their clarity, smell, texture, and the presence of any foreign particles. The texture of the prepared gels was tested by rubbing them between two fingers to check their grittiness and stickiness.

Water separation from the gel is known as syneresis, which is a common problem associated with jellies during their storage [32–34] (Brinker and Scherer, 2013). Iota and kappa carrageenan gels at two different concentrations (1% and 2.5% w/v) were stored at room temperature (25 ± 2 °C) and in the refrigerator (8 ± 3 °C) for 24 h to observe syneresis, if any [25].

2.5.2. Homogeneity

A homogeneity test was carried out to ensure the distribution uniformity of CBZ beads in the gel. Beads prepared from 5 mL alginate suspension were added into 5 mL or 10 mL 2.5% *w/v* iota carrageenan gel to yield a ratio of 1:1 or 1:2. Three 1 mL aliquots from the gel (upper, middle and lower regions) were individually dissolved in 100 mL of phosphate buffer (pH 6.8) under continuous shaking at 200 rpm using an incubator shaker (Innova 4000, GMI, Ramsey, MN, USA) at 37 for 4 h. The samples were filtered and analyzed at 286 nm using a spectrophotometer (Shimadzu UV-1800, Kyoto, Japan) [35].

2.5.3. Rheology

Iota carrageenan gelling agent was first tested for rheology using a HAAKE Mars rheometer (Thermo-Scientific, Waltham, MA, USA). The data were then digitally analyzed by Haake Rheo-Win 3.61.0000 software (Thermo-Scientific, Waltham, MA, USA). The test was conducted at 25 °C ± 0.05 °C using a PP35 Ti spindle of 35 mm diameter and 1 mm gap. The test was conducted at an increasing shear rate (γ) from 0.01 to 100 s^{-1} at 1 Hz frequency, then a constant shear rate of 100 s^{-1} for 30 s, then a decreasing shear rate from 100 to 0.015 in 120 s [36]. The results were represented graphically as apparent viscosity (η), and shear stress (τ) vs. shear rate (γ). The same test was repeated after loading the CBZ alginate beads in the gel vehicle. Rheological modelling for each of the gels was fitted to either the Herschel Bulkley or Ostwald De Waele model.

2.6. In Vitro Drug Release

The sustained release properties of the CBZ gel formulation were evaluated and compared with the commercially available 200 mg Tegretol®-XR sustained release tablet (Novartis), by calculating the similarity factor (F2) using Equation (3). In addition, the release profiles of CBZ powder, CBZ microparticles, and CBZ-alginate beads were also compared in order to observe the effect of each preparation step on the release properties.

$$f_2 = 50 \log \left\{ \left[1 + \frac{1}{\rho} \sum_{j=1}^{\rho} (u_{Tj} - u_{Rj})^2 \right]^{-\frac{1}{2}} \times 100 \right\}, \qquad (3)$$

where F2 is the similarity factor, R_t and T_t are the dissolved cumulative percentage of test and reference samples at selected (t) time points respectively, and n is the number of time points [37–39].

The release profile tests were conducted with a USP-II dissolution apparatus using a 900 mL volume of dissolution medium at 37 ± 0.5 °C and a rotating speed of 100 rpm. At a predetermined time, point (1, 3, 6, 12, and 24 h), 5 mL of dissolution medium was taken ($n = 3$) and replaced with an equal volume of fresh medium. The samples were filtered and analyzed spectrophotometrically at the wavelength of 286 nm.

For CBZ powder, CBZ microparticles and CBZ-alginate beads, the dissolution test was adopted from United States Pharmacopeia (USP), since these formulations can be considered solid dosage forms [40]. However, CBZ gel is a new dosage form not described in USP. Therefore, to compare it with commercial formulations, the dissolution was conducted using the two stage general dissolution method (HCl and phosphate buffer stages).

The Tegretol®-XR sustained release tablets containing 200 mg CBZ were immersed in HCl for the first 2 h, then the disintegrated tablet was filtered using Whatman filter paper no. 1. The tablet particles were collected easily, then transferred directly into phosphate buffer (pH 6.8) to continue the dissolution test for up to 24 h. For the CBZ gel, an amount containing 200 mg CBZ was immersed in HCl for 2 h. In another dissolution vessel, a similar quantity was added into the phosphate buffer pH 6.8 and the test was run for 24 h. The readings from 2 h were deducted from all subsequent readings.

2.7. Stability Study

The CBZ gel formulation, packed in glass containers, was evaluated for physical stability at 30 ± 2 °C with 70 ± 5% RH (real time stability conditions) and 40 ± 2 °C with 70 ± 5% RH (accelerated stability conditions) for 30 days (Countries, 2005). At different time points (0, 7, 15, and 30 days), various quality attributes were evaluated, including pH, physical appearance, syneresis, viscosity, and assay. The viscosity was evaluated using a Brookfield® viscometer (DVII+, Massachusetts, USA) with a spindle number (CPE51) at room temperature (25 °C ± 5 °C) and a rotating speed of 50 rpm [32].

2.8. Statistical Analysis

Statistical analysis was completed using a fractional factorial design for the preparation of all formulations, and a t-test for the stability study of the gel utilizing Minitab software (version 17.1.0; Minitab Inc., State College, PA, USA). When the p-value is less than 0.05 the null hypothesis will be rejected, and it will be considered as significant. When p-value is more than 0.05, the results will be considered as not significant and the null hypothesis will be accepted.

3. Results

3.1. CBZ-Loaded Microparticles

CBZ was successfully encapsulated in ethyl cellulose microparticles using the solvent evaporation method. The microparticles exhibited a particle size of 135.01 ± 0.61 µm with a monodisperse distribution (Figure 1), a span value of 1.28, and an encapsulation efficiency (EE) of 83.89 ± 3.98%. ATR-FTIR spectra confirmed the presence of CBZ in the microparticles, where CBZ peaks were clearly seen in the microparticle spectrum as presented in Figure 1c.

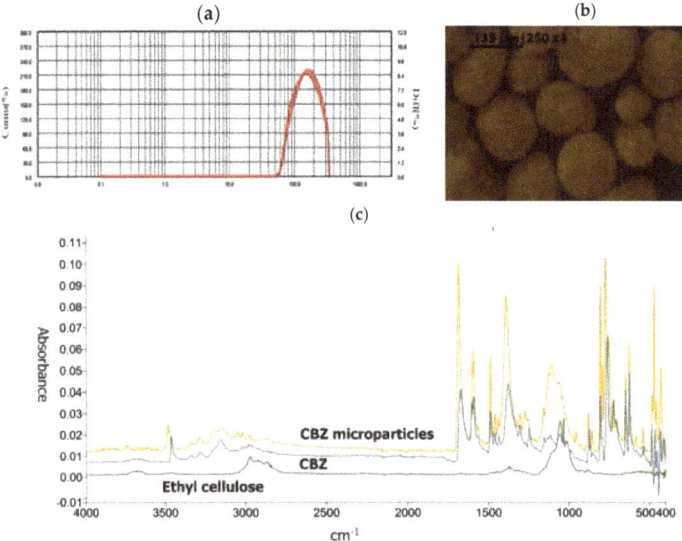

Figure 1. CBZ-loaded microparticle characterization. (**a**) Particle size distribution measured by laser diffraction, (**b**) morphology of the particles under a light microscope, (**c**) ATR-FTIR spectra of ethyl cellulose, CBZ and CBZ-loaded microparticles.

3.2. CBZ-Loaded Microparticles in Alginate Beads

Alginate beads were formed instantly upon contact of alginate solution containing CBZ-loaded microparticles with calcium chloride solution. The beads were spherical (Figure 2) with a size of 1.4 ± 0.05 mm and a sphericity factor of less than 0.05, which is considered spherical [41]. Spectrophotometric measurements revealed that only 0.38 ± 0.01% of the CBZ was un-encapsulated and dissolved in the calcium chloride solution. No CBZ-loaded microparticles were detected in the calcium chloride solution, whereby the turbidity of the solution did not change. This reveals that the encapsulation efficiency of CBZ in the beads was 99.62 ± 0.01%.

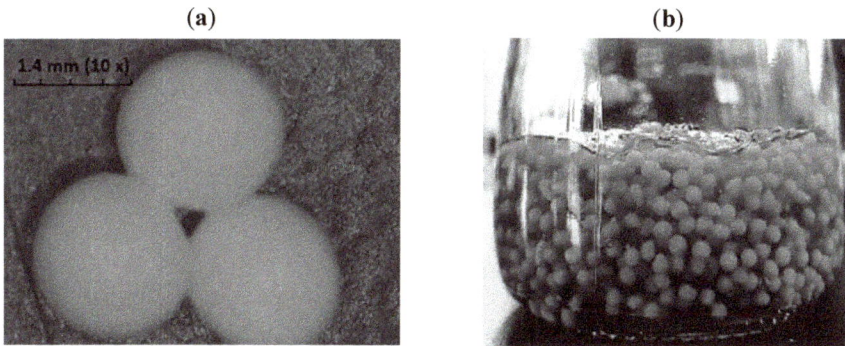

Figure 2. (a) CBZ-alginate beads, (b) CBZ-gel prepared at a 1:1 ratio of beads to iota carrageenan gel.

3.3. CBZ Oral Gel

3.3.1. Physical Appearance and Syneresis

CBZ gel prepared from iota carrageenan were transparent, non-sticky, of acceptable consistency, and without any feeling of grittiness. No syneresis was seen with any of the iota carrageenan gels, while all the kappa carrageenan gels exhibited syneresis except for the 2.5% gel stored in the refrigerator.

3.3.2. Homogeneity

Table 1 shows the assay results of CBZ from samples taken from different locations of the gel. The average value of the three locations was 100%. The ratio of 1:1 shows very close agreement between the three locations, while in the 1:2 ratio the CBZ was not homogenously distributed. The lower layer had a high concentration of CBZ compared to the upper layer due to precipitation of the CBZ-alginate beads in the bottom of the gel container.

Table 1. Homogeneity of CBZ gel.

Sample Location	Beads to Gel Ratio	CBZ Assay (%)
Up	(1:1)	100.9 ± 1.3
Middle	(1:1)	99.9 ± 1.1
Bottom	(1:1)	99.2 ± 1.9
Up	(1:2)	65.4 ± 2.4
Middle	(1:2)	96.5 ± 3.3
Bottom	(1:2)	138.0 ± 4.5

3.3.3. Rheology

The rheology profile for 2.5% *w/v* iota carrageenan gel exhibited a non-Newtonian profile, where the shear stress increased non-linearly with the shear rate. The gel fits the Herschel Bulkley model (R = 0.9981) with clear yield shear stress (Figure 3). However, after incorporating CBZ-alginate beads at a 1:1 loading ratio, the gel did not fit any model and exhibited a degree of thixotropy. The rheology profile of the gel containing the beads was disrupted with spikes. This was because the bead size was more than 1 mm and the gap between the upper and lower spindles was 1 mm. When the spindle rotated, it smashed and compressed the beads. Therefore, the measurement of gel rheology was interrupted with the presence of beads in the gel. The overall trend represents the gel where it appeared to have a shear thinning property with a degree of thixotropy, but the spikes in the graph came from the beads.

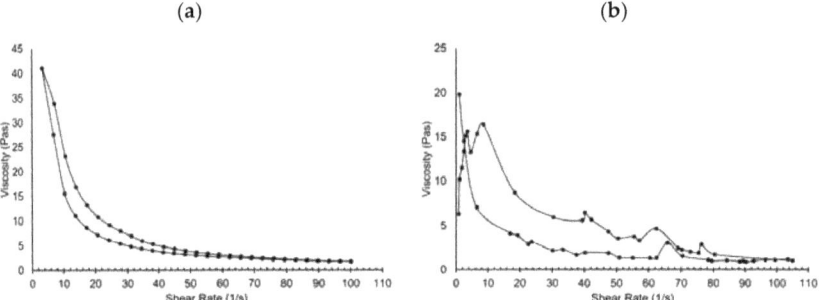

Figure 3. Rheology profile of 2.5% w/v iota-carrageenan gel, (**a**) without CBZ-alginate beads, (**b**) with CBZ-alginate beads.

3.4. In vitro Drug Release

CBZ oral gel exhibited a sustained release profile for 24 h (Figure 4). The release was comparable to the release from commercial Tegretol®-XR tablets, with a similarity factor of $f_2 = 74$. At t50 % the percentage of CBZ release from the microparticles was 71.05%, was 74.12% from the beads, was 68.94% from the gel, and was 68.25% from the commercial Tegretol®-XR tablets. These results revealed that the prepared CBZ gel was comparable to the commercial tablet.

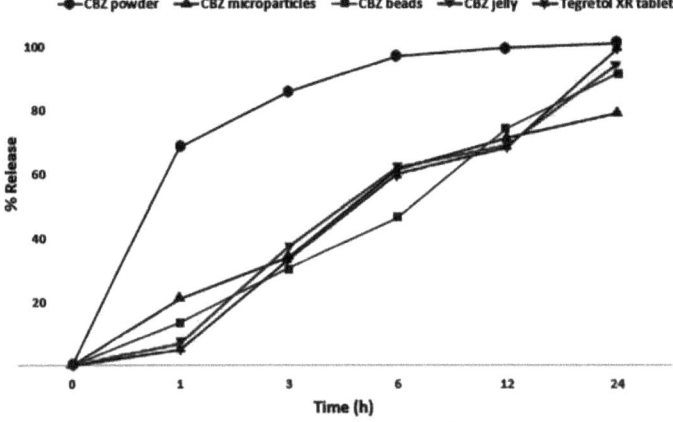

Figure 4. In vitro CBZ release (mean ± 1.86, $n = 3$) from CBZ gel in comparison with Tegretol®-XR tablets, CBZ powder, CBZ microparticles, and CBZ beads.

Release kinetic fitting is shown in Table 2. CBZ microparticles fitted best into the Higuchi model, suggesting a diffusion controlled mechanism. This was expected as the polymer used in the microparticle preparation was ethyl cellulose, which is not a fast degrading polymer. Therefore, the CBZ will release by diffusing through the microparticle matrix. On the other hand, CBZ beads and CBZ gel fitted best into first order kinetics. The presence of an alginate matrix around the microparticles, then the gel around the beads, slowed down the release.

Table 2. Fitting of the release profiles into different kinetic models.

Model	R2			
	CBZ Microparticles	CBZ Beads	CBZ Gel	CBZ Tablets (Tegretol®-XR)
Zero Order	0.7190	0.8828	0.8143	0.8601
First Order	0.8555	0.9968	0.9759	0.9301
Higuchi	0.9222	0.9842	0.9482	0.9591
Korsmeyer Peppas	0.6973	0.7677	0.8121	0.8457
Hixson Crowell	0.8116	0.9760	0.9527	0.9748

3.5. Stability Study

The appearance and texture of the gel in terms of stickiness did not change during the stability study (Table 3). No syneresis was observed within the stability period. The pH slightly dropped with time in both real time and accelerated conditions, but the change was not significantly different, with a p-value of 0.25. Viscosity of the gel stored at 40 °C decreased significantly, while no significant change was observed for the sample stored at 30 °C.

Table 3. Stability study of CBZ gel.

Test	Initial (0) Days	7 Days	15 Days	30 Days
Real Time Conditions (30 ± 2 °C/70 ± 5% RH)				
Appearance	Transparent with embedded white beads	No change	No change	No change
Syneresis	No	No	No	No
pH	5.7 ± 0.0	5.4 ± 0.1	5.1 ± 0.0	4.5 ± 0.5
Viscosity (mPa.s)	644 ± 271	552 ± 239	676 ± 173	899 ± 208
Accelerated Conditions (40 ± 2 °C/70 ± 5% RH)				
Appearance	Transparent with embedded white beads	No change	No change	No change
Syneresis	No	No	No	No
pH	5.8 ± 0.1	5.4 ± 0.0	4.6 ± 0.1	5.0 ± 1.8
Viscosity (mPa.s)	357 ± 37	325 ± 5	253 ± 92	180 ± 22

4. Discussion

CBZ was first encapsulated in microparticles using an ethyl cellulose polymer, a well-known polymer for sustained release formulations [42–46]. The microparticles exhibited good sustained release properties, comparable to those of commercial tablets that are given twice daily. However, CBZ-loaded microparticles precipitate when suspended in a liquid vehicle. In addition, microparticles, as relatively large particles, give an unpleasant gritty feeling.

To overcome the precipitation issue of the microparticles, gel was proposed as a vehicle for the microparticles. Gels have high viscosity and do not flow in the normal conditions of temperature and stress, so precipitation is avoided. However, the grittiness of the microparticles may not be overcome. In addition, CBZ may slowly leak out from the microparticles into the gel during long-term storage, resulting in loss of the sustained release properties. To solve this issue, another layer of coating was considered, using alginate beads. Upon crosslinking of alginate with calcium ions, rubbery gel beads are formed with no gritty texture. Alginate beads were prepared to encapsulate the CBZ-loaded microparticles. The beads were spherical in shape, within the recommended size for pediatric use (1–6 years old), and effectively entrapped the microparticles inside them. Since the targeted sustained release profile was obtained from the microparticles, the beads should have little effect on the release profile. The required or the target release profile was found to be similar to the release profile of commercial sustained release tablets, as stated in the United States Pharmacopeia (USP39)—10–35% in 3 h, 35–65% in 6 h, 65–90% in 12 h, and not less than (NLT) 75% in 24 h [47]. A kinetic release study showed that the all prepared formulations followed first order release mechanisms, as the coefficient correlation (R^2) was equal to 0.989 for the CBZ microparticles, 0.976 for the CBZ beads, 0.948 for the CBZ gel, and 0.948 for the Tegretol®-XR tablets. The first order model explained that the release of CBZ based on its dosage form was CBZ-concentration dependent. This means that the release of the drug can be increased when the concentration of that drug is increased in the dosage form over time [48–50]. The release study confirmed that the release of CBZ from the beads was comparable to that of the microparticles and was still similar to that of the commercial tablet.

The last step was to suspend the beads in the gel vehicle. This was performed at a temperature slightly higher than the solidifying temperature of the gelling agent. In comparing kappa and iota carrageenan at two concentrations, iota carrageenan gave the needed properties: no syneresis, homogenous, and with shear-thinning properties. During gel preparation the beads tended to precipitate due to the low viscosity of the hot gel. This is why homogeneity was better at a higher concentration of the beads, where the gel amount was just enough to suspend the beads. The shear-thinning property is needed for this medicated gel in order to allow easy dispensing. Iota carrageenan gel fits the Herschel-Bulkley model, which means it has yield stress—the state of the gel does not change until a specific stress is applied. The gel has high viscosity during storage to prevent bead precipitation, but the viscosity decreases upon applying stress like syringe withdrawal. This allows flexible dosing based on body weight, like a normal CBZ suspension. Similar to the beads, the iota carrageenan gel vehicle was found to have no significant effect on the release properties of CBZ-loaded microparticles. Consequently, the sustained release profile from the final formulation (CBZ-loaded microparticles-in-beads-in-gel) was similar to that of the FDA-approved Tegretol®-XR tablet.

The physical stability study showed that the gel formulation maintained its properties for 30 days when stored at 30 °C. However, the gel viscosity decreased when it was stored at 40 °C. This highlights the importance of storage conditions for this formulation. The pH of the gel was slightly acidic after preparation and showed a decreasing trend during the stability period. Using an ANOVA as the statistical analysis, the change in pH value was found to be not significant, possibly due to the large standard deviation of some points. The change in pH might be attributed to the fact that carrageenans are susceptible to acid-catalyzed hydrolysis [51]. Since the gel was slightly acidic after preparation, the hydrolysis of iota carrageenan might occur and accelerate at a higher temperature, leading to a further drop in pH. This explains the faster drop in pH under the accelerated stability condition (40 °C) compared to the real-time condition (30 °C). Such a change in pH is important to avoid. Iota carrageenan undergoes rapid and extensive loss of viscosity and gelation potential when solutions below pH 5 are heated. The loss of viscosity and gelation potential is primarily due to cleavage of the (1→3) glycosidic linkages [51]. For the gel dosage form, viscosity is critical and should be maintained. The pH of the formulation can be controlled by adding suitable buffering systems.

Based on these preliminary results of the stability study, the gel might need to be stored in the fridge (5 ± 3 °C). A scale up study is recommended to ensure suitability of the preparation method for large scale production. Further investigations are needed, but they are recommended to be done for a larger scale preparation.

5. Conclusions

A carbamazepine sustained release new dosage form designed for pediatric use was prepared and analyzed in this study. This dosage form was based on encapsulation of carbamazepine in microparticles to obtain the required sustained release profile. The microparticles were then embedded in alginate beads, which, in turn, were suspended in iota carrageenan gel. The developed formulation has the advantages of a suspension formulation, that is, flexible dosing and being easy to swallow. It also overcomes the issue of carbamazepine precipitation that is seen in the suspension formulation, which leads to overdose. Carbamazepine sustained release gel has the potential to make the advantages of a sustained release dosage form to pediatric patients accessible, especially children below six years old who have no current option for such a formulation.

6. Patents

The gel as dosage form was patented under the file number (PI 2017704458/Malaysia), under the patent name "A sustained-release drug composition".

Author Contributions: Conceptualization, A.A.D. and S.M.A.A.-M.; Methodology, S.M.M.; Formal Analysis, A.A.D. and S.M.M.; Investigation, S.M.M.; Data Curation, S.M.M. and B.C.; Writing—Original Draft Preparation, S.M.M.; Writing—Review & Editing, S.M.M., S.M.A.A.-M., B.C., H.A.H., and A.A.D.

Funding: This work was funded by IIUM Research Initiative Grant Scheme (Grant Number. P-RIGS18-026-0026).

Acknowledgments: The authors would like to thank Muhammad Taher and the department of pharmaceutical technology at IIUM for technical and facilitation support.

Conflicts of Interest: The authors report no conflict of interest.

References

1. Zajicek, A.; Fossler, M.J.; Barrett, J.S.; Worthington, J.H.; Ternik, R.; Charkoftaki, G.; Lum, S.; Breitkreutz, J.; Baltezor, M.; Macheras, P. A report from the pediatric formulations task force: Perspectives on the state of child-friendly oral dosage forms. *AAPS J.* **2013**, *15*, 1072–1081. [CrossRef]
2. Standing, J.F.; Tuleu, C. Paediatric formulations—Getting to the heart of the problem. *Int. J. Pharm.* **2005**, *300*, 56–66. [CrossRef]
3. Schiele, J.T.; Quinzler, R.; Klimm, H.-D.; Pruszydlo, M.G.; Haefeli, W.E. Difficulties swallowing solid oral dosage forms in a general practice population: Prevalence, causes, and relationship to dosage forms. *Eur. J. Clin. Pharmacol.* **2013**, *69*, 937–948. [CrossRef] [PubMed]
4. European Medicines Agency. *ICH E11 (R1) Guideline on Clinical Investigation of Medicinal Products in the Pediatric Population*; European Medicines Agency: Amsterdam, The Netherlands, 2017.
5. Nunn, T. *Age Appropriate Formulations—Paediatric Needs*; National Institute for Health Research: Southampton, UK, 2011.
6. Nunn, T.; Williams, J. Formulation of medicines for children. *Br. J. Clin. Pharmacol.* **2005**, *59*, 674–676. [CrossRef] [PubMed]
7. Wolters Kluwer Health, A.S.O. H.-S.P. Cerner Multum and Micromedex from Truven Health Carbamazepine. Available online: https://www.drugs.com/cdi/carbamazepine.html (accessed on 8 September 2018).
8. Yuan, H.G.; Kalfas, G.; Ray, W.H. Suspension polymerization. *J. Macromol. Sci. Part C Polym. Rev.* **1991**, *31*, 215–299. [CrossRef]
9. Costenbader, V.; Markson, S. School suspension: A study with secondary school students. *J. Sch. Psychol.* **1998**, *36*, 59–82. [CrossRef]
10. Bloomer, D.; Dupuis, L.; MacGregor, D.; Soldin, S. Palatability and relative bioavailability of an extemporaneous carbamazepine oral suspension. *Clin. Pharm.* **1987**, *6*, 646–649.
11. Richard, D.; Mycek, J.; Harvey, R.; Champe, P. Lippincott's illustrated reviews: Pharmacology. *Philadelphia* **2006**, *3*, 413–415.
12. Magalhães, J.; Rodrigues, A.T.; Roque, F.; Figueiras, A.; Falcão, A.; Herdeiro, M.T. Use of off-label and unlicenced drugs in hospitalised paediatric patients: A systematic review. *Eur. J. Clin. Pharmacol.* **2015**, *71*, 1–13. [CrossRef]
13. Ernest, T.B.; Elder, D.P.; Martini, L.G.; Roberts, M.; Ford, J.L. Developing paediatric medicines: Identifying the needs and recognizing the challenges. *J. Pharm. Pharmacol.* **2007**, *59*, 1043–1055. [CrossRef]

14. Krishnan, V.; Xu, X.; Barwe, S.P.; Yang, X.; Czymmek, K.; Waldman, S.A.; Mason, R.W.; Jia, X.; Rajasekaran, A.K. Dexamethasone-loaded block copolymer nanoparticles induce leukemia cell death and enhance therapeutic efficacy: A novel application in pediatric nanomedicine. *Mol. Pharm.* **2012**, *10*, 2199–2210. [CrossRef] [PubMed]
15. Dumont, M.F.; Yadavilli, S.; Sze, R.W.; Nazarian, J.; Fernandes, R. Manganese-containing Prussian blue nanoparticles for imaging of pediatric brain tumors. *Int. J. Nanomed.* **2014**, *9*, 2581.
16. Basha, R.; Sabnis, N.; Heym, K.; Bowman, W.P.; Lacko, A.G. Targeted nanoparticles for pediatric leukemia therapy. *Front. Oncol.* **2014**, *4*, 101. [CrossRef] [PubMed]
17. Machado, M.C.; Cheng, D.; Tarquinio, K.M.; Webster, T.J. Nanotechnology: Pediatric applications. *Pediatr. Res.* **2010**, *67*, 500. [CrossRef] [PubMed]
18. Deutschmann, A.; Schlagenhauf, A.; Leschnik, B.; Hoffmann, K.M.; Hauer, A.; Muntean, W. Increased procoagulant function of microparticles in pediatric inflammatory bowel disease: Role in increased thrombin generation. *J. Pediatr. Gastroenterol. Nutr.* **2013**, *56*, 401–407. [CrossRef] [PubMed]
19. Chicella, M.; Branim, B.; Lee, K.R.; Phelps, S.J. Comparison of microparticle enzyme and fluorescence polarization immunoassays in pediatric patients not receiving digoxin. *Ther. Drug Monit.* **1998**, *20*, 347–351. [CrossRef] [PubMed]
20. Elsayh, K.I.; Zahran, A.M.; El-Abaseri, T.B.; Mohamed, A.O.; El-Metwally, T.H. Hypoxia biomarkers, oxidative stress, and circulating microparticles in pediatric patients with thalassemia in Upper Egypt. *Clin. Appl. Thromb. Hemost.* **2014**, *20*, 536–545. [CrossRef] [PubMed]
21. Albertini, B.; Di Sabatino, M.; Melegari, C.; Passerini, N. Formulating SLMs as oral pulsatile system for potential delivery of melatonin to pediatric population. *Int. J. Pharm.* **2014**, *469*, 67–79. [CrossRef] [PubMed]
22. Roy, D.; Semsarilar, M.; Guthrie, J.T.; Perrier, S. Cellulose modification by polymer grafting: A review. *Chem. Soc. Rev.* **2009**, *38*, 2046–2064. [CrossRef] [PubMed]
23. Blakemore, W.R.; Harpell, A.R. Carrageenan. In *Food Stabilisers, Thickeners and Gelling Agents*; Blackwell Publishing: Hoboken, NJ, USA, 2009; pp. 73–94.
24. Sosnik, A. Alginate Particles as Platform for Drug Delivery by the Oral Route: State-of-the-Art. *ISRN Pharm.* **2014**, *2014*, 926157. [CrossRef] [PubMed]
25. Prakash, K.; Satyanarayana, V.; Nagiat, H.; Fathi, A.; Shanta, A.; Prameela, A. Formulation development and evaluation of novel oral jellies of carbamazepine using pectin, guar gum, and gellan gum. *Asian J. Pharm.* **2014**, *8*, 241. [CrossRef]
26. Imai, K. Alendronate sodium hydrate (oral jelly) for the treatment of osteoporosis: Review of a novel, easy to swallow formulation. *Clin. Interv. Aging* **2013**, *8*, 681. [CrossRef] [PubMed]
27. Miyazaki, S.; Takahashi, A.; Itoh, K.; Ishitani, M.; Dairaku, M.; Togashi, M.; Mikami, R.; Attwood, D. Preparation and evaluation of gel formulations for oral sustained delivery to dysphagic patients. *Drug Dev. Ind. Pharm.* **2009**, *35*, 780–787. [CrossRef] [PubMed]
28. Satyanarayana, A.D.; Kulkarni, K.P.; Shivakumar, G.H. Gels and jellies as a dosage form for dysphagia patients: A review. *Curr. Drug Ther.* **2011**, *6*, 79–86. [CrossRef]
29. Rosca, I.D.; Watari, F.; Uo, M. Microparticle formation and its mechanism in single and double emulsion solvent evaporation. *J. Control. Release* **2004**, *99*, 271–280. [CrossRef] [PubMed]
30. Chen, X.; Young, T.J.; Sarkari, M.; Williams, R.O., III; Johnston, K.P. Preparation of cyclosporine A nanoparticles by evaporative precipitation into aqueous solution. *Int. J. Pharm.* **2002**, *242*, 3–14. [CrossRef]
31. Craig, D.; Barker, S.; Banning, D.; Booth, S. An investigation into the mechanisms of self-emulsification using particle size analysis and low frequency dielectric spectroscopy. *Int. J. Pharm.* **1995**, *114*, 103–110. [CrossRef]
32. Suda, N.; Shinzato, R.; Kiyokawa, M.; Kaneuchi, M.; Sugawara, M.; Kohri, N. Development of acetylcysteine jelly for the prevention of radiocontrast-induced reductions in renal function and its evaluation. *Jpn. J. Pharm. Health Care Sci.* **2005**, *31*, 355–359. [CrossRef]
33. Christensen, B.E. Alginates as biomaterials in tissue engineering. In *Carbohydrate Chemistry: Chemical and Biological Approaches*; Royal Society of Chemistry: London, UK, 2011; Volume 37, pp. 227–258.
34. Brinker, C.J.; Scherer, G.W. *Sol-Gel Science: The Physics and Chemistry of Sol-Gel Processing*; Academic Press: Cambridge, MA, USA, 2013.
35. Garud, N.; Garud, A. Preparation and in-vitro evaluation of metformin microspheres using non-aqueous solvent evaporation technique. *Trop. J. Pharm. Res.* **2012**, *11*, 577–583. [CrossRef]

36. Watanabe, A.; Hanawa, T.; Sugihara, M. Application of glycerogelatin as oral dosage form for the elderly. *J. Pharm. Sci. Technol. Jpn.* **1994**, *54*, 77.
37. Shah, V.P.; Tsong, Y.; Sathe, P.; Liu, J.-P. In vitro dissolution profile comparison—Statistics and analysis of the similarity factor, f2. *Pharm. Res.* **1998**, *15*, 889–896. [CrossRef] [PubMed]
38. Liu, J.-P.; Ma, M.-C.; Chow, S.-C. Statistical evaluation of similarity factor f2 as a criterion for assessment of similarity between dissolution profiles. *Drug Inf. J.* **1997**, *31*, 1255–1271. [CrossRef]
39. Ocaña, J.; Frutos, G.; Sánchez, P. Using the similarity factor f2 in practice: A critical revision and suggestions for its standard error estimation. *Chemom. Intell. Lab. Syst.* **2009**, *99*, 49–56. [CrossRef]
40. Mawazi, S.M.; Hadi, H.A.B.; Al-Mahmood, S.M.A.; Doolaanea, A. Development and Validation of UV-VIS Spectroscopic Method of Assay of Carbamazepine in Microparticles. *Int. J. Appl. Pharm.* **2019**, *11*, 34–37. [CrossRef]
41. Chan, E.-S.; Lim, T.-K.; Voo, W.-P.; Pogaku, R.; Tey, B.T.; Zhang, Z. Effect of formulation of alginate beads on their mechanical behavior and stiffness. *Particuology* **2011**, *9*, 228–234. [CrossRef]
42. Zhang, G.; Pinnamaraju, P.; Ali, M.A. Water Insoluble Polymer Based Sustained Release Formulation. U.S. Patent 6251430B1, 26 June 2001.
43. Follonier, N.; Doelker, E.; Cole, E.T. Evaluation of hot-melt extrusion as a new technique for the production of polymer-based pellets for sustained release capsules containing high loadings of freely soluble drugs. *Drug Dev. Ind. Pharm.* **1994**, *20*, 1323–1339. [CrossRef]
44. Li, X.-Y.; Zheng, Z.-B.; Yu, D.-G.; Liu, X.-K.; Qu, Y.-L.; Li, H.-L. Electrosprayed sperical ethylcellulose nanoparticles for an improved sustained-release profile of anticancer drug. *Cellulose* **2017**, *24*, 5551–5564. [CrossRef]
45. Parida, P.; Mishra, S.C.; Sahoo, S.; Behera, A.; Nayak, B.P. Development and characterization of ethylcellulose based microsphere for sustained release of nifedipine. *J. Pharm. Anal.* **2016**, *6*, 341–344. [CrossRef]
46. Maulvi, F.A.; Soni, T.G.; Shah, D.O. Extended release of timolol from ethyl cellulose microparticles laden hydrogel contact lenses. *Open Pharm. Sci. J.* **2015**, *2*. [CrossRef]
47. Sandoz Inc. *Carbamazepine Extended-Release Tablets, USP*; Sandoz Inc.: Princeton, NJ, USA, 2016; pp. 2917–2921.
48. Gefter, J.; Zaks, B.; Kirmayer, D.; Lavy, E.; Steinberg, D.; Friedman, M. Chlorhexidine sustained-release varnishes for catheter coating–Dissolution kinetics and antibiofilm properties. *Eur. J. Pharm. Sci.* **2018**, *112*, 1–7. [CrossRef]
49. Higuchi, T. Mechanism of sustained-action medication. Theoretical analysis of rate of release of solid drugs dispersed in solid matrices. *J. Pharm. Sci.* **1963**, *52*, 1145–1149. [CrossRef] [PubMed]
50. Barzegar-Jalali, M.; Adibkia, K.; Valizadeh, H.; Shadbad, M.R.S.; Nokhodchi, A.; Omidi, Y.; Mohammadi, G.; Nezhadi, S.H.; Hasan, M. Kinetic analysis of drug release from nanoparticles. *J. Pharm. Pharm. Sci.* **2008**, *11*, 167–177. [CrossRef] [PubMed]
51. BeMiller, J. *Carrageenans*, 3rd ed.; Elsevier: Amsterdam, The Netherlands, 2019; p. 12.

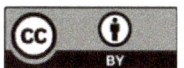

© 2019 by the authors. Licensee MDPI, Basel, Switzerland. This article is an open access article distributed under the terms and conditions of the Creative Commons Attribution (CC BY) license (http://creativecommons.org/licenses/by/4.0/).

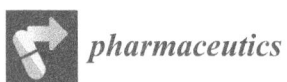

Review

Poloxamer Hydrogels for Biomedical Applications

Eleonora Russo * and Carla Villa

Department of Pharmacy, University of Genoa, Viale Benedetto XV, 16132 Genova, Italy; villa@difar.unige.it
* Correspondence: russo@difar.unige.it

Received: 31 October 2019; Accepted: 6 December 2019; Published: 10 December 2019

Abstract: This review article focuses on thermoresponsive hydrogels consisting of poloxamers which are of high interest for biomedical application especially in drug delivery for ophthalmic, injectable, transdermal, and vaginal administration. These hydrogels remain fluid at room temperature but become more viscous gel once they are exposed to body temperature. In this way, the gelling system remains at the topical level for a long time and the drug release is controlled and prolonged. Poloxamers are synthetic triblock copolymers of poly(ethylene oxide)-b-poly(propylene oxide)-b-poly(ethylene oxide) (PEO-PPO-PEO), also commercially known as Pluronics®, Synperonics® or Lutrol®. The different poloxamers cover a range of liquids, pastes, and solids, with molecular weights and ethylene oxide–propylene oxide weight ratios varying from 1100 to 14,000 and 1:9 to 8:2, respectively. Concentrated aqueous solutions of poloxamers form thermoreversible gels. In recent years this type of gel has arouse interest for tissue engineering. Finally, the use of poloxamers as biosurfactants is evaluated since they are able to form micelles in an aqueous environment above a concentration threshold known as critical micelle concentration (CMC). This property is exploited for drug delivery and different therapeutic applications.

Keywords: poloxamer; hydrogels; micelle; thermosensitive; biomedical; copolymer

---

1. Introduction

The word "hydrogel", according to Lee, Kwon and Park is due to an article published in 1894, but the first crosslinked network material that appeared in literature and that has been described by its typical hydrogel properties, was a polyhydroxyethylmethacrylate (HEMA) hydrogel developed much later, in 1960, by O. Wichterle and D. Lim, with the aim of using it in permanent contact applications with human tissues, i.e., as soft contact lenses [1].

Since then, hydrogels have been used as systems for drug controlled delivery, to facilitate the localized, sustained and prolonged release of a drug, thereby decreasing the number of administrations, avoiding side effects and following low doses [2].

The most widely studied environmentally responsive systems were temperature sensitive hydrogels, in which physical entanglements, hydrogen bonding, and hydrophobic interactions are the main features that constitute the crosslinks. Two different types of thermo-sensitive hydrogels exist that undergo gelation either by cooling below the upper critical gelation temperature (UCGT) or by heating above the lower critical gelation temperature (LCGT), respectively. Hydrogels with LCGT behavior and sol-to-gel transition at 37 °C have gained increasing attention in the biomedical field as carriers for cells, drugs, and biomolecules, since they allow encapsulation in mild conditions (temperature ≤ 37°C) [3].

Poloxamers and poloxamines are examples of these LCGT biocompatible thermoreversible hydrogels that were introduced in the 1950s by BASF (Iselin, NJ, USA) when they started being used for detergent development, but also in other areas, like agriculture, food, and paints [4].

Poloxamers or Pluronics® are a class of water-soluble nonionic triblock copolymers formed by polar (poly ethylene oxide) and non-polar (poly propylene oxide) blocks, which confer amphiphilic and surface active properties to the polymers. Their aqueous solutions undergo sol-to-gel transition with increasing the temperature above a LCGT; moreover, the coexistence of hydrophilic and hydrophobic monomers into block copolymers allows the formation of ordered structures in solution, the most common of these being the micelles. The formation of micelles in solution is a reversible and dynamic process useful for encapsulating hydrophobic drugs and delivering them into an aqueous environment.

They can be considered as smart polymers, for their stimuli-sensitive properties, due to the different behaviors of these polymers since they can modify their structure in function of pH, temperature and salt concentration [5]. For this reason, a variety of Pluronics is available on the market, differing for the molecular weight of the building blocks and for the hydrophobic–hydrophilic ratio, allowing the preparation of thermosensitive hydrogels with different properties, e.g., in terms of critical gelation concentration (CGC) and gelation time at physiological condition [3].

Thus, poloxamers represent a convenient choice in pharmaceutical technology and biomedical area due to their commercial availability, wide range of molecular weights, peculiar behavior and flexibility. Poloxamers are FDA approved and listed in the US and European Pharmacopoeia; they are non-toxic and non-irritant therefore they can be used as solubilizer, emulsifier, stabilizer, and administered through oral, parenteral, topical routes. As wetting agents, they are useful in ointments, suppository bases, and gels [6].

Poloxamer hydrogels use in drug release appeared at the beginning of the 1970s; they were a response in the search for new safer and faster treatments for the delivery of highly-effective therapeutic agents to a target cell, even if they have poor mechanical properties such as low tensile strength and low Young's modulus that limit their practical applications, sometimes even as medical device coatings [7].

Analysis of recent literature covering a range of treatment pathways and diseases, reveals a major emphasis on "smart" drug carriers developed with poloxamers. The different range of potential delivery methods is highlighted in this review by discussing how the poloxamer solution behavior enables multiple formulation processing routes, drug-encapsulating structures, and engagement with physiological barriers to drug passage.

The first research work concerned the treatment of thermal burns [8] followed by researches on the release of hormones [9], tetracycline [10], proteins [11], and more recently for norcantharidin delivery [12], heparin [13], and anti-HIV drugs [14]. In the last twenty years the numbers of papers related to poloxamer hydrogels for biomedical applications is exponentially increased (Figure 1).

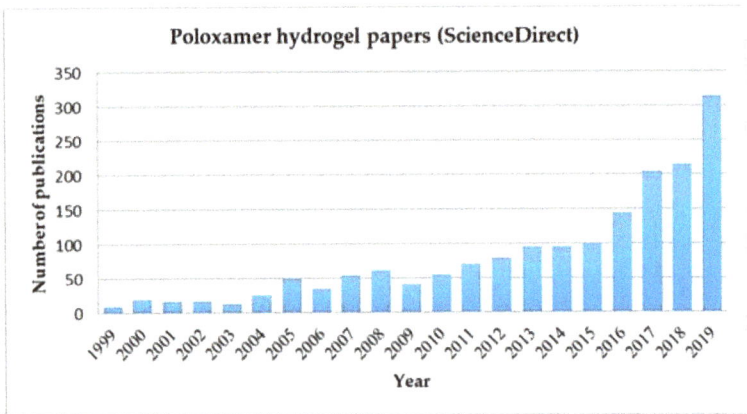

Figure 1. Histogram showing the increase in publications related to the keywords "poloxamer hydrogel" in Science Direct database during the past twenty years.

More recently such hydrogels have become especially attractive to the new field of "tissue engineering" as matrices for repairing and regenerating a wide variety of tissues and organs [15].

They have been successfully employed as scaffold-forming materials for cell printing technology, a computer-aided tissue engineering technology based on the layered deposition of cellularized hydrogels to form complex 3D constructs [16–18].

In this review the poloxamer hydrogels will be taken into consideration, giving an overview of their use as drug delivery systems (DDS) in different routes of administration, especially ophthalmic, transdermal, and vaginal ones. Finally, this paper focused on their potential in tissue and membrane regeneration, in the field of biomedical engineering and their application as micellar systems for gene delivery and cancer therapy.

2. Poloxamers

2.1. Poloxamers Properties

These polymers are synthetic triblock copolymers of poly(ethylene oxide)-b-poly(propylene oxide)-b-poly(ethylene oxide) (PEO-PPO-PEO) (Figure 2).

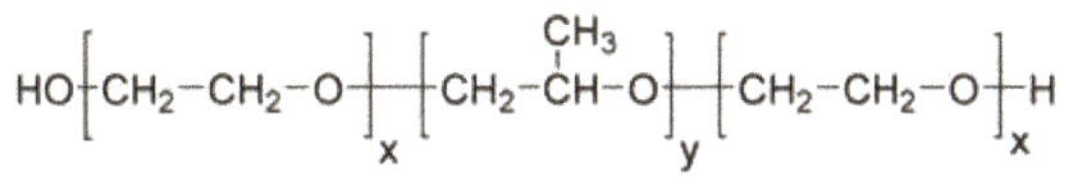

$$HO\left[CH_2-CH_2-O\right]_x\left[CH_2-\underset{CH_3}{CH}-O\right]_y\left[CH_2-CH_2-O\right]_x H$$

Figure 2. Chemical formula for poloxamers: x and y are the lengths of PEO and PPO: poly(ethylene oxide) and poly(propylene oxide) chains, respectively.

They are synthesized through the sequential addition of PO and EO monomers in the presence of an alkaline catalyst, such as sodium or potassium hydroxide, obtaining different copolymers with a different number of hydrophilic EO and hydrophobic PO units, which are also characterized by their distinct hydrophilic–lipophilic balance (HLB) value. Changes in the copolymer composition (PPO/PEO ratio) and molecular weight (PEO and PPO block length) during synthesis leads to macromolecular surface active agents with specific properties suitable in various technological areas.

Poloxamers appear in the form of liquids, pastes, and solids, depending on their molecular weights varying from 1100 to 14,000, offering a pool of more than 50 amphiphilic, water-soluble and polymorphic materials. Their water solubility is subjected by different ratio (1:9 to 8:2) between the chain of propylene oxide (PO) and ethylene oxide (EO) with hydrophobic and hydrophilic behavior, respectively [16]. These differences also alter the in vivo properties and interactions with cells and cell membranes, and provides high potential for the design of innovative nanomedicines and new biomaterials.

Poloxamers were the first block copolymers produced for industrial purposes, synthesized by Wyandotte Chemical Corporation in the late 1940s. Today they are commercially known by the trade names Pluronics®, Lutrol®, Kolliphor® (BASF), Antarox® (Rhodia), and Synperonics® (Croda).

The original manufacturer BASF introduced a specific nomenclature for Pluronics consisting of a letter indicating the morphism of each copolymer: L (for liquid), P (for paste) or F (for flakes) followed by a number referring to the molecular weight of the PPO block (the first one or two) and the weight fraction of the PEO block (the last one).

For example, P123 and F127 have the same molecular weight of PPO (in the order of 4000) but P123 has 30% of PEO and F127 70% of PEO [17].

The physicochemical characteristics and applications of Poloxamers were firstly reviewed extensively by Alexandridis and Hatton in 1995 [16]. In Figure 3, a 3D poloxamer modified pluronic grid showing the distribution of different copolymers, gathered according their physical state, is reported.

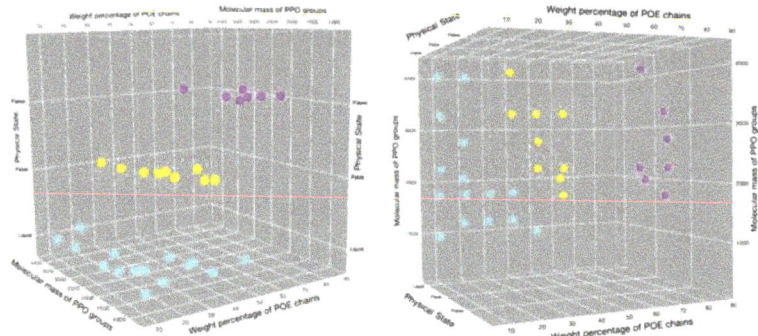

Figure 3. Poloxamers 3D distribution according to physical state (solid flakes = magenta; paste = yellow; liquid = blue), weight percentage of POE chains and molecular mass of the PPO groups (adapted from [16]).

The most significant physical properties of most common poloxamers, are reported in Table 1: average molecular weight, melting point expressed in °C, viscosity (Pa·s) measured at 25 °C, 60 °C, and 50 °C for pastes, liquids, and solids, respectively, surface tension at 0.1% at 25 °C (dyn cm^{-1}), hydrophilic–lipophilic balance (HLB) [4,17,19,20].

Table 1. Properties of the most common poloxamer poly(ethylene oxide)-b-poly(propylene oxide)-b-poly(ethylene oxide) (PEO-PPO-PEO) copolymers.

Poloxamer	Pluronic	PEO%	Average Molecular Weight	Melting Point (°C)	Viscosity (Pa·s)	Surface Tension (dyn cm^{-1})	HLB
P105	L35	50	1900	7	0.375	49	18–23
P108	F38	80	4700	48	0.260	52	>24
P122	L42	20	1630	−26	0.280	46	7–12
P123	L43	30	1850	−1	0.310	47	7–12
P124	L44	40	2200	16	0.440	45	12–18
P182	L62	20	2500	−4	0.450	43	1–7
P183	L63	30	2650	10	0.490	43	7–12
P184	L64	40	2900	16	0.850	43	12–18
P185	P65	50	3400	27	0.180	46	12–18
P188	F68	80	8400	52	1.000	50	>24
P212	L72	20	2750	−7	0.510	39	1–7
P215	P75	50	4150	27	0.250	43	12–18
P217	F77	70	6600	48	0.480	47	>24
P234	P84	40	4200	34	0.280	42	12–18
P235	P85	50	4600	34	0.310	42	12–18
P237	F87	70	7700	49	0.700	44	>24
P238	F88	80	11,400	54	2.300	48	>24
P288	F98	80	13,000	58	2.700	43	>24
P333	P103	30	4950	30	0.285	34	7–12
P334	P104	40	5900	32	0.390	33	12–18
P335	P105	50	6500	35	0.750	39	12–18
P338	F108	80	14,600	57	2.800	41	>24
P402	L122	20	5000	20	1.750	33	1–7
P403	P123	30	5750	31	0.350	34	7–12
P407	F127	70	12600	56	3.100	41	18–23

Commonly used poloxamers include P188 (F-68 grade), P237 (F-87 grade), P338 (F-108 grade), and P407 (F-127 grade) types, which are freely soluble in water.

2.2. Poloxamers Behavior

The aqueous solution properties of poloxamers have been intensely studied and thoroughly reviewed owing to their unique behavior and benefit to myriad applications.

In water solutions, the amphiphilic character of copolymers lead the macromolecule to self-aggregate into micelles with an inner core constituted by hydrophobic blocks and an outer shell constituted by hydrophilic units. They are nano-sized structures, normally between 10 and 200 nm that appears at the critical micellization concentration (CMC) and at critical micellization temperature (CMT). CMC value of poloxamer aqueous solutions decreases with increasing temperature and number of PEO segments, indicating that polymers with a larger hydrophobic (PPO) domain form micelles at lower concentrations and temperatures [21].

Poloxamer water solutions exhibit temperature sensitivity, in particular a "thermoreversible gelation" [21] for sufficiently concentrated samples; they show a sol-gel transition around 37 °C (physiological temperature) and gel-sol transition around 50 °C, being able to produce thermoreversible gels, some already approved by the Food and Drug Administration, which present great interest in food additives, drug delivery carriers in cosmetics, pharmaceutical ingredients, and tissue engineering [5,17]

Several mechanisms have been proposed for this behavior, the first one was related to the gel transition that was due to changes in micellar properties (Figure 4).

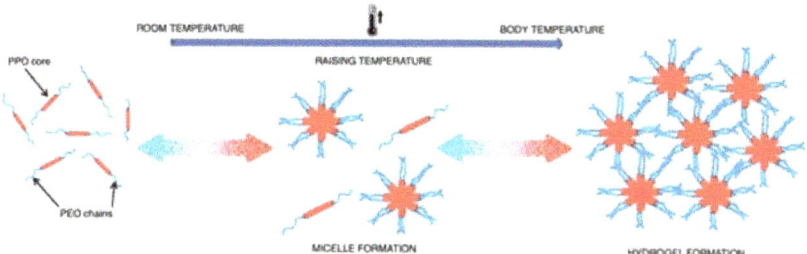

Figure 4. Schematic representation for hydrogel formation.

Thanks to their core–shell architecture, the hydrophobic core can act as a drug-loading site, creating a space for the encapsulation of hydrophobic drugs through the establishment of physical or chemical interactions. The properties of the outer shell and inner core have an influence in the drug release, that can promote an easier or sustained release of the drug. Due the properties above mentioned, polymeric micelles can transport several drugs, improving the circulation time, as well as the enhanced permeability and retention effect. Moreover, these systems exhibit low-risk of chronic toxicity since the polymeric micelles are disassembled in vivo, in single polymer chains that can be excreted by kidneys.

In order to prepare polymeric micelles for drug encapsulation, different methods can be used, however, the more common are the direct dissolution, dialysis, evaporation or film method, freeze-drying, microphase separation, and the oil-in-water emulsion [22].

The method depends, mostly, on the solubility of the copolymer and the drug in an aqueous medium. Some other aspects are also important to an efficient drug incorporation, such as copolymer characteristics, molecular weight and HLB. The structural and chemical characterization of polymeric micelles are important features to take into account in the development of these nanocarriers, since they have a direct influence on the efficiency of these drug release forms, in terms of size, polydispersion index, zeta potential, encapsulation efficiency (EE), and drug loading capacity (DL) [23].

Other researchers [24] discussed gelation as a function of thermodynamical parameters. The enthalpy of gelation depends on CMC and temperature, the value change in the case of poloxamers gelation is unfavorable unlike the gelatine gelation where a great enthalpy change occurred.

The useful concentration for gel formation is the same as for poloxamers with the same PPO/PEO ratio and it decreases with the increasing of polymer molecular weight, denoting the significance of this parameter. While the presence of electrolytes reduces gel transition temperature, enthalpy of gel formation is not significantly changed by the addition of other substances. This behavior suggests that entropy plays the major role in the gelation process.

For all these behaviors, the poloxamers were used for the study and for the development of innovative pharmaceutical forms in different administration routes.

3. Drug Delivery Systems (DDS)

Poloxamer sol-gel reversible hydrogels have attracted the attention for practical biomedical and pharmaceutical applications because of constituents solubility, biocompatibility with biological systems and easy administration of pharmaceutical formulations. The pharmaceutical and biomedical fields covered by the use of poloxamers including solubilization of hydrophobic drugs, controlled release, biomacromolecule delivery (e.g., proteins and genes) and tissue engineering.

Most applications involve the use of Poloxamer P407 and include delivery of protein/peptide drugs [25], such as insulin [26], interleukin-2 [27], epidermal growth factor [28], bone morphogenic protein [29], fibroblastic growth factor, and endothelial cell growth factor [30].

In recent years these hydrogels have been used as carriers for most routes of administration, the most interesting are discussed below.

3.1. Poloxamers for Oftalmic Administration

The thermoreversible gels have shown a growing interest at ocular level because they combine peculiar characteristics: i.e., the formulation when applied is sol (it performs like eye drops) and becomes gel with body temperature (it performs like ointment) increasing the in situ residence time.

The most well-known ocular drug delivery system is eye drops, but they have a short residence time because they are quickly drained through the nasolacrimal route resulting in frequent dosage regimen which leads to an increase in side effects and poor patient compliance.

Poloxamers P407 and P188 are among the most commonly used in this case for their good water solubility, solution clearness, optimal viscosity, and ocular tissue safety.

Recent works have focused on the best formulation to obtain a hydrogel with useful features for ocular administration and without toxicity. About this point Al Khateb et al. [31] studied two formulations containing poloxamers, i.e., P407 and P188, with different gelation properties depending on concentration solutions and the ratio of their mixtures. Transparent gels were obtained only in the case of 20% w/w P407 and P188 solutions. Furthermore, these preparations were non-toxic or irritating to the corneal mucosa and then suitable for application in ocular drug delivery.

Fathalla Z.M.A. et al. [32] studied the blend of the same two poloxamers for a controlled ocular delivery of ketorolac tromethamine (KT). The most promising gel formulations, loaded with KT, were those containing the mixtures of P407:P188 23:10 w/v% and 23:15 w/v% respectively. These gels do not present toxicity and do not irritate the conjunctiva and cornea.

In recent years other polymers have been added to poloxamers-based gels to obtain different drug release characteristics and to modify the rheological properties.

Among these works, Yu et al. [33] has to be remembered for the synthesis of a cross-linked hydrogel system containing carboxymethyl chitosan (CMC) and poloxamer P407, where the presence of CMC with biological properties could improve hydrogel biocompatibility. This formulation, containing nepafenac (NP) as a model drug, showed good rheological properties at gelation temperature (32–33 °C) and a sustained release of NP from hydrogel, so as to be considered a pH–temperature-responsive ophthalmic drug delivery system.

Another approach, with good results, involved the introduction of various colloidal carrier systems to easily load poorly soluble drugs into poloxamers hydrogels.

Lou et al. [34] incorporated curcumin-loaded albumin nanoparticles into a hydrogel based on a mixture of P407/P188 for local ocular administration, to treat diabetic retinopathy. This formulation, which became a gel when exposed to eye temperature, may be applied as eye drops. Nanoparticles provided the sustained drug release while the presence of hydrogel prolonged the in situ residence time.

Finally, Almeda et al. [35] reported the combination of lipid nanoparticles and a thermoresponsive polymer with mucomimetic properties (poloxamer P407). The incorporated nanoparticles showed an average size below 200 nm, a good positive zeta potential and an efficiency of ibuprofen encapsulation of about 90%. The optimal poloxamer concentration in thermoreversible gel was 15% (w/w) Pluronic® F-127. The formulation did not present a relevant cytotoxicity and showed a sustained release of ibuprofen over several hours. The strategy proposed in this work can be successfully applied to increase bioavailability and therapeutic efficacy of conventional eyedrops.

3.2. Poloxamers for Transdermal Administration

Transdermal drug delivery is a valid alternative to the oral and parenteral route because it offers several advantages: Avoidance the hepatic first pass, good compliance by the patient, and easy access. The most studied formulations for this route contained poloxamer P407, as a polymer, and as drugs those with anti-inflammatory [36,37], analgesic [38], local anesthetic [39], and cardiac [40,41] activity, rarely are present preparations containing big molecules such as arginine, vasopressin, and insulin [42,43].

Generally in these topical preparations it is necessary to introduce an enhancer substance which is able to facilitate the passage through the stratum corneum (thickness of 10 to 15 µm) which is the main barrier to drug penetration.

In the last decade the penetration enhancers have been replaced by the microneedles (MNs) that have the capacity to permeate the stratum corneum and infuse the active ingredient in the deep areas of the skin.

Microneedles are needles similar to the ones useful for hypodermic injections but they present different sizes: from 1–100 microns in length and 1 micron in diameter (Figure 5). They are manufactured with silicon [44,45], metals such as stainless steel, palladium, nickel and titanium [46–48], carbohydrates including galactose, maltose, and polysaccharide [49–51], glass [52], ceramics [53], and various other polymers [54,55]. MNs are fabricated in backing that can be applied to the substrate like a patch carrying different drugs by penetrating through the skin, mucosal tissue and sclera [56–59]. Their dissolution has to be taken into consideration because it can influence drug delivery [60,61].

One of the most recent researches regards sol-gel transition property of poloxamers to obtain in situ forming hydrogel microneedles, for the delivery of methotrexate to treat solid tumors [62]. The use of this drug by transdermal route is generally limited by its relatively high molecular weight and hydrophilicity. For this purpose four formulations were prepared with two different methotrexate concentrations (0.2% and 0.4% w/w) with poloxamer P407 (20% w/w) and without, using the last one as a control, replacing the polymer with deionized water. In this study, it was confirmed the sol-gel transition of the formulations at skin temperature (32 °C), maintaining skin barrier function and skin viscoelastic properties after administration of the formulations. In vitro drug diffusion studies, using a Franz cell, showed that the formulations containing methotrexate (0.2% and 0.4%) without P407 released overall drug after 22 and 35 h respectively, while the one with P407 after 72 h. For this reason it is possible to conclude that the poloxamer-based formulations provided a steady and sustained delivery.

In an even more recent work, the formation of depots of thermoreversible poloxamers in skin micropores using MNs to transdermal drug delivery has been reported for the first time [63]. Sodium fluorescein (FS) was used as model drug to study in vitro permeation at different concentrations. In order to crate pores into the skin and to overcome the stratum corneum MNs have been used, then the drug loaded poloxamer solution was applied to fill pores, subsequently an in situ gelation at skin temperature of 32 °C occurred.

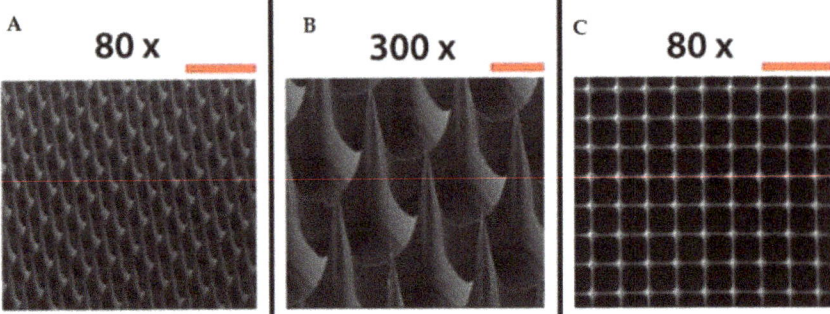

Figure 5. Scanning electron microscopy images of microneedle arrays imaged from a lateral view (**A**,**B**) and from the top side (**C**). Scale bars represent 500 μm (80×) (**A**,**C**) and 100 μm (300×) (**B**) (adapted from [64]).

For this goal poloxamers P407, P237, and P338 were used at different concentrations (from 15 to 30% w/w in water) loading different amounts of fluorescein.

The formulations were characterized for their rheological properties and in situ gel formation. The distribution of FS in skin tissue was tracked by confocal laser microscopic analysis with higher intensity of FS in MN-treated skin tissues. The in vitro fluorescein release studies were carried out using vertical Franz diffusion cells. The release profiles indicated that the concentration of fluorescein (0.1%, 0.3%, and 0.5% w/w) was a variable parameter that significantly affects drug release as well as the type of poloxamer used. In particular P338 and P237 0.1–0.3% FS-loaded formulations provided a total drug release during 16 h while 0.5% FS-loaded provided a release for 20 h. Moreover, for a longer time (about 24 h), the release from P407 formulations was comparable. All the poloxamers depots started dissolving according to the dominant hydrophilic interactions and gels did not remain intact. It was concluded that P407 provided the best release for a longer duration and it was selected as the best drug delivery for in vitro permeation assays. These studies confirmed that drug loading is not a limitation and permeation of FS after MN treatment was found in more controlled manner and for a long time when compared to a permeation across untreated skin sample.

3.3. Poloxamers for Vaginal Administration

Another interesting pathway exploited in drug delivery systems is the vaginal route, allowing both the systemic and local absorption of drugs poorly absorbed after oral administration [65–67]. The vagina has a vast network of blood vessels that make easy the systemic absorption, avoiding deactivation at gastrointestinal level and hepatic first pass. Mucoadhesive pharmaceutical forms have been studied for this district due to the presence of mucus which increases permeability. The thermoreversible systems, appropriately modified with polymers that promote mucoadhesion, allow to obtain a sustained drug release and a good bioavailability without altering the vaginal physiology [68].

After application of poloxamers for vaginal administration occurring gelation favored a long permanence of drugs on the administration site to promote a drug controlled release [69]. Vaginal drug delivery is based on the exploitation of polymers which are able not only to gelify at physiological temperature but also to adhere to the vaginal mucosa improving the in situ residence time.

A brief description of recent reports in the literature, based on poloxamer formulations by vaginal route, is given below.

In the first work [70] the authors investigated a novel amphotericin B (AmB) release system in the form of nanosuspension loaded into a poloxamer P407/P188 hydrogel. P407 (20% w/w) and P188 (5% w/w) were dissolved in AmB nanosuspension, the AmB NPs thermogel were characterized regarding nanoparticle features (particle size, zeta potential, morphology) and gel behavior (rheology, stability, in vitro drug release, and in vitro and in vivo anti-Candida efficiency). The nanosuspension-gel combination has been necessary because nanoparticles alone tended to aggregate while they were more stable in the poloxamer hydrogel. When compared with other biodegradable thermosensitive hydrogel, such as polyester-based gels, poloxamer were not capable of an in vivo degradation. This property is really suitable for vaginal delivery because it means grater safety in use. Another very important element in the development of vaginal formulations was mucoadhesion; poloxamers have lower adhesion properties compared to compounds such as Carbopol, the addition of some bioadhesive materials into P407/P188 thermogel would be a feasible path [71–73]. Finally, the in vivo anti-Candida assay showed a better antifungal efficiency of AmB in the thermoreversible gel when compared with commercial effervescent tablets at the same drug dose (2.5 mg/Kg).

A second paper [74] described a novel vaginal delivery strategy consisting of two pharmaceutical forms placed together to give an expansible thermal gelling aerosol foam (ETGFA) that combined the advantages of foam and gel penetration and carrier retention in vaginal canal, respectively.

ETGA was prepared adding an optimized amount of P407 (18–22% w/w) and P188 (0–5% w/w), achieved by evaluating the gelation temperature, the adhesive agents (arabic gum, sodium carboxymethyl cellulose, sodium alginate, and xanthan gum) and silver nanoparticles to obtain a drug concentration of 1% w/w. To study a better performance in foam expansion and duration, propane/butane 80/20 v/v and dimethyl ether were compared as propellants. The formulation was characterized in regards of rheology, foam expansion, adhesiveness and drug release. ETGA showed a better extended drug release (over 4 h) dose –dependent antimicrobial effects on the vaginal flora and no tissue irritation when compared to a commercial antimicrobial gel. These results indicated that ETGA could be a suitable formulation for vaginal drug delivery.

4. Tissue Regeneration Scaffolders

Tissue engineering, in this last decade, has emerged in the biomedical field because it allows researchers to create specific devices that represent in vivo tissues that can be replaced or increased to address current therapeutic challenges [75].

Poloxamers have received special attention for tissue regeneration based on their biocompatibility, low cytotoxicity, and good rheological properties [76].

In particular, the area the most explored deals with regeneration of bone tissue. The use of growth factors such as bone morphogenetic protein-2 (BMP-2) for bone repair has been reported [77,78] but it is very expensive and easily loose its integrity. Recently, other compounds that have received interest were statins because they altered bone metabolism through different mechanisms [79–81]. Their bioavailability after oral administration was low and a real bone healing cannot be expected. For this reason different delivery systems for local delivery of statins have been evaluated. The study of incorporation of rosuvastatin (RSV)-loaded chitosan/chondroitin sulfate nanoparticles into a thermosensitive hydrogel is reported below [82]. At first this research considered nanoparticles preparation and optimization, thereafter it dealt with the characterization of thermosensible hydrogels.

Gel formulation consisted of poloxamer P407 (18–20% w/v), hyaluronic acid (HA) 1–3% w/v and hydroxypropyl methylcellulose (2% w/v) to stabilize the formulation itself.

HA [83] and P407 had also positive effects on articular cartilage, simulating the regenerative process within the joint. The study showed that gel provided a low viscosity at 4 °C and gelification at 35 °C; drug release from nanoparticles, inserted into the hydrogel, was around 60% after 48 h, while it was completely released from nanoparticles alone within 12 h. This behavior indicated that the drug release was controlled and sustained.

Moreover, the hydrogel formulation showed an improvement in osteoblast viability and proliferation due to the used polymer and the biological properties of the nanoparticle delivery system.

Another paper [84] reported the design of a cryogel scaffold for the regeneration of an intervertebral disc tissue (nucleus pulposus NP). NP is located inside the vertebral discs and has the function of absorbing the pressure exerted on the spine and keeping the vertebrae separated. The symptoms of NP degeneration are pain and limited mobility of the extremities. It is composed of up to 90% water, type II collagen and proteoglycans [85]. This study focused on the preparation of a novel gelatin-P407 cryogel (in different ratio: 1:1,2:1, 4:1,5:1, 7:1, or 10:1 respectively) as an alternative to the spinal fusion procedure. The composite hydrogel was tested by the following assays: Pore analysis, swelling potential, stability, mechanical integrity and cellular infiltration. The inclusion of P407 in the cryogel was designed to increase swelling ratio, due its hydrophilic nature, since in the NP degradation there is a rapid water loss. All sample presented a high swelling ratio after 24 h, mechanical durability and stability for 28 days in a body-like environment. The 7:1 and 10:1 gel scaffolds showed the most ideal pore diameters and a profuse cell infiltration after only 14 days.

In recent years, 3D printing technology has become important in the biomedical field and in particular the use of thermoreversible gels that with their sol-gel characteristics can be very useful in tissue regeneration [86].

The principle on which the 3D printer is based is to lay a filament of polymeric material which is deposited layer upon layer until the desired system is obtained in 3 dimensions.

Bioprinting systems can be classified into three types: Laser based, jetting based, and extrusion based; recent techniques such as magnetic bioprinting and electrohydrodynamic jetting have been used in tissue engineering.

Hydrogels requirements for 3D bioprinting of ideal engineered tissues should be the following [87]: High porosity, rapid gelation, shape retention, and immunological issue avoidance.

Thermoreversible hydrogels have been successfully applied thanks to their gelation characteristics as they quickly pass from sol-gel state and are also easily extruded from 3D printers [88].

P407 showed good printability [86] but it was not suitable for long-term cell viability. As reported by the recent work [89] it is used, combined with gelatin to create a biocompatible hydrogel for vascular channels, for molds, exploiting its excellent rheological behavior, under shear stress, and its elasticity.

In addition to bioprintability, biological properties of hydrogels played a crucial role in successful tissues regeneration [90]. One of the major disadvantages of available hydrogel materials was that they do not facilitate differentiation of cells into multiple linkages. Despite this, thermoresponsive hydrogels may be very useful for tissue engineering applications and they will become part of the advancement in bio printing technology.

5. Poloxamer as Micellar Systems

Polymeric micelles generated by poloxamers with peculiar characteristics and under specific conditions are exploited as nanometric drug carriers [91]. They have taken hold in recent years as they are able to solubilize poorly water-soluble drugs [36] and decrease undesirable cellular interactions [92,93]. In this review chapter, two recent applications (gene delivery and cancer therapy) of poloxamer micelles have been taken into account.

The development of gene delivery carriers has emerged as a promising technology in transporting genes directly to the target site as therapeutic factors [94]. Current gene transfer vectors used in regenerative medicine approaches included no viral [95] and viral vehicles [96]. The complexation of DNA with cationic polymers (polyplexes) or lipids (lipoplexes) protected DNA against degradation by nucleases and serum components creating a less negative surface charge. They can be designed to target specific cell types through receptor–ligand interactions [97], but these systems exhibited aggregation tendency, a low transfection efficiency and short time transgene expression levels [98]. The use of poloxamers has been described as a tool to increase efficiency of viral gene transfer, obtaining a localized delivery into targets or protecting the vectors.

In the last decade many works that focused the attention on gene delivery were published; the most recent and significant studies are here summarized.

Many researchers have studied the recombinant adeno-associated viral (rAAV) carriers as adapted gene transfer vectors to direct human cartilagine in regenerative medicine [99–101]. However, their use is limited cause their rapid neutralization by the presence of antibodies or heparin which prevent their binding to the viral receptor, present on the cell surface. In this regard, based on the use of polymeric biocompatible materials the combining of direct rAAV-mediated gene transfer with tissue engineering approaches, may offer efficient alternatives.

In this study [102] the possibility of providing rAAV to cartilage regenerative cells via self-assembled poloxamers was evaluated. The formulations consisted of P188 and P407 (2% w/v i.e., above CMC)/rAAV or poloxamine/rAAV were directly incubated within monolayer cultures of hMSCs, cartilagine regenerative cells. At thisoptimized concentration the two poloxamers were more efficient in increasing gene expression over time than a treatment lacking them.

The highest rAAV gene transfer occurred when the PEO/PPO ratio was shifted to hydrophilicity (HLB > 24) using a concentration above CMC (2%) (89.5–94.6% efficiencies with up to 2.7-fold increase in transgene expression for at least 21 days, suggesting that micelles may be better carriers than unimers).

In another paper [103], lentiviral vectors (LV) used for the transduction of human and nonhuman cells were taken into consideration. The optimal transduction conditions for efficient LV gene delivery into target cells depended on a number of factors, including cell density, purity of lentiviral preparation, virus transduction units (TU), multiplicity of infection (MOI) and presence of adjuvants that facilitate transduction [104–106]. These researches identified and validated novel adjuvants for improving transduction efficiency, in particular five representatives poloxamers (P402, P235, P188, P407, and P338). P338 proved to be the best choice since it produced low toxicity and effective viral transduction, especially in difficult-to-transduce cells of T-cell origin.

Further application strategies with poloxamer regard cancer therapy [4]. Poloxamers have gained interest in the field of oncology because of their ability to developed stable systems with the capability of efficient drugs encapsulation and deliver. They usually present small sizes and self-assembling behavior in micellar systems in an aqueous medium, good stability in physiological medium and they avoid the deactivation by RES organs improving consequently drug bioavailability [22,107].

In this biomedical and pharmaceutical area the most recent works in the literature are reported. The first one concerned the use of poloxamer micelles containing a dye (CyFaP) as photo-acoustic imaging (PAI) contrast for mammary neoplastic tissue [108]. In this formulation, dye was inserted in P407 (10% w/v) micelle dropwise under constant stirring. Serum stability studies, cell viability assays, deep tissue penetration and in vivo biodistribution studies were performed. This work has shown that poloxamer micelles are effective for PAI as they penetrate more deeply into breast cancer tissue and are also useful for lymphatic mapping.

The second work [109] explored the anticancer activity of Salinomycin (SAL), an antibiotic isolated from Streptomyces albus [110], that has recently been reported as being effective against tumor cells and mainly to inhibit growth of a specific cancer cell sub-population: CSC. The main goal of the research was the encapsulation of SAL into an innovative poloxamer micelles (PM) system and a further evaluation of in vitro PM-SAL delivery in bacterial and in eukaryotic tumor cells. PM formulations containing P407 and SAL in different amounts were defined with a two multivariate experimental design (DoE) to get the best preparation conditions. Micelles were characterized for size by dynamic light scattering, for their zeta potential and for the encapsulation efficiency. Their in vitro activity was conducted in bacterial cell culture and A549 (adenocarcinoma cell line) cell culture. In conclusion, these micelles seem to be able to deliver SAL into human cancer cells promoting a high drug intracellular accumulation, greatly decreasing toxicity on healthy cells.

Finally, a combined study between radiation therapy and systemic chemotherapeutics to provide both local radiosensitization and systemic control of tumor disease has been reported [111,112]. This study showed the development of a single micelles formulation consisting of multiple poloxamers (MPMs) containing PARP (poly ADP- ribose polymerase) inhibitor talazoparib (Tal) and PI3K (phosphoinositol-3-kinase) inhibitor buparlisib (Bup). When administered during a radiotherapy cycle, that would increase the therapeutic activity of the two drugs in a preclinical model [113]. The performed formulation was made of poloxamer mixture (P103 and P407) obtaining micelles (MPMs) via a modified nanoprecipitation method [114]. MPMs were characterized by dynamic light scattering, to determine size, zeta potential and polydispersity, and by transmission electron microscopy (TEM).

It was also observed that MPMs modulate drug release depending on pH; this behavior is a very useful tool, as the change in pH at tumor level (pH 6.8) would result in a faster release than what occurs when they are circulating in the blood stream (pH 7.4). Furthermore, metabolic assays confirmed that the use of both Tal and Bup synergistically enhanced in vitro cytotoxicity. The in vitro therapeutic activity of the two drugs was studied by a colony-forming assay and a DNA damage assay.

In vivo experiments have shown that the administration of this new MPMs formulation during the course of radiotherapy gave promising results into the enhanced tumor control. The results of this study confirmed that it is important to carry on the development and advancement of combination therapies, especially with the aim of enhancing the outcomes of patients in late-stage and metastatic disease.

6. Summary

Poloxamers are peculiar synthetic tri-block copolymers composed of two poly(ethylene oxide) units and a poly(propylene oxide) one with amphiphilic properties. The dual character, confers to the copolymers interesting properties that can be controlled and changed by different PPO/PEO ratios. These polymers exhibit thermogelling behavior at strategical physiological temperatures.

The most used and studied poloxamer P407, at a concentration of 20% w/w in water, is able to convert the solution to a clear gel by warming the system from room (25 °C) to body temperature (near 37 °C). This thermoresponsive feature has made it attractive for several applications including injectable and topical pharmaceutical formulations, where the material may flow through an applicator or syringe before forming a gel upon contact with the body (35–37 °C).

Because of their biocompatibility and nontoxicity poloxamers have been widely utilized in biomedical applications. In this review their usefulness as thermoreversible hydrogels in the most significant routes of administration (i.e., ocular, transdermic and vaginal route) was reported. Moreover, the latest frontiers have been highlighted for what concerns poloxamers employed in tissue engineering and in gene and cancer therapy.

Funding: This research received no external funding.

Conflicts of Interest: The authors declare no conflict of interest.

References

1. Wichterle, O.; Lim, D. Hydrophilic Gels for Biological Use. *Nature* **1960**, *185*, 117–118. [CrossRef]
2. Buwalda, S.J.; Boere, K.W.; Dijkstra, P.J.; Feijen, J.; Vermonden, T.; Hennink, W.E. Hydrogels in a historical perspective: From simple networks to smart materials. *J. Control. Release* **2014**, *190*, 254–273. [CrossRef] [PubMed]
3. Gioffredi, E.; Boffito, M.; Calzone, S.; Giannitelli, S.M.; Rainer, A.; Trombetta, M.; Mozetic, P.; Chiono, V. Pluronic F127 hydrogel characterization and biofabrication in cellularized constructs for tissue engineering applications. *Procedia Cirp* **2016**, *49*, 125–132. [CrossRef]
4. Almeida, M.; Magalhães, M.; Veiga, F.; Figueiras, A. Poloxamers, poloxamines and polymeric micelles: Definition, structure and therapeutic applications in cancer. *J. Polym. Res.* **2018**, *25*, 31. [CrossRef]
5. Aguilar, M.R.; Elvira, C.; Gallardo, A.; Vázquez, B.; Román, J.S. Smart Polymers and Their Applications as Biomaterials. In *Topics in Tissue Engineering*; Ashammakhi, N., Reis, R.L., Chiellini, E., Eds.; Biomaterials and Tissue Engineering Group: Oulu, Finland, 2007; Volume 3.
6. Johnston, T.P.; Palmer, W.K. Mechanism of poloxamer 407-induced hypertriglyceridemia in the rat. *Biochem. Pharm.* **1993**, *46*, 1037–1042. [CrossRef]
7. Li, J.; Stachowski, M.; Zhang, Z. Application of responsive polymers in implantable medical devices and biosensors. In *Switchable and Responsive Surfaces and Materials for Biomedical Applications*; Woodhead Publishing: Sawston, UK; Cambridge, UK, 2015.
8. Nalbandian, R.M.; Henry, R.L.; Wilks, H.S. Artificial skin. II. Pluronic F-127 Silver nitrate or silver lactate gel in the treatment of thermal burns. *J. Biomed. Mater. Res.* **1972**, *6*, 583–590. [CrossRef] [PubMed]

9. Law, T.; Florence, A.T.; Whateley, T.L. Some chemically modified poloxamer hydrogels-controlled release of prostaglandin-e2 and testosterone. *Int. J. Pharm.* **1986**, *33*, 65–69. [CrossRef]
10. Esposito, E.; Carotta, V.; Scabbia, A.; Trombelli, L.; D'Antona, P.; Menegatti, E.; Nastruzzi, C. Comparative analysis of tetracycline-containing dental gels: Poloxamer- and monoglyceride-based formulations. *Int. J. Pharm.* **1996**, *142*, 9–23. [CrossRef]
11. Stratton, L.P.; Dong, A.; Manning, M.C.; Carpenter, J.F. Drug delivery matrix containing native protein precipitates suspended in a poloxamer gel. *J. Pharm. Sci.* **1997**, *86*, 1006–1010. [CrossRef]
12. Xie, M.H.; Ge, M.; Peng, J.B.; Jiang, X.R.; Wang, D.S.; Ji, L.Q.; Ying, Y.; Wang, Z. In-vivo anti-tumor activity of a novel poloxamer-based thermosensitive in situ gel for sustained delivery of norcantharidin. *Pharm. Dev. Technol.* **2019**, *24*, 623–629. [CrossRef]
13. He, C.; Ji, H.; Qian, Y.; Wang, Q.; Liu, X.; Zhao, W.; Zhao, C. Heparin-based and heparin-inspired hydrogels: Size-effect, gelation and biomedical applications. *J. Mater. Chem. B* **2019**, *7*, 1186–1208. [CrossRef]
14. Tian, W.; Han, S.; Huang, X.; Han, M.; Cao, J.; Liang, Y.; Sun, Y. LDH hybrid thermosensitive hydrogel for intravaginal delivery of anti-HIV drugs. *Artif. Cells Nanomed. Biotechnol.* **2019**, *47*, 1234–1240. [CrossRef] [PubMed]
15. Hoffman, A.S. Hydrogels for biomedical applications. *Adv. Drug Deliv. Rev.* **2012**, *64*, 18–23. [CrossRef]
16. Alexandridis, P.; Hatton, T.A. Poly(ethylene oxide)-poly(propylene oxide)-poly (ethylene oxide) block copolymer surfactants in aqueous solutions and at interfaces: Thermodynamics, structure, dynamics, and modeling. *Colloids Surf. A Physicochem. Eng. Asp.* **1995**, *96*, 1–46. [CrossRef]
17. Singh-Joy, S.D.; McLain, V.C. Safety Assessment of Poloxamers 101, 105, 108, 122, 123, 124, 181, 182, 183, 184, 185, 188, 212, 215, 217, 231, 234, 235, 237, 238, 282, 284, 288, 331, 333, 334, 335, 338, 401, 402, 403, and 407, Poloxamer 105 Benzoate, and Poloxamer 182 Dibenzoate as Used in Cosmetics. *Int. J. Toxicol.* **2008**, *27*, 93–128.
18. Pitto-Barry, A.; Barry, N.P. Pluronic®block-copolymers in medicine: From chemical and biological versatility to rationalization and clinical advances. *Polym. Chem.* **2014**, *5*, 3281–3496. [CrossRef]
19. Jeong, B.; Kim, S.W.; Bae, Y.H. Thermosensitive sol–gel reversible hydrogels. *Adv. Drug Deliv. Rev.* **2012**, *64*, 154–162. [CrossRef]
20. Devi, D.R.; Sandhya, P.; Hari, B.V. Poloxamer: A novel functional molecule for drug delivery and gene therapy. *J. Pharm. Sci. Res.* **2013**, *5*, 159–165.
21. Alexandridis, P.; Holzwarth, J.F.; Hatton, T.A. Micellization of Poly(Ethylene Oxide)-Poly(Propylene Oxide)-Poly(Ethylene Oxide) Triblock Copolymers in Aqueous-Solutions-Thermodynamics of Copolymer Association. *Macromolecules* **1994**, *27*, 2414–2425. [CrossRef]
22. Simões, S.M.; Figueiras, A.R.; Veiga, F.; Concheiro, A.; Alvarez-Lorenzo, C. Polymeric micelles for oral drug administration enabling loco regional and systemic treatments. *Expert Opin. Drug Deliv.* **2015**, *12*, 297–318. [CrossRef]
23. Ahmad, Z.; Shah, A.; Siddiq, M.; Kraatz, H.B. Polymeric micelles as drug delivery vehicles. *RSC Adv.* **2014**, *4*, 17028–17038. [CrossRef]
24. Vadnere, M.; Amidon, G.L.; Lindenbaum, S.; Haslam, J.L. Thermodynamic studies on the gel-sol transition of some pluronic polyols. *Int. J. Pharm.* **1984**, *22*, 207. [CrossRef]
25. Cho, C.W.; Cho, Y.S.; Lee, H.K.; Yeom, Y.I.; Park, S.N.; Yoon, D.Y. Improvement of receptor-mediated gene delivery to HepG2 cells using an amphiphilic gelling agent. *Biotechnol. Appl. Biochem.* **2000**, *32*, 21–26. [CrossRef] [PubMed]
26. Morishita, M.; Barichello, J.M.; Takayama, K.; Chiba, Y.; Tokwa, S.; Nagai, T. Pluronic F-127 gels incorporating highly purified unsaturated fatty acids for buccal delivery of insulin. *Int. J. Pharm.* **2001**, *212*, 289–293. [CrossRef]
27. Johnston, T.P.; Punjabi, M.A.; Froelich, C.J. Sustained delivery of interleukin-2 from a Poloxamer 407 gel matrix following intraperitoneal injection in mice. *Pharm. Res.* **1992**, *9*, 425–434. [CrossRef]
28. DiBiase, M.D.; Rhodes, C.T. Investigations of epidermal growth factor in semisolid formulations. *Pharm. Acta Helv.* **1991**, *66*, 165–169.
29. Clokie, C.M.; Urist, M.R. Bone morphogenic protein excipients: Comparative observations on poloxamer. *Plast. Reconstr. Surg.* **2000**, *105*, 628–637. [CrossRef]
30. Hom, D.B.; Medhi, K.; Assefa, G.; Juhn, S.K.; Johnston, T.P. Vascular effects of sustained-release fibroblast growth factors. *Ann. Otol. Rhinol. Laryngol.* **1996**, *105*, 109–116. [CrossRef]

31. Al Khateb, K.; Ozhmukhametova, E.K.; Mussin, M.N.; Seilkhanov, S.K.; Rakhypbekov, T.K.; Lau, W.M.; Khutoryanskiy, V.V. In situ gelling systems based on Pluronic F127/Pluronic F68 formulations for ocular drug delivery. *Int. J. Pharm.* **2016**, *502*, 70–79. [CrossRef]
32. Fathalla, Z.M.; Vangala, A.; Longman, M.; Khaled, K.A.; Hussein, A.K.; El-Garhy, O.H.; Alany, R.G. Poloxamer-based thermoresponsive ketorolac tromethamine in situ gel preparations: Design, characterisation, toxicity and transcorneal permeation studies. *Eur. J. Pharm. Biopharm.* **2017**, *114*, 119–134. [CrossRef]
33. Yu, S.; Zhang, X.; Tan, G.; Tian, L.; Liu, D.; Liu, Y.; Yang, X.; Pan, W. A novel pH-induced thermosensitive hydrogel composed of carboxymethyl chitosan and poloxamer cross-linked by glutaraldehyde for ophthalmic drug delivery. *Carbohydr. Polym.* **2017**, *155*, 208–217. [CrossRef] [PubMed]
34. Lou, J.; Hu, W.; Tian, R.; Zhang, H.; Jia, Y.; Zhang, J.; Zhang, L. Optimization and evaluation of a thermoresponsive ophthalmic in situ gel containing curcumin-loaded albumin nanoparticles. *Int. J. Nanomed.* **2014**, *9*, 2517–2525.
35. Almeida, H.; Lobão, P.; Frigerio, C.; Fonseca, J.; Silva, R.; Sousa Lobo, J.M.; Amaral, M.H. Preparation, characterization and biocompatibility studies of thermoresponsive eyedrops based on the combination of nanostructured lipid carriers (NLC) and the polymer Pluronic F-127 for controlled delivery of ibuprofen. *Pharm. Dev. Technol.* **2017**, *22*, 336–349. [CrossRef] [PubMed]
36. Cafaggi, S.; Russo, E.; Caviglioli, G.; Parodi, B.; Stefani, R.; Sillo, G.; Leardi, R.; Bignardi, G. Poloxamer 407 as a solubilising agent for tolfenamic acid and as a base for a gel formulation. *Eur. J. Pharm. Sci.* **2008**, *35*, 19–29. [CrossRef] [PubMed]
37. Ur-Rehman, T.; Tavelin, S.; Gröbner, G. Effect of DMSO on micellization, gelation and drugrelease profile of Poloxamer 407. *Int. J. Pharm.* **2010**, *394*, 92–98. [CrossRef] [PubMed]
38. Liaw, J.; Lin, Y.C. Evaluation of poly(ethylene oxide)–poly(propylene oxide)–poly(ethylene oxide) (PEO–PPO–PEO) gels as a release vehicle for percutaneous fentanyl. *J. Control. Release* **2000**, *68*, 273–282. [CrossRef]
39. Shin, S.C.; Cho, C.W.; Yang, K.H. Development of lidocaine gels for enhanced local anesthetic action. *Int. J. Pharm.* **2004**, *287*, 73–78. [CrossRef]
40. Suedee, R.; Bodhibukkana, C.; Tangthong, N.; Amnuaikit, C.; Kaewnopparat, S.; Srichana, T. Development of a reservoir-type transdermal enantioselective-controlled delivery system for racemic propranolol using a molecularly imprinted polymer composite membrane. *J. Control. Release* **2008**, *129*, 170–178. [CrossRef]
41. Stamatialis, D.F.; Rolevink, H.H.M.; Koops, G.H. Transdermal timolol delivery from a Pluronic gel. *J. Control. Release* **2006**, *116*, 53–65. [CrossRef]
42. Nair, V.; Panchagnula, R. Poloxamer gel as vehicle for transdermal iontophoretic delivery of arginine vasopressin: Evaluation of in vivo performance in rats. *Pharm. Res.* **2003**, *47*, 555–562. [CrossRef]
43. Pillai, O.; Panchagnula, R. Transdermal delivery of insulin from poloxamer gel: Ex vivo and in vivo skin permeation studies in rat using iontophoresis and chemical enhancers. *J. Control. Release* **2003**, *89*, 127–140. [CrossRef]
44. Donnelly, R.F.; Morrow, D.I.; McCarron, P.A.; Woolfson, A.D.; Morrissey, A.; Juzenas, P.; Juzeniene, A.; Iani, V.; McCarthy, H.O.; Moan, J. Microneedle-mediated intradermal delivery of 5-aminolevulinic acid: Potential for enhanced topical photodynamic therapy. *J. Control. Release* **2008**, *129*, 154–162. [CrossRef] [PubMed]
45. Khanna, P.; Flam, B.R.; Osborn, B.; Strom, J.A.; Bhansali, S. Skin penetration and fracture strength testing of silicon dioxide microneedles. *Sens. Actuators A* **2011**, *170*, 180–186. [CrossRef]
46. Chandrasekaran, S.; Brazzle, J.D.; Frazier, A.B. Surface micromachined metallic microneedles. *J. Microelectromech. Syst.* **2003**, *12*, 281–288. [CrossRef]
47. Gill, H.S.; Prausnitz, M.R. Coating formulations for microneedles. *Pharm. Res.* **2007**, *24*, 1369–1380. [CrossRef] [PubMed]
48. Parker, E.R.; Rao, M.P.; Turner, K.L.; Meinhart, C.D.; MacDonald, N.C. Bulk micromachined titanium microneedles. *J. Microelectromech. Syst.* **2007**, *16*, 289–295. [CrossRef]
49. Donnelly, R.F.; Morrow, D.I.; Singh, T.R.; Migalska, K.; McCarron, P.A. Processing difficulties and instability of carbohydrate microneedle arrays. *Drug Deliv. Ind. Pharm.* **2009**, *35*, 1242–1254. [CrossRef]
50. Lee, K.; Lee, C.Y.; Jung, H. Dissolving microneedles for transdermal drug administration prepared by stepwise controlled drawing of maltose. *Biomaterials* **2011**, *32*, 3134–3140. [CrossRef]
51. Li, G.; Badkar, A.; Nema, S.; Kolli, C.S.; Banga, A.K. In vitro transdermal delivery of therapeutic antibodies using maltose microneedles. *Int. J. Pharm.* **2009**, *368*, 109–115. [CrossRef]

52. Wang, P.M.; Cornwell, M.; Hill, J.; Prausnitz, M.R. Precise microinjection into skin using hollow microneedles. *J. Investig. Derm.* **2006**, *126*, 1080–1087. [CrossRef]
53. Bystrova, S.; Luttge, R. Micromolding for ceramic microneedle arrays. *Microelectron. Eng.* **2011**, *88*, 1681–1684. [CrossRef]
54. Ito, Y.; Murano, H.; Hamasaki, N.; Fukushima, K.; Takada, K. Incidence of low bioavailability of leuprolide acetate after percutaneous administration to rats by dissolving microneedles. *Int. J. Pharm.* **2011**, *407*, 126–131. [CrossRef]
55. Noh, Y.W.; Kim, T.H.; Baek, J.S.; Park, H.H.; Lee, S.S.; Han, M.; Shin, S.C.; Cho, C.W. In vitro characterization of the invasiveness of polymer microneedle against skin. *Int. J. Pharm.* **2010**, *397*, 201–205. [CrossRef]
56. Sachdeva, V.; Banga, A.K. Microneedles and their applications. *Recent Pat. Drug Deliv. Formul.* **2011**, *5*, 95–132. [CrossRef]
57. Thakur, R.R.S.; Fallows, S.J.; McMillan, H.L.; Donnelly, R.F.; Jones, D.S. Microneedle-mediated intrascleral delivery of in situ forming thermoresponsive implants for sustained ocular drug delivery. *J. Pharm Pharm. Pharmacol.* **2014**, *66*, 584–595. [CrossRef]
58. Gilger, B.C.; Abarca, E.M.; Salmon, J.H.; Patel, S. Treatment of acute posterior uveitis in a porcine model by injection of triamcinolone acetonide into the suprachoroidal space using microneedles. *Investig. Ophthalmol. Vis. Sci.* **2013**, *54*, 2483–2492. [CrossRef]
59. Patel, S.R.; Lin, A.S.; Edelhauser, H.F.; Prausnitz, M.R. Suprachoroidal drug delivery to the back of the eye using hollow microneedles. *Pharm. Res.* **2011**, *28*, 166–176. [CrossRef]
60. Roxhed, N.; Griss, P.; Stemme, G. Membrane-sealed hollow microneedles and related administration schemes for transdermal drug delivery. *Biomed. Microdevices* **2008**, *10*, 271–279. [CrossRef]
61. Ovsianikov, A.; Chichkov, B.; Mente, P.; Monteiro-Riviere, N.A.; Doraiswamy, A.; Narayan, R.J. Two photon polymerization of polymer–ceramic hybrid materials for transdermal drug delivery. *Int. J. Appl. Ceram Technol.* **2007**, *4*, 22–29. [CrossRef]
62. Sivaraman, A.; Banga, A.K. Novel in situ forming hydrogel microneedles for transdermal drug delivery. *Drug Deliv. Transl. Res.* **2017**, *7*, 16–26. [CrossRef]
63. Khan, S.; Minhas, M.U.; Tekko, I.A.; Donnelly, R.F.; Thakur, R.R.S. Evaluation of microneedles-assisted in situ depot forming poloxamer gels for sustained transdermal drug delivery. *Drug Deliv. Transl. Res.* **2019**, *9*, 764–782. [CrossRef] [PubMed]
64. Leone, M.; van Oorschot, B.H.; Nejadnik, M.R.; Bocchino, A.; Rosato, M.; Kersten, G.; O'Mahony, C.; Bouwstra, J.; van der Maaden, K. Universal applicator for digitally-controlled pressing force and impact velocity insertion of microneedles into skin. *Pharmaceutics* **2018**, *10*, 211. [CrossRef] [PubMed]
65. Sahoo, C.K.; Nayak, P.K.; Sarangi, D.K.; Sahoo, T.K. Intra vaginal drug delivery system: An overview. *Am. J. Adv. Drug Deliv.* **2013**, *1*, 43–55.
66. Ndesendo, V.M.; Pillay, V.; Choonara, Y.E.; Buchmann, E.; Bayever, D.N.; Meyer, L.C. A review of current intravaginal drug delivery approaches employed for the prophylaxis of HIV/AIDS and prevention of sexually transmitted infections. *AAPS Pharmscitech* **2008**, *9*, 505–520. [CrossRef] [PubMed]
67. Hussain, A.; Ahsan, F. The vagina as a route for systemic drug delivery. *J. Control. Release* **2005**, *103*, 301–313. [CrossRef] [PubMed]
68. Taurin, S.; Almomen, A.A.; Pollak, T.; Kim, S.J.; Maxwell, J.; Peterson, C.M.; Owen, S.C.; Janát-Amsbury, M.M. Thermosensitive hydrogels a versatile concept adapted to vaginal drug delivery. *J. Drug Target.* **2018**, *26*, 533–550. [CrossRef] [PubMed]
69. Caramella, C.M.; Rossi, S.; Ferrari, F.; Bonferoni, M.C.; Sandri, G. Mucoadhesive and thermogelling systems for vaginal drug delivery. *Adv. Drug Deliv. Rev.* **2015**, *92*, 39–52. [CrossRef]
70. Ci, T.; Yuan, L.; Bao, X.; Hou, Y.; Wu, H.; Sun, H.; Cao, D.; Ke, X. Development and anti-Candida evaluation of the vaginal delivery system of amphotericin B nanosuspension-loaded thermogel. *J. Drug Target.* **2018**, *26*, 829–839. [CrossRef]
71. Ibrahim, E.S.; Ismail, S.; Fetih, G.; Shaaban, O.; Hassanein, K.; Abdellah, N. Development and characterization of thermosensitive pluronic-based metronidazole in situ gelling formulations for vaginal application. *Acta Pharma.* **2012**, *62*, 59–70. [CrossRef]
72. Xuan, J.-J.; Yan, Y.D.; Oh, D.H.; Choi, Y.K.; Yong, C.S.; Choi, H.G. Development of thermosensitive injectable hydrogel with sustained release of doxorubicin: Rheological characterization and in vivo evaluation in rats. *Drug Deliv.* **2011**, *18*, 305–311. [CrossRef]

73. Hani, U.; Shivakamuar, H.G. Development of miconazole nitrate thermosensitive bioadhesive vaginal gel for vaginal candidiasis. *Am. J. Adv. Drug Deliv.* **2013**, *3*, 358–368.
74. Mei, L.; Chen, J.; Yu, S.; Huang, Y.; Xie, Y.; Wang, H.; Pan, X.; Wu, C. Expansible thermal gelling foam aerosol for vaginal drug delivery. *Drug Deliv.* **2017**, *24*, 1325–1337. [CrossRef] [PubMed]
75. Holland, I.; Logan, J.; Shi, J.; McCormick, C.; Liu, D.; Shu, W. 3D biofabrication for tubular tissue engineering. *Bio-Des. Manuf.* **2018**, *1*, 89–100. [CrossRef] [PubMed]
76. Doğan, A.; Yalvaç, M.E.; Şahin, F.; Kabanov, A.V.; Palotás, A.; Rizvanov, A.A. Differentiation of human stem cells is promoted by amphiphilic pluronic block copolymers. *Int. J. Nanomed.* **2012**, *7*, 4849–4860.
77. Bessa, P.C.; Casal, M.; Reis, R.L. Bone morphogenetic proteins in tissue engineering: The road from laboratory to clinic, part II (BMP delivery). *J. Tissue Eng. Regen. Med.* **2008**, *2*, 81–96. [CrossRef]
78. Gittens, S.A.; Uludag, H. Growth factor delivery for bone tissue engineering. *J. Drug Target.* **2001**, *9*, 407–429. [CrossRef]
79. Han, Q.Q.; Du, Y.; Yang, P.S. The role of small molecules in bone regeneration. *Future Med. Chem.* **2013**, *5*, 1671–1684. [CrossRef]
80. Laurencin, C.T.; Ashe, K.M.; Henry, N.; Kan, H.M.; Lo, K.W.-H. Delivery of small molecules for bone regenerative engineering: Preclinical studies and potential clinical applications. *Drug Discov. Today* **2014**, *19*, 794–800. [CrossRef]
81. Zhang, Y.; Bradley, A.D.; Wang, D.; Reinhardt, R.A. Statins, bone metabolism and treatment of bone catabolic diseases. *Pharm. Res.* **2014**, *88*, 53–61. [CrossRef]
82. Rezazadeh, M.; Parandeh, M.; Akbari, V.; Ebrahimi, Z.; Taheri, A. Incorporation of rosuvastatin-loaded chitosan/chondroitin sulfate nanoparticles into a thermosensitive hydrogel for bone tissue engineering: Preparation, characterization, and cellular behavior. *Pharm. Dev. Technol.* **2019**, *24*, 357–367. [CrossRef]
83. Muzzarelli, R.A.; Greco, F.; Busilacchi, A.; Sollazzo, V.; Gigante, A. Chitosan, hyaluronan and chondroitin sulfate in tissue engineering for cartilage regeneration: A review. *Carbohydr. Polym.* **2012**, *89*, 723–739. [CrossRef] [PubMed]
84. Temofeew, A.; Hixon, K.R.; McBride-Gagyi, S.H.; Scott, A. Sell The fabrication of cryogel scaffolds incorporated with poloxamer 407 for potential use in the regeneration of the nucleus pulposus. *J. Mater. Sci. Mater. Med.* **2017**, *28*, 36–47. [CrossRef] [PubMed]
85. Pattappa, G.; Li, Z.; Peroglio, M.; Wismer, N.; Alini, M.; Grad, S. Diversity of intervertebral disc cells: Phenoztype and function. *J. Anat.* **2012**, *221*, 480–496. [CrossRef] [PubMed]
86. Suntornnond, R.; An, J.; Chua, C.K. Bioprinting of Thermoresponsive Hydrogels for Next Generation Tissue Engineering: A Review. *Macromol. Mater. Eng.* **2017**, *302*, 1600266. [CrossRef]
87. Chung, J.H.; Naficy, S.; Yue, Z.; Kapsa, R.; Quigley, A.; Moulton, S.E.; Wallace, G.G. Bio-ink properties and printability for extrusion printing living cells. *Biomater. Sci.* **2013**, *1*, 763. [CrossRef]
88. Nicmodeus, G.D.; Bryant, S.J. Cell encapsulation in biodegradable hydrogels for tissue engineering applications. *Tissue Eng Part B Rev.* **2008**, *14*, 149–165.
89. Kolesky, D.B.; Truby, R.L.; Gladman, A.S.; Busbee, T.A.; Homan, K.A.; Lewis, J.A. 3D Bioprinting of Vascularized, Heterogeneous Cell-Laden Tissue Constructs. *Adv. Mater.* **2013**, *25*, 3124–3130. [CrossRef]
90. Hospodiuk, M.; Dey, M.; Sosnoski, D.; Ozbolat, I.T. The bioink: A comprehensive review on bioprintable materials. *Biotechnol. Adv.* **2017**, *35*, 217–239. [CrossRef]
91. Aliabadi, H.M.; Lavasanifar, A. Polymeric micelles for drug delivery. *Expert Opin. Drug Deliv.* **2006**, *3*, 139–162. [CrossRef]
92. Kabanov, A.V.; Lemieux, P.; Vinogradov, S.; Alakhov, V. Pluronic block copolymers: Novel functional molecules for gene therapy. *Adv. Drug Deliv. Rev.* **2002**, *54*, 223–233. [CrossRef]
93. Anderson, R.A. Micelle formation by oxyethylene-oxypropylene polymers. *Pharm. Acta Helv.* **1972**, *47*, 304–308. [PubMed]
94. Rey-Rico, A.; Cucchiarini, M. Controlled release strategies for raav-mediated gene delivery. *Acta Biomater.* **2016**, *29*, 1–10. [CrossRef] [PubMed]
95. Niidome, T.; Huang, L. Gene therapy progress and prospects: Nonviral vectors. *Gene Ther.* **2002**, *9*, 1647–1652. [CrossRef] [PubMed]
96. Rey-Rico, A.; Cucchiarini, M. Recent tissue engineering-based advances for effective rAAV-mediated gene transfer in the musculoskeletal system. *Bioengineered* **2016**, *7*, 175–188. [CrossRef]

97. De Laporte, L.; Cruz Rea, J.; Shea, L.D. Design of modular non-viral gene therapy vectors. *Biomaterials* **2006**, *27*, 947–954. [CrossRef]
98. Wang, W.; Li, W.; Ma, N.; Steinhoff, G. Non-viral gene delivery methods. *Curr. Pharm. Biotechnol.* **2013**, *14*, 46–60.
99. Cucchiarini, M.; Madry, H. Gene therapy for cartilage defects. *J. Gene Med.* **2005**, *7*, 1495–1509. [CrossRef]
100. Madry, H.; Cucchiarini, M. Advances and challenges in gene-based approaches for osteoarthritis. *J. Gene Med.* **2013**, *15*, 343–355. [CrossRef]
101. Johnstone, B.; Alini, M.; Cucchiarini, M.; Dodge, G.R.; Eglin, D.; Guilak, F.; Madry, H.; Mata, A.; Mauck, R.L.; Semino, C.E.; et al. Tissue engineering for articular cartilage repair—The state of the art. *Eur. Cell Mater.* **2013**, *25*, 248–267. [CrossRef]
102. Rey-Rico, A.; Venkatesan, J.K.; Frisch, J.; Rial-Hermida, I.; Schmitt, G.; Concheiro, A.; Madry, H.; Alvarez-Lorenzo, C.; Cucchiarini, M. PEO–PPO–PEO micelles as effective rAAV-mediated gene delivery systems to target human mesenchymal stem cells without altering their differentiation potency. *Acta Biomater.* **2015**, *27*, 42–52. [CrossRef]
103. Höfig, I.; Atkinson, M.J.; Mall, S.; Krackhardt, A.M.; Thirion, C.; Anastasov, N. Poloxamer synperonic F108 improves cellular transduction with lentiviral vectors. *J. Gene Med.* **2012**, *14*, 549–560. [CrossRef] [PubMed]
104. Millington, M.; Aendt, A.; Boyd, M.; Applegate, T.; Shen, S. Towards a clinically relevant lentiviral transduction protocol for primary human CD34 haematopoietic stem/progenitor cells. *PLoS ONE* **2009**, *4*, 6461. [CrossRef] [PubMed]
105. Birmingham, A.; Anderson, E.; Sullivan, K.; Reynolds, A.; Boese, Q.; Leake, D.; Karpilow, J.; Khvorova, A. A protocol for designing siRNAs with high functionality and specificity. *Nat. Protoc.* **2007**, *9*, 2068–2078. [CrossRef] [PubMed]
106. Takahashi, K.; Tanabe, K.; Ohnuki, M.; Narita, M.; Ichisaka, T.; Tomoda, K.; Yamanaka, S. Induction of pluripotent stem cells from adult human fibroblasts by defined factors. *Cell* **2007**, *131*, 861–872. [CrossRef] [PubMed]
107. Alvarez-Lorenzo, C.; Rey-Rico, A.; Sosnik, A.; Taboada, P.; Concheiro, A. Poloxamine-based nanomaterials for drug delivery. *Front. Biosci.* **2012**, *337*, 303–305. [CrossRef] [PubMed]
108. Chitgupi, U.; Nyayapathi, N.; Kim, J.; Wang, D.; Sun, B.; Li, C.; Carter, K.; Huang, W.C.; Kim, C.; Xia, J.; et al. Surfactant-Stripped Micelles for NIR-II Photoacoustic Imaging through 12 cm of Breast Tissue and Whole Human Breasts. *Adv. Mater.* **2019**, *31*, 1–10. [CrossRef]
109. Sousa, C.; Gouveia, L.F.; Kreutzer, B.; Silva-Lima, B.; Maphasa, R.E.; Dube, A.; Videira, M. Polymeric Micellar Formulation Enhances Antimicrobial and Anticancer Properties of Salinomycin. *Pharm. Res.* **2019**, *36*, 83. [CrossRef]
110. Naujokat, C.; Steinhart, R. Salinomycin as a drug for targeting human cancer stem cells. *J. Biomed. Biotechnol.* **2012**, *20*, 44–46. [CrossRef]
111. Steel, G.G.; Peckham, M.J. Exploitable Mechanisms in Combined Radiotherapy-Chemotherapy: The Concept of Additivity. *Int. J. Radiat. Oncol. Biol. Phys.* **1979**, *5*, 85–91. [CrossRef]
112. Seiwert, T.Y.; Salama, J.K.; Vokes, E.E. The Concurrent Chemoradiation Paradigm—General Principles. *Nat. Rev. Clin. Oncol.* **2007**, *4*, 86–100. [CrossRef]
113. DuRoss, A.N.; Neufeld, M.J.; Landry, M.R.; Rosch, J.G.; Eaton, C.T.; Sahay, G.; Thomas, C.R., Jr.; Sun, C. Micellar Formulation of Talazoparib and Buparlisib for Enhanced DNA Damage in Breast Cancer Chemoradiotherapy. *ACS Appl. Mater. Interfaces* **2019**, *11*, 12342–12356. [CrossRef] [PubMed]
114. Fessi, H.; Puisieux, F.; Devissaguet, J.P.; Ammoury, N.; Benita, S. Nanocapsule Formation by Interfacial Polymer Deposition Following Solvent Displacement. *Int. J. Pharm.* **1989**, *55*, R1–R4. [CrossRef]

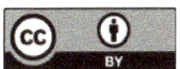

© 2019 by the authors. Licensee MDPI, Basel, Switzerland. This article is an open access article distributed under the terms and conditions of the Creative Commons Attribution (CC BY) license (http://creativecommons.org/licenses/by/4.0/).

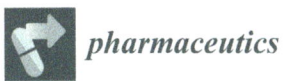

Review
Poloxamer Hydrogels for Biomedical Applications

Eleonora Russo * and Carla Villa

Department of Pharmacy, University of Genoa, Viale Benedetto XV, 16132 Genova, Italy; villa@difar.unige.it
* Correspondence: russo@difar.unige.it

Received: 31 October 2019; Accepted: 6 December 2019; Published: 10 December 2019

Abstract: This review article focuses on thermoresponsive hydrogels consisting of poloxamers which are of high interest for biomedical application especially in drug delivery for ophthalmic, injectable, transdermal, and vaginal administration. These hydrogels remain fluid at room temperature but become more viscous gel once they are exposed to body temperature. In this way, the gelling system remains at the topical level for a long time and the drug release is controlled and prolonged. Poloxamers are synthetic triblock copolymers of poly(ethylene oxide)-b-poly(propylene oxide)-b-poly(ethylene oxide) (PEO-PPO-PEO), also commercially known as Pluronics®, Synperonics® or Lutrol®. The different poloxamers cover a range of liquids, pastes, and solids, with molecular weights and ethylene oxide–propylene oxide weight ratios varying from 1100 to 14,000 and 1:9 to 8:2, respectively. Concentrated aqueous solutions of poloxamers form thermoreversible gels. In recent years this type of gel has arouse interest for tissue engineering. Finally, the use of poloxamers as biosurfactants is evaluated since they are able to form micelles in an aqueous environment above a concentration threshold known as critical micelle concentration (CMC). This property is exploited for drug delivery and different therapeutic applications.

Keywords: poloxamer; hydrogels; micelle; thermosensitive; biomedical; copolymer

---

1. Introduction

The word "hydrogel", according to Lee, Kwon and Park is due to an article published in 1894, but the first crosslinked network material that appeared in literature and that has been described by its typical hydrogel properties, was a polyhydroxyethylmethacrylate (HEMA) hydrogel developed much later, in 1960, by O. Wichterle and D. Lim, with the aim of using it in permanent contact applications with human tissues, i.e., as soft contact lenses [1].

Since then, hydrogels have been used as systems for drug controlled delivery, to facilitate the localized, sustained and prolonged release of a drug, thereby decreasing the number of administrations, avoiding side effects and following low doses [2].

The most widely studied environmentally responsive systems were temperature sensitive hydrogels, in which physical entanglements, hydrogen bonding, and hydrophobic interactions are the main features that constitute the crosslinks. Two different types of thermo-sensitive hydrogels exist that undergo gelation either by cooling below the upper critical gelation temperature (UCGT) or by heating above the lower critical gelation temperature (LCGT), respectively. Hydrogels with LCGT behavior and sol-to-gel transition at 37 °C have gained increasing attention in the biomedical field as carriers for cells, drugs, and biomolecules, since they allow encapsulation in mild conditions (temperature ≤ 37°C) [3].

Poloxamers and poloxamines are examples of these LCGT biocompatible thermoreversible hydrogels that were introduced in the 1950s by BASF (Iselin, NJ, USA) when they started being used for detergent development, but also in other areas, like agriculture, food, and paints [4].

Poloxamers or Pluronics® are a class of water-soluble nonionic triblock copolymers formed by polar (poly ethylene oxide) and non-polar (poly propylene oxide) blocks. which confer amphiphilic and surface active properties to the polymers. Their aqueous solutions undergo sol-to-gel transition with increasing the temperature above a LCGT; moreover, the coexistence of hydrophilic and hydrophobic monomers into block copolymers allows the formation of ordered structures in solution, the most common of these being the micelles. The formation of micelles in solution is a reversible and dynamic process useful for encapsulating hydrophobic drugs and delivering them into an aqueous environment.

They can be considered as smart polymers, for their stimuli-sensitive properties, due to the different behaviors of these polymers since they can modify their structure in function of pH, temperature and salt concentration [5]. For this reason, a variety of Pluronics is available on the market, differing for the molecular weight of the building blocks and for the hydrophobic–hydrophilic ratio, allowing the preparation of thermosensitive hydrogels with different properties, e.g., in terms of critical gelation concentration (CGC) and gelation time at physiological condition [3].

Thus, poloxamers represent a convenient choice in pharmaceutical technology and biomedical area due to their commercial availability, wide range of molecular weights, peculiar behavior and flexibility. Poloxamers are FDA approved and listed in the US and European Pharmacopoeia; they are non-toxic and non-irritant therefore they can be used as solubilizer, emulsifier, stabilizer, and administered through oral, parenteral, topical routes. As wetting agents, they are useful in ointments, suppository bases, and gels [6].

Poloxamer hydrogels use in drug release appeared at the beginning of the 1970s; they were a response in the search for new safer and faster treatments for the delivery of highly-effective therapeutic agents to a target cell, even if they have poor mechanical properties such as low tensile strength and low Young's modulus that limit their practical applications, sometimes even as medical device coatings [7].

Analysis of recent literature covering a range of treatment pathways and diseases, reveals a major emphasis on "smart" drug carriers developed with poloxamers. The different range of potential delivery methods is highlighted in this review by discussing how the poloxamer solution behavior enables multiple formulation processing routes, drug-encapsulating structures, and engagement with physiological barriers to drug passage.

The first research work concerned the treatment of thermal burns [8] followed by researches on the release of hormones [9], tetracycline [10], proteins [11], and more recently for norcantharidin delivery [12], heparin [13], and anti-HIV drugs [14]. In the last twenty years the numbers of papers related to poloxamer hydrogels for biomedical applications is exponentially increased (Figure 1).

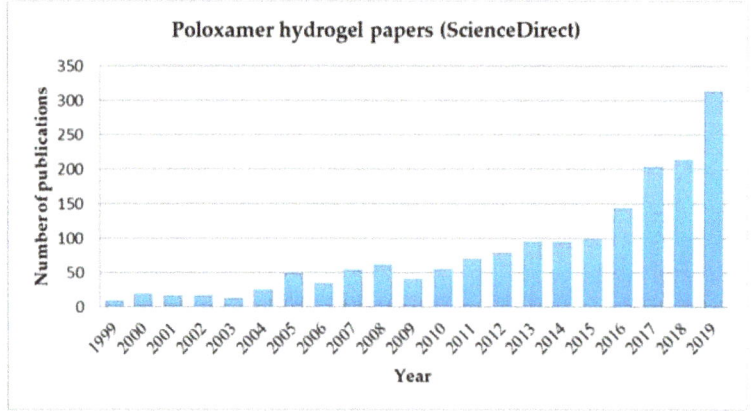

Figure 1. Histogram showing the increase in publications related to the keywords "poloxamer hydrogel" in Science Direct database during the past twenty years.

More recently such hydrogels have become especially attractive to the new field of "tissue engineering" as matrices for repairing and regenerating a wide variety of tissues and organs [15].

They have been successfully employed as scaffold-forming materials for cell printing technology, a computer-aided tissue engineering technology based on the layered deposition of cellularized hydrogels to form complex 3D constructs [16–18].

In this review the poloxamer hydrogels will be taken into consideration, giving an overview of their use as drug delivery systems (DDS) in different routes of administration, especially ophthalmic, transdermal, and vaginal ones. Finally, this paper focused on their potential in tissue and membrane regeneration, in the field of biomedical engineering and their application as micellar systems for gene delivery and cancer therapy.

2. Poloxamers

2.1. Poloxamers Properties

These polymers are synthetic triblock copolymers of poly(ethylene oxide)-b-poly(propylene oxide)-b-poly(ethylene oxide) (PEO-PPO-PEO) (Figure 2).

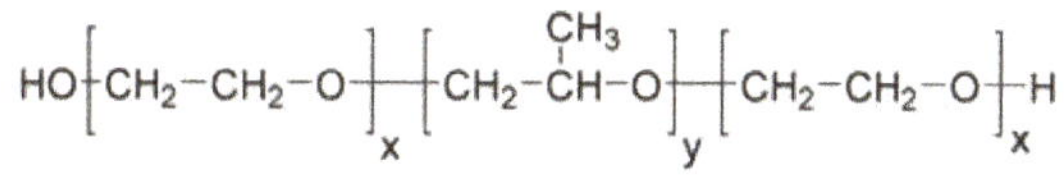

$$HO\text{-}[CH_2\text{-}CH_2\text{-}O]_x\text{-}[CH_2\text{-}CH(CH_3)\text{-}O]_y\text{-}[CH_2\text{-}CH_2\text{-}O]_x\text{-}H$$

Figure 2. Chemical formula for poloxamers: x and y are the lengths of PEO and PPO: poly(ethylene oxide) and poly(propylene oxide) chains, respectively.

They are synthesized through the sequential addition of PO and EO monomers in the presence of an alkaline catalyst, such as sodium or potassium hydroxide, obtaining different copolymers with a different number of hydrophilic EO and hydrophobic PO units, which are also characterized by their distinct hydrophilic–lipophilic balance (HLB) value. Changes in the copolymer composition (PPO/PEO ratio) and molecular weight (PEO and PPO block length) during synthesis leads to macromolecular surface active agents with specific properties suitable in various technological areas.

Poloxamers appear in the form of liquids, pastes, and solids, depending on their molecular weights varying from 1100 to 14,000, offering a pool of more than 50 amphiphilic, water-soluble and polymorphic materials. Their water solubility is subjected by different ratio (1:9 to 8:2) between the chain of propylene oxide (PO) and ethylene oxide (EO) with hydrophobic and hydrophilic behavior, respectively [16]. These differences also alter the in vivo properties and interactions with cells and cell membranes, and provides high potential for the design of innovative nanomedicines and new biomaterials.

Poloxamers were the first block copolymers produced for industrial purposes, synthesized by Wyandotte Chemical Corporation in the late 1940s. Today they are commercially known by the trade names Pluronics®, Lutrol®, Kolliphor® (BASF), Antarox® (Rhodia), and Synperonics® (Croda).

The original manufacturer BASF introduced a specific nomenclature for Pluronics consisting of a letter indicating the morphism of each copolymer: L (for liquid), P (for paste) or F (for flakes) followed by a number referring to the molecular weight of the PPO block (the first one or two) and the weight fraction of the PEO block (the last one).

For example, P123 and F127 have the same molecular weight of PPO (in the order of 4000) but P123 has 30% of PEO and F127 70% of PEO [17].

The physicochemical characteristics and applications of Poloxamers were firstly reviewed extensively by Alexandridis and Hatton in 1995 [16]. In Figure 3, a 3D poloxamer modified pluronic grid showing the distribution of different copolymers, gathered according their physical state, is reported.

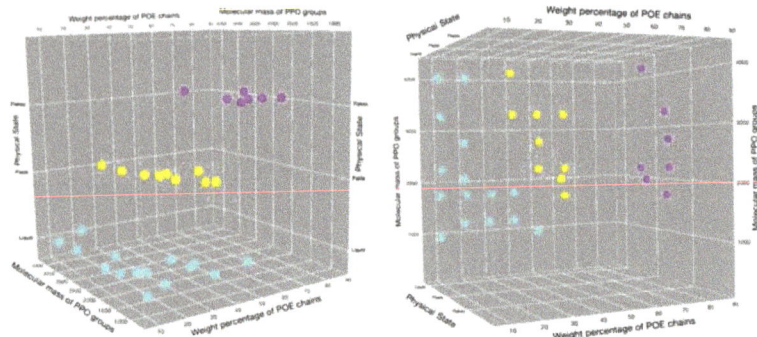

Figure 3. Poloxamers 3D distribution according to physical state (solid flakes = magenta; paste = yellow; liquid = blue), weight percentage of POE chains and molecular mass of the PPO groups (adapted from [16]).

The most significant physical properties of most common poloxamers, are reported in Table 1: average molecular weight, melting point expressed in °C, viscosity (Pa·s) measured at 25 °C, 60 °C, and 50 °C for pastes, liquids, and solids, respectively, surface tension at 0.1% at 25 °C (dyn cm^{-1}), hydrophilic–lipophilic balance (HLB) [4,17,19,20].

Table 1. Properties of the most common poloxamer poly(ethylene oxide)-b-poly(propylene oxide)-b-poly(ethylene oxide) (PEO-PPO-PEO) copolymers.

Poloxamer	Pluronic	PEO%	Average Molecular Weight	Melting Point (°C)	Viscosity (Pa·s)	Surface Tension (dyn cm^{-1})	HLB
P105	L35	50	1900	7	0.375	49	18–23
P108	F38	80	4700	48	0.260	52	>24
P122	L42	20	1630	−26	0.280	46	7–12
P123	L43	30	1850	−1	0.310	47	7–12
P124	L44	40	2200	16	0.440	45	12–18
P182	L62	20	2500	−4	0.450	43	1–7
P183	L63	30	2650	10	0.490	43	7–12
P184	L64	40	2900	16	0.850	43	12–18
P185	P65	50	3400	27	0.180	46	12–18
P188	F68	80	8400	52	1.000	50	>24
P212	L72	20	2750	−7	0.510	39	1–7
P215	P75	50	4150	27	0.250	43	12–18
P217	F77	70	6600	48	0.480	47	>24
P234	P84	40	4200	34	0.280	42	12–18
P235	P85	50	4600	34	0.310	42	12–18
P237	F87	70	7700	49	0.700	44	>24
P238	F88	80	11,400	54	2.300	48	>24
P288	F98	80	13,000	58	2.700	43	>24
P333	P103	30	4950	30	0.285	34	7–12
P334	P104	40	5900	32	0.390	33	12–18
P335	P105	50	6500	35	0.750	39	12–18
P338	F108	80	14,600	57	2.800	41	>24
P402	L122	20	5000	20	1.750	33	1–7
P403	P123	30	5750	31	0.350	34	7–12
P407	F127	70	12600	56	3.100	41	18–23

Commonly used poloxamers include P188 (F-68 grade), P237 (F-87 grade), P338 (F-108 grade), and P407 (F-127 grade) types, which are freely soluble in water.

2.2. Poloxamers Behavior

The aqueous solution properties of poloxamers have been intensely studied and thoroughly reviewed owing to their unique behavior and benefit to myriad applications.

In water solutions, the amphiphilic character of copolymers lead the macromolecule to self-aggregate into micelles with an inner core constituted by hydrophobic blocks and an outer shell constituted by hydrophilic units. They are nano-sized structures, normally between 10 and 200 nm that appears at the critical micellization concentration (CMC) and at critical micellization temperature (CMT). CMC value of poloxamer aqueous solutions decreases with increasing temperature and number of PEO segments, indicating that polymers with a larger hydrophobic (PPO) domain form micelles at lower concentrations and temperatures [21].

Poloxamer water solutions exhibit temperature sensitivity, in particular a "thermoreversible gelation" [21] for sufficiently concentrated samples; they show a sol-gel transition around 37 °C (physiological temperature) and gel-sol transition around 50 °C, being able to produce thermoreversible gels, some already approved by the Food and Drug Administration, which present great interest in food additives, drug delivery carriers in cosmetics, pharmaceutical ingredients, and tissue engineering [5,17]

Several mechanisms have been proposed for this behavior, the first one was related to the gel transition that was due to changes in micellar properties (Figure 4).

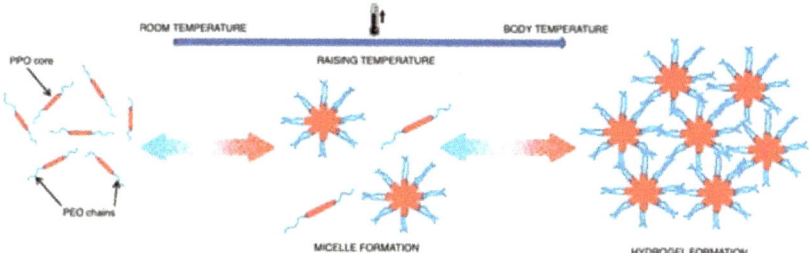

Figure 4. Schematic representation for hydrogel formation.

Thanks to their core–shell architecture, the hydrophobic core can act as a drug-loading site, creating a space for the encapsulation of hydrophobic drugs through the establishment of physical or chemical interactions. The properties of the outer shell and inner core have an influence in the drug release, that can promote an easier or sustained release of the drug. Due the properties above mentioned, polymeric micelles can transport several drugs, improving the circulation time, as well as the enhanced permeability and retention effect. Moreover, these systems exhibit low-risk of chronic toxicity since the polymeric micelles are disassembled in vivo, in single polymer chains that can be excreted by kidneys.

In order to prepare polymeric micelles for drug encapsulation, different methods can be used, however, the more common are the direct dissolution, dialysis, evaporation or film method, freeze-drying, microphase separation, and the oil-in-water emulsion [22].

The method depends, mostly, on the solubility of the copolymer and the drug in an aqueous medium. Some other aspects are also important to an efficient drug incorporation, such as copolymer characteristics, molecular weight and HLB. The structural and chemical characterization of polymeric micelles are important features to take into account in the development of these nanocarriers, since they have a direct influence on the efficiency of these drug release forms, in terms of size, polydispersion index, zeta potential, encapsulation efficiency (EE), and drug loading capacity (DL) [23].

Other researchers [24] discussed gelation as a function of thermodynamical parameters. The enthalpy of gelation depends on CMC and temperature, the value change in the case of poloxamers gelation is unfavorable unlike the gelatine gelation where a great enthalpy change occurred.

The useful concentration for gel formation is the same as for poloxamers with the same PPO/PEO ratio and it decreases with the increasing of polymer molecular weight, denoting the significance of this parameter. While the presence of electrolytes reduces gel transition temperature, enthalpy of gel formation is not significantly changed by the addition of other substances. This behavior suggests that entropy plays the major role in the gelation process.

For all these behaviors, the poloxamers were used for the study and for the development of innovative pharmaceutical forms in different administration routes.

3. Drug Delivery Systems (DDS)

Poloxamer sol-gel reversible hydrogels have attracted the attention for practical biomedical and pharmaceutical applications because of constituents solubility, biocompatibility with biological systems and easy administration of pharmaceutical formulations. The pharmaceutical and biomedical fields covered by the use of poloxamers including solubilization of hydrophobic drugs, controlled release, biomacromolecule delivery (e.g., proteins and genes) and tissue engineering.

Most applications involve the use of Poloxamer P407 and include delivery of protein/peptide drugs [25], such as insulin [26], interleukin-2 [27], epidermal growth factor [28], bone morphogenic protein [29], fibroblastic growth factor, and endothelial cell growth factor [30].

In recent years these hydrogels have been used as carriers for most routes of administration, the most interesting are discussed below.

3.1. Poloxamers for Oftalmic Administration

The thermoreversible gels have shown a growing interest at ocular level because they combine peculiar characteristics: i.e., the formulation when applied is sol (it performs like eye drops) and becomes gel with body temperature (it performs like ointment) increasing the in situ residence time.

The most well-known ocular drug delivery system is eye drops, but they have a short residence time because they are quickly drained through the nasolacrimal route resulting in frequent dosage regimen which leads to an increase in side effects and poor patient compliance.

Poloxamers P407 and P188 are among the most commonly used in this case for their good water solubility, solution clearness, optimal viscosity, and ocular tissue safety.

Recent works have focused on the best formulation to obtain a hydrogel with useful features for ocular administration and without toxicity. About this point Al Khateb et al. [31] studied two formulations containing poloxamers, i.e., P407 and P188, with different gelation properties depending on concentration solutions and the ratio of their mixtures. Transparent gels were obtained only in the case of 20% w/w P407 and P188 solutions. Furthermore, these preparations were non-toxic or irritating to the corneal mucosa and then suitable for application in ocular drug delivery.

Fathalla Z.M.A. et al. [32] studied the blend of the same two poloxamers for a controlled ocular delivery of ketorolac tromethamine (KT). The most promising gel formulations, loaded with KT, were those containing the mixtures of P407:P188 23:10 w/v% and 23:15 w/v% respectively. These gels do not present toxicity and do not irritate the conjunctiva and cornea.

In recent years other polymers have been added to poloxamers-based gels to obtain different drug release characteristics and to modify the rheological properties.

Among these works, Yu et al. [33] has to be remembered for the synthesis of a cross-linked hydrogel system containing carboxymethyl chitosan (CMC) and poloxamer P407, where the presence of CMC with biological properties could improve hydrogel biocompatibility. This formulation, containing nepafenac (NP) as a model drug, showed good rheological properties at gelation temperature (32–33 °C) and a sustained release of NP from hydrogel, so as to be considered a pH–temperature-responsive ophthalmic drug delivery system.

Another approach, with good results, involved the introduction of various colloidal carrier systems to easily load poorly soluble drugs into poloxamers hydrogels.

Lou et al. [34] incorporated curcumin-loaded albumin nanoparticles into a hydrogel based on a mixture of P407/P188 for local ocular administration, to treat diabetic retinopathy. This formulation, which became a gel when exposed to eye temperature, may be applied as eye drops. Nanoparticles provided the sustained drug release while the presence of hydrogel prolonged the in situ residence time.

Finally, Almeda et al. [35] reported the combination of lipid nanoparticles and a thermoresponsive polymer with mucomimetic properties (poloxamer P407). The incorporated nanoparticles showed an average size below 200 nm, a good positive zeta potential and an efficiency of ibuprofen encapsulation of about 90%. The optimal poloxamer concentration in thermoreversible gel was 15% (w/w) Pluronic® F-127. The formulation did not present a relevant cytotoxicity and showed a sustained release of ibuprofen over several hours. The strategy proposed in this work can be successfully applied to increase bioavailability and therapeutic efficacy of conventional eyedrops.

3.2. Poloxamers for Transdermal Administration

Transdermal drug delivery is a valid alternative to the oral and parenteral route because it offers several advantages: Avoidance the hepatic first pass, good compliance by the patient, and easy access. The most studied formulations for this route contained poloxamer P407, as a polymer, and as drugs those with anti-inflammatory [36,37], analgesic [38], local anesthetic [39], and cardiac [40,41] activity, rarely are present preparations containing big molecules such as arginine, vasopressin, and insulin [42,43].

Generally in these topical preparations it is necessary to introduce an enhancer substance which is able to facilitate the passage through the stratum corneum (thickness of 10 to 15 µm) which is the main barrier to drug penetration.

In the last decade the penetration enhancers have been replaced by the microneedles (MNs) that have the capacity to permeate the stratum corneum and infuse the active ingredient in the deep areas of the skin.

Microneedles are needles similar to the ones useful for hypodermic injections but they present different sizes: from 1–100 microns in length and 1 micron in diameter (Figure 5). They are manufactured with silicon [44,45], metals such as stainless steel, palladium, nickel and titanium [46–48], carbohydrates including galactose, maltose, and polysaccharide [19–51], glass [52], ceramics [53], and various other polymers [54,55]. MNs are fabricated in backing that can be applied to the substrate like a patch carrying different drugs by penetrating through the skin, mucosal tissue and sclera [56–59]. Their dissolution has to be taken into consideration because it can influence drug delivery [60,61].

One of the most recent researches regards sol-gel transition property of poloxamers to obtain in situ forming hydrogel microneedles, for the delivery of methotrexate to treat solid tumors [62]. The use of this drug by transdermal route is generally limited by its relatively high molecular weight and hydrophilicity. For this purpose four formulations were prepared with two different methotrexate concentrations (0.2% and 0.4% w/w) with poloxamer P407 (20% w/w) and without, using the last one as a control, replacing the polymer with deionized water. In this study, it was confirmed the sol-gel transition of the formulations at skin temperature (32 °C), maintaining skin barrier function and skin viscoelastic properties after administration of the formulations. In vitro drug diffusion studies, using a Franz cell, showed that the formulations containing methotrexate (0.2% and 0.4%) without P407 released overall drug after 22 and 35 h respectively, while the one with P407 after 72 h. For this reason it is possible to conclude that the poloxamer-based formulations provided a steady and sustained delivery.

In an even more recent work, the formation of depots of thermoreversible poloxamers in skin micropores using MNs to transdermal drug delivery has been reported for the first time [63]. Sodium fluorescein (FS) was used as model drug to study in vitro permeation at different concentrations. In order to crate pores into the skin and to overcome the stratum corneum MNs have been used, then the drug loaded poloxamer solution was applied to fill pores, subsequently an in situ gelation at skin temperature of 32 °C occurred.

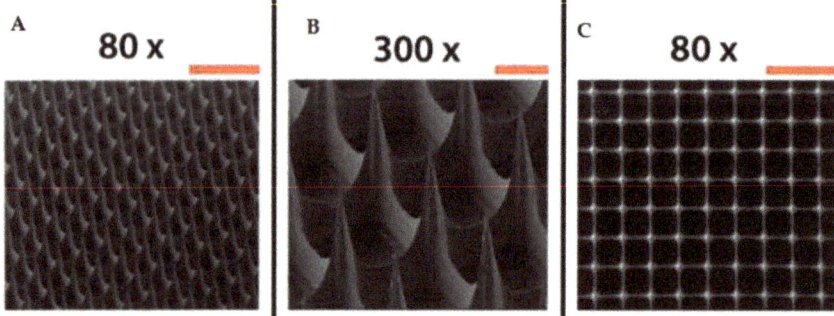

Figure 5. Scanning electron microscopy images of microneedle arrays imaged from a lateral view (**A,B**) and from the top side (**C**). Scale bars represent 500 μm (80×) (**A,C**) and 100 μm (300×) (**B**) (adapted from [64]).

For this goal poloxamers P407, P237, and P338 were used at different concentrations (from 15 to 30% w/w in water) loading different amounts of fluorescein.

The formulations were characterized for their rheological properties and in situ gel formation. The distribution of FS in skin tissue was tracked by confocal laser microscopic analysis with higher intensity of FS in MN-treated skin tissues. The in vitro fluorescein release studies were carried out using vertical Franz diffusion cells. The release profiles indicated that the concentration of fluorescein (0.1%, 0.3%, and 0.5% w/w) was a variable parameter that significantly affects drug release as well as the type of poloxamer used. In particular P338 and P237 0.1–0.3% FS-loaded formulations provided a total drug release during 16 h while 0.5% FS-loaded provided a release for 20 h. Moreover, for a longer time (about 24 h), the release from P407 formulations was comparable. All the poloxamers depots started dissolving according to the dominant hydrophilic interactions and gels did not remain intact. It was concluded that P407 provided the best release for a longer duration and it was selected as the best drug delivery for in vitro permeation assays. These studies confirmed that drug loading is not a limitation and permeation of FS after MN treatment was found in more controlled manner and for a long time when compared to a permeation across untreated skin sample.

3.3. Poloxamers for Vaginal Administration

Another interesting pathway exploited in drug delivery systems is the vaginal route, allowing both the systemic and local absorption of drugs poorly absorbed after oral administration [65–67]. The vagina has a vast network of blood vessels that make easy the systemic absorption, avoiding deactivation at gastrointestinal level and hepatic first pass. Mucoadhesive pharmaceutical forms have been studied for this district due to the presence of mucus which increases permeability. The thermoreversible systems, appropriately modified with polymers that promote mucoadhesion, allow to obtain a sustained drug release and a good bioavailability without altering the vaginal physiology [68].

After application of poloxamers for vaginal administration occurring gelation favored a long permanence of drugs on the administration site to promote a drug controlled release [69]. Vaginal drug delivery is based on the exploitation of polymers which are able not only to gelify at physiological temperature but also to adhere to the vaginal mucosa improving the in situ residence time.

A brief description of recent reports in the literature, based on poloxamer formulations by vaginal route, is given below.

In the first work [70] the authors investigated a novel amphotericin B (AmB) release system in the form of nanosuspension loaded into a poloxamer P407/P188 hydrogel. P407 (20% w/w) and P188 (5% w/w) were dissolved in AmB nanosuspension, the AmB NPs thermogel were characterized regarding nanoparticle features (particle size, zeta potential, morphology) and gel behavior (rheology, stability, in vitro drug release, and in vitro and in vivo anti-Candida efficiency). The nanosuspension-gel combination has been necessary because nanoparticles alone tended to aggregate while they were more stable in the poloxamer hydrogel. When compared with other biodegradable thermosensitive hydrogel, such as polyester-based gels, poloxamer were not capable of an in vivo degradation. This property is really suitable for vaginal delivery because it means grater safety in use. Another very important element in the development of vaginal formulations was mucoadhesion; poloxamers have lower adhesion properties compared to compounds such as Carbopol, the addition of some bioadhesive materials into P407/P188 thermogel would be a feasible path [71–73]. Finally, the in vivo anti-Candida assay showed a better antifungal efficiency of AmB in the thermoreversible gel when compared with commercial effervescent tablets at the same drug dose (2.5 mg/Kg).

A second paper [74] described a novel vaginal delivery strategy consisting of two pharmaceutical forms placed together to give an expansible thermal gelling aerosol foam (ETGFA) that combined the advantages of foam and gel penetration and carrier retention in vaginal canal, respectively.

ETGA was prepared adding an optimized amount of P407 (18–22% w/w) and P188 (0–5% w/w), achieved by evaluating the gelation temperature, the adhesive agents (arabic gum, sodium carboxymethyl cellulose, sodium alginate, and xanthan gum) and silver nanoparticles to obtain a drug concentration of 1% w/w. To study a better performance in foam expansion and duration, propane/butane 80/20 v/v and dimethyl ether were compared as propellants. The formulation was characterized in regards of rheology, foam expansion, adhesiveness and drug release. ETGA showed a better extended drug release (over 4 h) dose –dependent antimicrobial effects on the vaginal flora and no tissue irritation when compared to a commercial antimicrobial gel. These results indicated that ETGA could be a suitable formulation for vaginal drug delivery.

4. Tissue Regeneration Scaffolders

Tissue engineering, in this last decade, has emerged in the biomedical field because it allows researchers to create specific devices that represent in vivo tissues that can be replaced or increased to address current therapeutic challenges [75].

Poloxamers have received special attention for tissue regeneration based on their biocompatibility, low cytotoxicity, and good rheological properties [76].

In particular, the area the most explored deals with regeneration of bone tissue. The use of growth factors such as bone morphogenetic protein-2 (BMP-2) for bone repair has been reported [77,78] but it is very expensive and easily loose its integrity. Recently, other compounds that have received interest were statins because they altered bone metabolism through different mechanisms [79–81]. Their bioavailability after oral administration was low and a real bone healing cannot be expected. For this reason different delivery systems for local delivery of statins have been evaluated. The study of incorporation of rosuvastatin (RSV)-loaded chitosan/chondroitin sulfate nanoparticles into a thermosensitive hydrogel is reported below [82]. At first this research considered nanoparticles preparation and optimization, thereafter it dealt with the characterization of thermosensible hydrogels.

Gel formulation consisted of poloxamer P407 (18–20% w/v), hyaluronic acid (HA) 1–3% w/v and hydroxypropyl methylcellulose (2% w/v) to stabilize the formulation itself.

HA [83] and P407 had also positive effects on articular cartilage, simulating the regenerative process within the joint. The study showed that gel provided a low viscosity at 4 °C and gelification at 35 °C; drug release from nanoparticles, inserted into the hydrogel, was around 60% after 48 h, while it was completely released from nanoparticles alone within 12 h. This behavior indicated that the drug release was controlled and sustained.

Moreover, the hydrogel formulation showed an improvement in osteoblast viability and proliferation due to the used polymer and the biological properties of the nanoparticle delivery system.

Another paper [84] reported the design of a cryogel scaffold for the regeneration of an intervertebral disc tissue (nucleus pulposus NP). NP is located inside the vertebral discs and has the function of absorbing the pressure exerted on the spine and keeping the vertebrae separated. The symptoms of NP degeneration are pain and limited mobility of the extremities. It is composed of up to 90% water, type II collagen and proteoglycans [85]. This study focused on the preparation of a novel gelatin-P407 cryogel (in different ratio: 1:1,2:1, 4:1,5:1, 7:1, or 10:1 respectively) as an alternative to the spinal fusion procedure. The composite hydrogel was tested by the following assays: Pore analysis, swelling potential, stability, mechanical integrity and cellular infiltration. The inclusion of P407 in the cryogel was designed to increase swelling ratio, due its hydrophilic nature, since in the NP degradation there is a rapid water loss. All sample presented a high swelling ratio after 24 h, mechanical durability and stability for 28 days in a body-like environment. The 7:1 and 10:1 gel scaffolds showed the most ideal pore diameters and a profuse cell infiltration after only 14 days.

In recent years, 3D printing technology has become important in the biomedical field and in particular the use of thermoreversible gels that with their sol-gel characteristics can be very useful in tissue regeneration [86].

The principle on which the 3D printer is based is to lay a filament of polymeric material which is deposited layer upon layer until the desired system is obtained in 3 dimensions.

Bioprinting systems can be classified into three types: Laser based, jetting based, and extrusion based; recent techniques such as magnetic bioprinting and electrohydrodynamic jetting have been used in tissue engineering.

Hydrogels requirements for 3D bioprinting of ideal engineered tissues should be the following [87]: High porosity, rapid gelation, shape retention, and immunological issue avoidance.

Thermoreversible hydrogels have been successfully applied thanks to their gelation characteristics as they quickly pass from sol-gel state and are also easily extruded from 3D printers [88].

P407 showed good printability [86] but it was not suitable for long-term cell viability. As reported by the recent work [89] it is used, combined with gelatin to create a biocompatible hydrogel for vascular channels, for molds, exploiting its excellent rheological behavior, under shear stress, and its elasticity.

In addition to bioprintability, biological properties of hydrogels played a crucial role in successful tissues regeneration [90]. One of the major disadvantages of available hydrogel materials was that they do not facilitate differentiation of cells into multiple linkages. Despite this, thermoresponsive hydrogels may be very useful for tissue engineering applications and they will become part of the advancement in bio printing technology.

5. Poloxamer as Micellar Systems

Polymeric micelles generated by poloxamers with peculiar characteristics and under specific conditions are exploited as nanometric drug carriers [91]. They have taken hold in recent years as they are able to solubilize poorly water-soluble drugs [36] and decrease undesirable cellular interactions [92,93]. In this review chapter, two recent applications (gene delivery and cancer therapy) of poloxamer micelles have been taken into account.

The development of gene delivery carriers has emerged as a promising technology in transporting genes directly to the target site as therapeutic factors [94]. Current gene transfer vectors used in regenerative medicine approaches included no viral [95] and viral vehicles [96]. The complexation of DNA with cationic polymers (polyplexes) or lipids (lipoplexes) protected DNA against degradation by nucleases and serum components creating a less negative surface charge. They can be designed to target specific cell types through receptor–ligand interactions [97], but these systems exhibited aggregation tendency, a low transfection efficiency and short time transgene expression levels [98]. The use of poloxamers has been described as a tool to increase efficiency of viral gene transfer, obtaining a localized delivery into targets or protecting the vectors.

In the last decade many works that focused the attention on gene delivery were published; the most recent and significant studies are here summarized.

Many researchers have studied the recombinant adeno-associated viral (rAAV) carriers as adapted gene transfer vectors to direct human cartilagine in regenerative medicine [99–101]. However, their use is limited cause their rapid neutralization by the presence of antibodies or heparin which prevent their binding to the viral receptor, present on the cell surface. In this regard, based on the use of polymeric biocompatible materials the combining of direct rAAV-mediated gene transfer with tissue engineering approaches, may offer efficient alternatives.

In this study [102] the possibility of providing rAAV to cartilage regenerative cells via self-assembled poloxamers was evaluated. The formulations consisted of P188 and P407 (2% w/v i.e., above CMC)/rAAV or poloxamine/rAAV were directly incubated within monolayer cultures of hMSCs, cartilagine regenerative cells. At thisoptimized concentration the two poloxamers were more efficient in increasing gene expression over time than a treatment lacking them.

The highest rAAV gene transfer occurred when the PEO/PPO ratio was shifted to hydrophilicity (HLB > 24) using a concentration above CMC (2%) (89.5–94.6% efficiencies with up to 2.7-fold increase in transgene expression for at least 21 days, suggesting that micelles may be better carriers than unimers).

In another paper [103], lentiviral vectors (LV) used for the transduction of human and nonhuman cells were taken into consideration. The optimal transduction conditions for efficient LV gene delivery into target cells depended on a number of factors, including cell density, purity of lentiviral preparation, virus transduction units (TU), multiplicity of infection (MOI) and presence of adjuvants that facilitate transduction [104–106]. These researches identified and validated novel adjuvants for improving transduction efficiency, in particular five representatives poloxamers (P402, P235, P188, P407, and P338). P338 proved to be the best choice since it produced low toxicity and effective viral transduction, especially in difficult-to-transduce cells of T-cell origin.

Further application strategies with poloxamer regard cancer therapy [4]. Poloxamers have gained interest in the field of oncology because of their ability to developed stable systems with the capability of efficient drugs encapsulation and deliver. They usually present small sizes and self-assembling behavior in micellar systems in an aqueous medium, good stability in physiological medium and they avoid the deactivation by RES organs improving consequently drug bioavailability [22,107].

In this biomedical and pharmaceutical area the most recent works in the literature are reported. The first one concerned the use of poloxamer micelles containing a dye (CyFaP) as photo-acoustic imaging (PAI) contrast for mammary neoplastic tissue [108]. In this formulation, dye was inserted in P407 (10% w/v) micelle dropwise under constant stirring. Serum stability studies, cell viability assays, deep tissue penetration and in vivo biodistribution studies were performed. This work has shown that poloxamer micelles are effective for PAI as they penetrate more deeply into breast cancer tissue and are also useful for lymphatic mapping.

The second work [109] explored the anticancer activity of Salinomycin (SAL), an antibiotic isolated from Streptomyces albus [110], that has recently been reported as being effective against tumor cells and mainly to inhibit growth of a specific cancer cell sub-population: CSC. The main goal of the research was the encapsulation of SAL into an innovative poloxamer micelles (PM) system and a further evaluation of in vitro PM-SAL delivery in bacterial and in eukaryotic tumor cells. PM formulations containing P407 and SAL in different amounts were defined with a two multivariate experimental design (DoE) to get the best preparation conditions. Micelles were characterized for size by dynamic light scattering, for their zeta potential and for the encapsulation efficiency. Their in vitro activity was conducted in bacterial cell culture and A549 (adenocarcinoma cell line) cell culture. In conclusion, these micelles seem to be able to deliver SAL into human cancer cells promoting a high drug intracellular accumulation, greatly decreasing toxicity on healthy cells.

Finally, a combined study between radiation therapy and systemic chemotherapeutics to provide both local radiosensitization and systemic control of tumor disease has been reported [111,112]. This study showed the development of a single micelles formulation consisting of multiple poloxamers (MPMs) containing PARP (poly ADP- ribose polymerase) inhibitor talazoparib (Tal) and PI3K (phosphoinositol-3-kinase) inhibitor buparlisib (Bup). When administered during a radiotherapy cycle, that would increase the therapeutic activity of the two drugs in a preclinical model [113]. The performed formulation was made of poloxamer mixture (P103 and P407) obtaining micelles (MPMs) via a modified nanoprecipitation method [114]. MPMs were characterized by dynamic light scattering, to determine size, zeta potential and polydispersity, and by transmission electron microscopy (TEM).

It was also observed that MPMs modulate drug release depending on pH; this behavior is a very useful tool, as the change in pH at tumor level (pH 6.8) would result in a faster release than what occurs when they are circulating in the blood stream (pH 7.4). Furthermore, metabolic assays confirmed that the use of both Tal and Bup synergistically enhanced in vitro cytotoxicity. The in vitro therapeutic activity of the two drugs was studied by a colony-forming assay and a DNA damage assay.

In vivo experiments have shown that the administration of this new MPMs formulation during the course of radiotherapy gave promising results into the enhanced tumor control. The results of this study confirmed that it is important to carry on the development and advancement of combination therapies, especially with the aim of enhancing the outcomes of patients in late-stage and metastatic disease.

6. Summary

Poloxamers are peculiar synthetic tri-block copolymers composed of two poly(ethylene oxide) units and a poly(propylene oxide) one with amphiphilic properties. The dual character, confers to the copolymers interesting properties that can be controlled and changed by different PPO/PEO ratios. These polymers exhibit thermogelling behavior at strategical physiological temperatures.

The most used and studied poloxamer P407, at a concentration of 20% w/w in water, is able to convert the solution to a clear gel by warming the system from room (25 °C) to body temperature (near 37 °C). This thermoresponsive feature has made it attractive for several applications including injectable and topical pharmaceutical formulations, where the material may flow through an applicator or syringe before forming a gel upon contact with the body (35–37 °C).

Because of their biocompatibility and nontoxicity poloxamers have been widely utilized in biomedical applications. In this review their usefulness as thermoreversible hydrogels in the most significant routes of administration (i.e., ocular, transdermic and vaginal route) was reported. Moreover, the latest frontiers have been highlighted for what concerns poloxamers employed in tissue engineering and in gene and cancer therapy.

Funding: This research received no external funding.

Conflicts of Interest: The authors declare no conflict of interest.

References

1. Wichterle, O.; Lim, D. Hydrophilic Gels for Biological Use. *Nature* **1960**, *185*, 117–118. [CrossRef]
2. Buwalda, S.J.; Boere, K.W.; Dijkstra, P.J.; Feijen, J.; Vermonden, T.; Hennink, W.E. Hydrogels in a historical perspective: From simple networks to smart materials. *J. Control. Release* **2014**, *190*, 254–273. [CrossRef] [PubMed]
3. Gioffredi, E.; Boffito, M.; Calzone, S.; Giannitelli, S.M.; Rainer, A.; Trombetta, M.; Mozetic, P.; Chiono, V. Pluronic F127 hydrogel characterization and biofabrication in cellularized constructs for tissue engineering applications. *Procedia Cirp* **2016**, *49*, 125–132. [CrossRef]
4. Almeida, M.; Magalhães, M.; Veiga, F.; Figueiras, A. Poloxamers, poloxamines and polymeric micelles: Definition, structure and therapeutic applications in cancer. *J. Polym. Res.* **2018**, *25*, 31. [CrossRef]
5. Aguilar, M.R.; Elvira, C.; Gallardo, A.; Vázquez, B.; Román, J.S. Smart Polymers and Their Applications as Biomaterials. In *Topics in Tissue Engineering*; Ashammakhi, N., Reis, R.L., Chiellini, E., Eds.; Biomaterials and Tissue Engineering Group: Oulu, Finland, 2007; Volume 3.
6. Johnston, T.P.; Palmer, W.K. Mechanism of poloxamer 407-induced hypertriglyceridemia in the rat. *Biochem. Pharm.* **1993**, *46*, 1037–1042. [CrossRef]
7. Li, J.; Stachowski, M.; Zhang, Z. Application of responsive polymers in implantable medical devices and biosensors. In *Switchable and Responsive Surfaces and Materials for Biomedical Applications*; Woodhead Publishing: Sawston, UK; Cambridge, UK, 2015.
8. Nalbandian, R.M.; Henry, R.L.; Wilks, H.S. Artificial skin. II. Pluronic F-127 Silver nitrate or silver lactate gel in the treatment of thermal burns. *J. Biomed. Mater. Res.* **1972**, *6*, 583–590. [CrossRef] [PubMed]

9. Law, T.; Florence, A.T.; Whateley, T.L. Some chemically modified poloxamer hydrogels-controlled release of prostaglandin-e2 and testosterone. *Int. J. Pharm.* **1986**, *33*, 65–69. [CrossRef]
10. Esposito, E.; Carotta, V.; Scabbia, A.; Trombelli, L.; D'Antona, P.; Menegatti, E.; Nastruzzi, C. Comparative analysis of tetracycline-containing dental gels: Poloxamer- and monoglyceride-based formulations. *Int. J. Pharm.* **1996**, *142*, 9–23. [CrossRef]
11. Stratton, L.P.; Dong, A.; Manning, M.C.; Carpenter, J.F. Drug delivery matrix containing native protein precipitates suspended in a poloxamer gel. *J. Pharm. Sci.* **1997**, *86*, 1006–1010. [CrossRef]
12. Xie, M.H.; Ge, M.; Peng, J.B.; Jiang, X.R.; Wang, D.S.; Ji, L.Q.; Ying, Y.; Wang, Z. In-vivo anti-tumor activity of a novel poloxamer-based thermosensitive in situ gel for sustained delivery of norcantharidin. *Pharm. Dev. Technol.* **2019**, *24*, 623–629. [CrossRef]
13. He, C.; Ji, H.; Qian, Y.; Wang, Q.; Liu, X.; Zhao, W.; Zhao, C. Heparin-based and heparin-inspired hydrogels: Size-effect, gelation and biomedical applications. *J. Mater. Chem. B* **2019**, *7*, 1186–1208. [CrossRef]
14. Tian, W.; Han, S.; Huang, X.; Han, M.; Cao, J.; Liang, Y.; Sun, Y. LDH hybrid thermosensitive hydrogel for intravaginal delivery of anti-HIV drugs. *Artif. Cells Nanomed. Biotechnol.* **2019**, *47*, 1234–1240. [CrossRef] [PubMed]
15. Hoffman, A.S. Hydrogels for biomedical applications. *Adv. Drug Deliv. Rev.* **2012**, *64*, 18–23. [CrossRef]
16. Alexandridis, P.; Hatton, T.A. Poly(ethylene oxide)-poly(propylene oxide)-poly (ethylene oxide) block copolymer surfactants in aqueous solutions and at interfaces: Thermodynamics, structure, dynamics, and modeling. *Colloids Surf. A Physicochem. Eng. Asp.* **1995**, *96*, 1–46. [CrossRef]
17. Singh-Joy, S.D.; McLain, V.C. Safety Assessment of Poloxamers 101, 105, 108, 122, 123, 124, 181, 182, 183, 184, 185, 188, 212, 215, 217, 231, 234, 235, 237, 238, 282, 284, 288, 331, 333, 334, 335, 338, 401, 402, 403, and 407, Poloxamer 105 Benzoate, and Poloxamer 182 Dibenzoate as Used in Cosmetics. *Int. J. Toxicol.* **2008**, *27*, 93–128.
18. Pitto-Barry, A.; Barry, N.P. Pluronic®block-copolymers in medicine: From chemical and biological versatility to rationalization and clinical advances. *Polym. Chem.* **2014**, *5*, 3281–3496. [CrossRef]
19. Jeong, B.; Kim, S.W.; Bae, Y.H. Thermosensitive sol–gel reversible hydrogels. *Adv. Drug Deliv. Rev.* **2012**, *64*, 154–162. [CrossRef]
20. Devi, D.R.; Sandhya, P.; Hari, B.V. Poloxamer: A novel functional molecule for drug delivery and gene therapy. *J. Pharm. Sci. Res.* **2013**, *5*, 159–165.
21. Alexandridis, P.; Holzwarth, J.F.; Hatton, T.A. Micellization of Poly(Ethylene Oxide)-Poly(Propylene Oxide)-Poly(Ethylene Oxide) Triblock Copolymers in Aqueous-Solutions-Thermodynamics of Copolymer Association. *Macromolecules* **1994**, *27*, 2414–2425. [CrossRef]
22. Simões, S.M.; Figueiras, A.R.; Veiga, F.; Concheiro, A.; Alvarez-Lorenzo, C. Polymeric micelles for oral drug administration enabling loco regional and systemic treatments. *Expert Opin. Drug Deliv.* **2015**, *12*, 297–318. [CrossRef]
23. Ahmad, Z.; Shah, A.; Siddiq, M.; Kraatz, H.B. Polymeric micelles as drug delivery vehicles. *RSC Adv.* **2014**, *4*, 17028–17038. [CrossRef]
24. Vadnere, M.; Amidon, G.L.; Lindenbaum, S.; Haslam, J.L. Thermodynamic studies on the gel-sol transition of some pluronic polyols. *Int. J. Pharm.* **1984**, *22*, 207. [CrossRef]
25. Cho, C.W.; Cho, Y.S.; Lee, H.K.; Yeom, Y.I.; Park, S.N.; Yoon, D.Y. Improvement of receptor-mediated gene delivery to HepG2 cells using an amphiphilic gelling agent. *Biotechnol. Appl. Biochem.* **2000**, *32*, 21–26. [CrossRef] [PubMed]
26. Morishita, M.; Barichello, J.M.; Takayama, K.; Chiba, Y.; Tokwa, S.; Nagai, T. Pluronic F-127 gels incorporating highly purified unsaturated fatty acids for buccal delivery of insulin. *Int. J. Pharm.* **2001**, *212*, 289–293. [CrossRef]
27. Johnston, T.P.; Punjabi, M.A.; Froelich, C.J. Sustained delivery of interleukin-2 from a Poloxamer 407 gel matrix following intraperitoneal injection in mice. *Pharm. Res.* **1992**, *9*, 425–434. [CrossRef]
28. DiBiase, M.D.; Rhodes, C.T. Investigations of epidermal growth factor in semisolid formulations. *Pharm. Acta Helv.* **1991**, *66*, 165–169.
29. Clokie, C.M.; Urist, M.R. Bone morphogenic protein excipients: Comparative observations on poloxamer. *Plast. Reconstr. Surg.* **2000**, *105*, 628–637. [CrossRef]
30. Hom, D.B.; Medhi, K.; Assefa, G.; Juhn, S.K.; Johnston, T.P. Vascular effects of sustained-release fibroblast growth factors. *Ann. Otol. Rhinol. Laryngol.* **1996**, *105*, 109–116. [CrossRef]

31. Al Khateb, K.; Ozhmukhametova, E.K.; Mussin, M.N.; Seilkhanov, S.K.; Rakhypbekov, T.K.; Lau, W.M.; Khutoryanskiy, V.V. In situ gelling systems based on Pluronic F127/Pluronic F68 formulations for ocular drug delivery. *Int. J. Pharm.* **2016**, *502*, 70–79. [CrossRef]
32. Fathalla, Z.M.; Vangala, A.; Longman, M.; Khaled, K.A.; Hussein, A.K.; El-Garhy, O.H.; Alany, R.G. Poloxamer-based thermoresponsive ketorolac tromethamine in situ gel preparations: Design, characterisation, toxicity and transcorneal permeation studies. *Eur. J. Pharm. Biopharm.* **2017**, *114*, 119–134. [CrossRef]
33. Yu, S.; Zhang, X.; Tan, G.; Tian, L.; Liu, D.; Liu, Y.; Yang, X.; Pan, W. A novel pH-induced thermosensitive hydrogel composed of carboxymethyl chitosan and poloxamer cross-linked by glutaraldehyde for ophthalmic drug delivery. *Carbohydr. Polym.* **2017**, *155*, 208–217. [CrossRef] [PubMed]
34. Lou, J.; Hu, W.; Tian, R.; Zhang, H.; Jia, Y.; Zhang, J.; Zhang, L. Optimization and evaluation of a thermoresponsive ophthalmic in situ gel containing curcumin-loaded albumin nanoparticles. *Int. J. Nanomed.* **2014**, *9*, 2517–2525.
35. Almeida, H.; Lobão, P.; Frigerio, C.; Fonseca, J.; Silva, R.; Sousa Lobo, J.M.; Amaral, M.H. Preparation, characterization and biocompatibility studies of thermoresponsive eyedrops based on the combination of nanostructured lipid carriers (NLC) and the polymer Pluronic F-127 for controlled delivery of ibuprofen. *Pharm. Dev. Technol.* **2017**, *22*, 336–349. [CrossRef] [PubMed]
36. Cafaggi, S.; Russo, E.; Caviglioli, G.; Parodi, B.; Stefani, R.; Sillo, G.; Leardi, R.; Bignardi, G. Poloxamer 407 as a solubilising agent for tolfenamic acid and as a base for a gel formulation. *Eur. J. Pharm. Sci.* **2008**, *35*, 19–29. [CrossRef] [PubMed]
37. Ur-Rehman, T.; Tavelin, S.; Gröbner, G. Effect of DMSO on micellization, gelation and drugrelease profile of Poloxamer 407. *Int. J. Pharm.* **2010**, *394*, 92–98. [CrossRef] [PubMed]
38. Liaw, J.; Lin, Y.C. Evaluation of poly(ethylene oxide)–poly(propylene oxide)–poly(ethylene oxide) (PEO–PPO–PEO) gels as a release vehicle for percutaneous fentanyl. *J. Control. Release* **2000**, *68*, 273–282. [CrossRef]
39. Shin, S.C.; Cho, C.W.; Yang, K.H. Development of lidocaine gels for enhanced local anesthetic action. *Int. J. Pharm.* **2004**, *287*, 73–78. [CrossRef]
40. Suedee, R.; Bodhibukkana, C.; Tangthong, N.; Amnuaikit, C.; Kaewnopparat, S.; Srichana, T. Development of a reservoir-type transdermal enantioselective-controlled delivery system for racemic propranolol using a molecularly imprinted polymer composite membrane. *J. Control. Release* **2008**, *129*, 170–178. [CrossRef]
41. Stamatialis, D.F.; Rolevink, H.H.M.; Koops, G.H. Transdermal timolol delivery from a Pluronic gel. *J. Control. Release* **2006**, *116*, 53–65. [CrossRef]
42. Nair, V.; Panchagnula, R. Poloxamer gel as vehicle for transdermal iontophoretic delivery of arginine vasopressin: Evaluation of in vivo performance in rats. *Pharm. Res.* **2003**, *47*, 555–562. [CrossRef]
43. Pillai, O.; Panchagnula, R. Transdermal delivery of insulin from poloxamer gel: Ex vivo and in vivo skin permeation studies in rat using iontophoresis and chemical enhancers. *J. Control. Release* **2003**, *89*, 127–140. [CrossRef]
44. Donnelly, R.F.; Morrow, D.I.; McCarron, P.A.; Woolfson, A.D.; Morrissey, A.; Juzenas, P.; Juzeniene, A.; Iani, V.; McCarthy, H.O.; Moan, J. Microneedle-mediated intradermal delivery of 5-aminolevulinic acid: Potential for enhanced topical photodynamic therapy. *J. Control. Release* **2008**, *129*, 154–162. [CrossRef] [PubMed]
45. Khanna, P.; Flam, B.R.; Osborn, B.; Strom, J.A.; Bhansali, S. Skin penetration and fracture strength testing of silicon dioxide microneedles. *Sens. Actuators A* **2011**, *170*, 180–186. [CrossRef]
46. Chandrasekaran, S.; Brazzle, J.D.; Frazier, A.B. Surface micromachined metallic microneedles. *J. Microelectromech. Syst.* **2003**, *12*, 281–288. [CrossRef]
47. Gill, H.S.; Prausnitz, M.R. Coating formulations for microneedles. *Pharm. Res.* **2007**, *24*, 1369–1380. [CrossRef] [PubMed]
48. Parker, E.R.; Rao, M.P.; Turner, K.L.; Meinhart, C.D.; MacDonald, N.C. Bulk micromachined titanium microneedles. *J. Microelectromech. Syst.* **2007**, *16*, 289–295. [CrossRef]
49. Donnelly, R.F.; Morrow, D.I.; Singh, T.R.; Migalska, K.; McCarron, P.A. Processing difficulties and instability of carbohydrate microneedle arrays. *Drug Deliv. Ind. Pharm.* **2009**, *35*, 1242–1254. [CrossRef]
50. Lee, K.; Lee, C.Y.; Jung, H. Dissolving microneedles for transdermal drug administration prepared by stepwise controlled drawing of maltose. *Biomaterials* **2011**, *32*, 3134–3140. [CrossRef]
51. Li, G.; Badkar, A.; Nema, S.; Kolli, C.S.; Banga, A.K. In vitro transdermal delivery of therapeutic antibodies using maltose microneedles. *Int. J. Pharm.* **2009**, *368*, 109–115. [CrossRef]

52. Wang, P.M.; Cornwell, M.; Hill, J.; Prausnitz, M.R. Precise microinjection into skin using hollow microneedles. *J. Investig. Derm.* **2006**, *126*, 1080–1087. [CrossRef]
53. Bystrova, S.; Luttge, R. Micromolding for ceramic microneedle arrays. *Microelectron. Eng.* **2011**, *88*, 1681–1684. [CrossRef]
54. Ito, Y.; Murano, H.; Hamasaki, N.; Fukushima, K.; Takada, K. Incidence of low bioavailability of leuprolide acetate after percutaneous administration to rats by dissolving microneedles. *Int. J. Pharm.* **2011**, *407*, 126–131. [CrossRef]
55. Noh, Y.W.; Kim, T.H.; Baek, J.S.; Park, H.H.; Lee, S.S.; Han, M.; Shin, S.C.; Cho, C.W. In vitro characterization of the invasiveness of polymer microneedle against skin. *Int. J. Pharm.* **2010**, *397*, 201–205. [CrossRef]
56. Sachdeva, V.; Banga, A.K. Microneedles and their applications. *Recent Pat. Drug Deliv. Formul.* **2011**, *5*, 95–132. [CrossRef]
57. Thakur, R.R.S.; Fallows, S.J.; McMillan, H.L.; Donnelly, R.F.; Jones, D.S. Microneedle-mediated intrascleral delivery of in situ forming thermoresponsive implants for sustained ocular drug delivery. *J. Pharm Pharm. Pharmacol.* **2014**, *66*, 584–595. [CrossRef]
58. Gilger, B.C.; Abarca, E.M.; Salmon, J.H.; Patel, S. Treatment of acute posterior uveitis in a porcine model by injection of triamcinolone acetonide into the suprachoroidal space using microneedles. *Investig. Ophthalmol. Vis. Sci.* **2013**, *54*, 2483–2492. [CrossRef]
59. Patel, S.R.; Lin, A.S.; Edelhauser, H.F.; Prausnitz, M.R. Suprachoroidal drug delivery to the back of the eye using hollow microneedles. *Pharm. Res.* **2011**, *28*, 166–176. [CrossRef]
60. Roxhed, N.; Griss, P.; Stemme, G. Membrane-sealed hollow microneedles and related administration schemes for transdermal drug delivery. *Biomed. Microdevices* **2008**, *10*, 271–279. [CrossRef]
61. Ovsianikov, A.; Chichkov, B.; Mente, P.; Monteiro-Riviere, N.A.; Doraiswamy, A.; Narayan, R.J. Two photon polymerization of polymer–ceramic hybrid materials for transdermal drug delivery. *Int. J. Appl. Ceram Technol.* **2007**, *4*, 22–29. [CrossRef]
62. Sivaraman, A.; Banga, A.K. Novel in situ forming hydrogel microneedles for transdermal drug delivery. *Drug Deliv. Transl. Res.* **2017**, *7*, 16–26. [CrossRef]
63. Khan, S.; Minhas, M.U.; Tekko, I.A.; Donnelly, R.F.; Thakur, R.R.S. Evaluation of microneedles-assisted in situ depot forming poloxamer gels for sustained transdermal drug delivery. *Drug Deliv. Transl. Res.* **2019**, *9*, 764–782. [CrossRef] [PubMed]
64. Leone, M.; van Oorschot, B.H.; Nejadnik, M.R.; Bocchino, A.; Rosato, M.; Kersten, G.; O'Mahony, C.; Bouwstra, J.; van der Maaden, K. Universal applicator for digitally-controlled pressing force and impact velocity insertion of microneedles into skin. *Pharmaceutics* **2018**, *10*, 211. [CrossRef] [PubMed]
65. Sahoo, C.K.; Nayak, P.K.; Sarangi, D.K.; Sahoo, T.K. Intra vaginal drug delivery system: An overview. *Am. J. Adv. Drug Deliv.* **2013**, *1*, 43–55.
66. Ndesendo, V.M.; Pillay, V.; Choonara, Y.E.; Buchmann, E.; Bayever, D.N.; Meyer, L.C. A review of current intravaginal drug delivery approaches employed for the prophylaxis of HIV/AIDS and prevention of sexually transmitted infections. *AAPS Pharmscitech* **2008**, *9*, 505–520. [CrossRef] [PubMed]
67. Hussain, A.; Ahsan, F. The vagina as a route for systemic drug delivery. *J. Control. Release* **2005**, *103*, 301–313. [CrossRef] [PubMed]
68. Taurin, S.; Almomen, A.A.; Pollak, T.; Kim, S.J.; Maxwell, J.; Peterson, C.M.; Owen, S.C.; Janát-Amsbury, M.M. Thermosensitive hydrogels a versatile concept adapted to vaginal drug delivery. *J. Drug Target.* **2018**, *26*, 533–550. [CrossRef] [PubMed]
69. Caramella, C.M.; Rossi, S.; Ferrari, F.; Bonferoni, M.C.; Sandri, G. Mucoadhesive and thermogelling systems for vaginal drug delivery. *Adv. Drug Deliv. Rev.* **2015**, *92*, 39–52. [CrossRef]
70. Ci, T.; Yuan, L.; Bao, X.; Hou, Y.; Wu, H.; Sun, H.; Cao, D.; Ke, X. Development and anti-Candida evaluation of the vaginal delivery system of amphotericin B nanosuspension-loaded thermogel. *J. Drug Target.* **2018**, *26*, 829–839. [CrossRef]
71. Ibrahim, E.S.; Ismail, S.; Fetih, G.; Shaaban, O.; Hassanein, K.; Abdellah, N. Development and characterization of thermosensitive pluronic-based metronidazole in situ gelling formulations for vaginal application. *Acta Pharma.* **2012**, *62*, 59–70. [CrossRef]
72. Xuan, J.-J.; Yan, Y.D.; Oh, D.H.; Choi, Y.K.; Yong, C.S.; Choi, H.G. Development of thermosensitive injectable hydrogel with sustained release of doxorubicin: Rheological characterization and in vivo evaluation in rats. *Drug Deliv.* **2011**, *18*, 305–311. [CrossRef]

73. Hani, U.; Shivakamuar, H.G. Development of miconazole nitrate thermosensitive bioadhesive vaginal gel for vaginal candidiasis. *Am. J. Adv. Drug Deliv.* **2013**, *3*, 358–368.
74. Mei, L.; Chen, J.; Yu, S.; Huang, Y.; Xie, Y.; Wang, H.; Pan, X.; Wu, C. Expansible thermal gelling foam aerosol for vaginal drug delivery. *Drug Deliv.* **2017**, *24*, 1325–1337. [CrossRef] [PubMed]
75. Holland, I.; Logan, J.; Shi, J.; McCormick, C.; Liu, D.; Shu, W. 3D biofabrication for tubular tissue engineering. *Bio-Des. Manuf.* **2018**, *1*, 89–100. [CrossRef] [PubMed]
76. Doğan, A.; Yalvaç, M.E.; Şahin, F.; Kabanov, A.V.; Palotás, A.; Rizvanov, A.A. Differentiation of human stem cells is promoted by amphiphilic pluronic block copolymers. *Int. J. Nanomed.* **2012**, *7*, 4849–4860.
77. Bessa, P.C.; Casal, M.; Reis, R.L. Bone morphogenetic proteins in tissue engineering: The road from laboratory to clinic, part II (BMP delivery). *J. Tissue Eng. Regen. Med.* **2008**, *2*, 81–96. [CrossRef]
78. Gittens, S.A.; Uludag, H. Growth factor delivery for bone tissue engineering. *J. Drug Target.* **2001**, *9*, 407–429. [CrossRef]
79. Han, Q.Q.; Du, Y.; Yang, P.S. The role of small molecules in bone regeneration. *Future Med. Chem.* **2013**, *5*, 1671–1684. [CrossRef]
80. Laurencin, C.T.; Ashe, K.M.; Henry, N.; Kan, H.M.; Lo, K.W.-H. Delivery of small molecules for bone regenerative engineering: Preclinical studies and potential clinical applications. *Drug Discov. Today* **2014**, *19*, 794–800. [CrossRef]
81. Zhang, Y.; Bradley, A.D.; Wang, D.; Reinhardt, R.A. Statins, bone metabolism and treatment of bone catabolic diseases. *Pharm. Res.* **2014**, *88*, 53–61. [CrossRef]
82. Rezazadeh, M.; Parandeh, M.; Akbari, V.; Ebrahimi, Z.; Taheri, A. Incorporation of rosuvastatin-loaded chitosan/chondroitin sulfate nanoparticles into a thermosensitive hydrogel for bone tissue engineering: Preparation, characterization, and cellular behavior. *Pharm. Dev. Technol.* **2019**, *24*, 357–367. [CrossRef]
83. Muzzarelli, R.A.; Greco, F.; Busilacchi, A.; Sollazzo, V.; Gigante, A. Chitosan, hyaluronan and chondroitin sulfate in tissue engineering for cartilage regeneration: A review. *Carbohydr. Polym.* **2012**, *89*, 723–739. [CrossRef] [PubMed]
84. Temofeew, A.; Hixon, K.R.; McBride-Gagyi, S.H.; Scott, A. Sell The fabrication of cryogel scaffolds incorporated with poloxamer 407 for potential use in the regeneration of the nucleus pulposus. *J. Mater. Sci. Mater. Med.* **2017**, *28*, 36–47. [CrossRef] [PubMed]
85. Pattappa, G.; Li, Z.; Peroglio, M.; Wismer, N.; Alini, M.; Grad, S. Diversity of intervertebral disc cells: Phenoztype and function. *J. Anat.* **2012**, *221*, 480–496. [CrossRef] [PubMed]
86. Suntornnond, R.; An, J.; Chua, C.K. Bioprinting of Thermoresponsive Hydrogels for Next Generation Tissue Engineering: A Review. *Macromol. Mater. Eng.* **2017**, *302*, 1600266. [CrossRef]
87. Chung, J.H.; Naficy, S.; Yue, Z.; Kapsa, R.; Quigley, A.; Moulton, S.E.; Wallace, G.G. Bio-ink properties and printability for extrusion printing living cells. *Biomater. Sci.* **2013**, *1*, 763. [CrossRef]
88. Nicmodeus, G.D.; Bryant, S.J. Cell encapsulation in biodegradable hydrogels for tissue engineering applications. *Tissue Eng Part B Rev.* **2008**, *14*, 149–165.
89. Kolesky, D.B.; Truby, R.L.; Gladman, A.S.; Busbee, T.A.; Homan, K.A.; Lewis, J.A. 3D Bioprinting of Vascularized, Heterogeneous Cell-Laden Tissue Constructs. *Adv. Mater.* **2013**, *25*, 3124–3130. [CrossRef]
90. Hospodiuk, M.; Dey, M.; Sosnoski, D.; Ozbolat, I.T. The bioink: A comprehensive review on bioprintable materials. *Biotechnol. Adv.* **2017**, *35*, 217–239. [CrossRef]
91. Aliabadi, H.M.; Lavasanifar, A. Polymeric micelles for drug delivery. *Expert Opin. Drug Deliv.* **2006**, *3*, 139–162. [CrossRef]
92. Kabanov, A.V.; Lemieux, P.; Vinogradov, S.; Alakhov, V. Pluronic block copolymers: Novel functional molecules for gene therapy. *Adv. Drug Deliv. Rev.* **2002**, *54*, 223–233. [CrossRef]
93. Anderson, R.A. Micelle formation by oxyethylene-oxypropylene polymers. *Pharm. Acta Helv.* **1972**, *47*, 304–308. [PubMed]
94. Rey-Rico, A.; Cucchiarini, M. Controlled release strategies for raav-mediated gene delivery. *Acta Biomater.* **2016**, *29*, 1–10. [CrossRef] [PubMed]
95. Niidome, T.; Huang, L. Gene therapy progress and prospects: Nonviral vectors. *Gene Ther.* **2002**, *9*, 1647–1652. [CrossRef] [PubMed]
96. Rey-Rico, A.; Cucchiarini, M. Recent tissue engineering-based advances for effective rAAV-mediated gene transfer in the musculoskeletal system. *Bioengineered* **2016**, *7*, 175–188. [CrossRef]

97. De Laporte, L.; Cruz Rea, J.; Shea, L.D. Design of modular non-viral gene therapy vectors. *Biomaterials* **2006**, *27*, 947–954. [CrossRef]
98. Wang, W.; Li, W.; Ma, N.; Steinhoff, G. Non-viral gene delivery methods. *Curr. Pharm. Biotechnol.* **2013**, *14*, 46–60.
99. Cucchiarini, M.; Madry, H. Gene therapy for cartilage defects. *J. Gene Med.* **2005**, *7*, 1495–1509. [CrossRef]
100. Madry, H.; Cucchiarini, M. Advances and challenges in gene-based approaches for osteoarthritis. *J. Gene Med.* **2013**, *15*, 343–355. [CrossRef]
101. Johnstone, B.; Alini, M.; Cucchiarini, M.; Dodge, G.R.; Eglin, D.; Guilak, F.; Madry, H.; Mata, A.; Mauck, R.L.; Semino, C.E.; et al. Tissue engineering for articular cartilage repair—The state of the art. *Eur. Cell Mater.* **2013**, *25*, 248–267. [CrossRef]
102. Rey-Rico, A.; Venkatesan, J.K.; Frisch, J.; Rial-Hermida, I.; Schmitt, G.; Concheiro, A.; Madry, H.; Alvarez-Lorenzo, C.; Cucchiarini, M. PEO–PPO–PEO micelles as effective rAAV-mediated gene delivery systems to target human mesenchymal stem cells without altering their differentiation potency. *Acta Biomater.* **2015**, *27*, 42–52. [CrossRef]
103. Höfig, I.; Atkinson, M.J.; Mall, S.; Krackhardt, A.M.; Thirion, C.; Anastasov, N. Poloxamer synperonic F108 improves cellular transduction with lentiviral vectors. *J. Gene Med.* **2012**, *14*, 549–560. [CrossRef] [PubMed]
104. Millington, M.; Aendt, A.; Boyd, M.; Applegate, T.; Shen, S. Towards a clinically relevant lentiviral transduction protocol for primary human CD34 haematopoietic stem/progenitor cells. *PLoS ONE* **2009**, *4*, 6461. [CrossRef] [PubMed]
105. Birmingham, A.; Anderson, E.; Sullivan, K.; Reynolds, A.; Boese, Q.; Leake, D.; Karpilow, J.; Khvorova, A. A protocol for designing siRNAs with high functionality and specificity. *Nat. Protoc.* **2007**, *9*, 2068–2078. [CrossRef] [PubMed]
106. Takahashi, K.; Tanabe, K.; Ohnuki, M.; Narita, M.; Ichisaka, T.; Tomoda, K.; Yamanaka, S. Induction of pluripotent stem cells from adult human fibroblasts by defined factors. *Cell* **2007**, *131*, 861–872. [CrossRef] [PubMed]
107. Alvarez-Lorenzo, C.; Rey-Rico, A.; Sosnik, A.; Taboada, P.; Concheiro, A. Poloxamine-based nanomaterials for drug delivery. *Front. Biosci.* **2012**, *337*, 303–305. [CrossRef] [PubMed]
108. Chitgupi, U.; Nyayapathi, N.; Kim, J.; Wang, D.; Sun, B.; Li, C.; Carter, K.; Huang, W.C.; Kim, C.; Xia, J.; et al. Surfactant-Stripped Micelles for NIR-II Photoacoustic Imaging through 12 cm of Breast Tissue and Whole Human Breasts. *Adv. Mater.* **2019**, *31*, 1–10. [CrossRef]
109. Sousa, C.; Gouveia, L.F.; Kreutzer, B.; Silva-Lima, B.; Maphasa, R.E.; Dube, A.; Videira, M. Polymeric Micellar Formulation Enhances Antimicrobial and Anticancer Properties of Salinomycin. *Pharm. Res.* **2019**, *36*, 83. [CrossRef]
110. Naujokat, C.; Steinhart, R. Salinomycin as a drug for targeting human cancer stem cells. *J. Biomed. Biotechnol.* **2012**, *20*, 44–46. [CrossRef]
111. Steel, G.G.; Peckham, M.J. Exploitable Mechanisms in Combined Radiotherapy-Chemotherapy: The Concept of Additivity. *Int. J. Radiat. Oncol. Biol. Phys.* **1979**, *5*, 85–91. [CrossRef]
112. Seiwert, T.Y.; Salama, J.K.; Vokes, E.E. The Concurrent Chemoradiation Paradigm—General Principles. *Nat. Rev. Clin. Oncol.* **2007**, *4*, 86–100. [CrossRef]
113. DuRoss, A.N.; Neufeld, M.J.; Landry, M.R.; Rosch, J.G.; Eaton, C.T.; Sahay, G.; Thomas, C.R., Jr.; Sun, C. Micellar Formulation of Talazoparib and Buparlisib for Enhanced DNA Damage in Breast Cancer Chemoradiotherapy. *ACS Appl. Mater. Interfaces* **2019**, *11*, 12342–12356. [CrossRef] [PubMed]
114. Fessi, H.; Puisieux, F.; Devissaguet, J.P.; Ammoury, N.; Benita, S. Nanocapsule Formation by Interfacial Polymer Deposition Following Solvent Displacement. *Int. J. Pharm.* **1989**, *55*, R1–R4. [CrossRef]

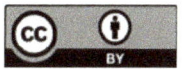

© 2019 by the authors. Licensee MDPI, Basel, Switzerland. This article is an open access article distributed under the terms and conditions of the Creative Commons Attribution (CC BY) license (http://creativecommons.org/licenses/by/4.0/).

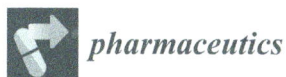

Review

Strategies for Hyaluronic Acid-Based Hydrogel Design in Drug Delivery

Sonia Trombino [†], Camilla Servidio [†], Federica Curcio and Roberta Cassano *

Department of Pharmacy, Health and Nutritional Science, University of Calabria, Arcavacata, 87036 Rende, Italy
* Correspondence: roberta.cassano@unical.it; Tel./Fax: +39-984-493227
† These authors contributed equally to this work.

Received: 5 July 2019; Accepted: 5 August 2019; Published: 12 August 2019

Abstract: Hyaluronic acid (HA) is a natural, linear, endogenous polysaccharide that plays important physiological and biological roles in the human body. Nowadays, among biopolymers, HA is emerging as an appealing starting material for hydrogels design due to its biocompatibility, native biofunctionality, biodegradability, non-immunogenicity, and versatility. Since HA is not able to form gels alone, chemical modifications, covalent crosslinking, and gelling agents are always needed in order to obtain HA-based hydrogels. Therefore, in the last decade, different strategies for the design of physical and chemical HA hydrogels have been developed, such as click chemistry reactions, enzymatic and disulfide crosslinking, supramolecular assembly via inclusion complexation, and so on. HA-based hydrogels turn out to be versatile platforms, ranging from static to smart and stimuli-responsive systems, and for these reasons, they are widely investigated for biomedical applications like drug delivery, tissue engineering, regenerative medicine, cell therapy, and diagnostics. Furthermore, the overexpression of HA receptors on various tumor cells makes these platforms promising drug delivery systems for targeted cancer therapy. The aim of the present review is to highlight and discuss recent advances made in the last years on the design of chemical and physical HA-based hydrogels and their application for biomedical purposes, in particular, drug delivery. Notable attention is given to HA hydrogel-based drug delivery systems for targeted therapy of cancer and osteoarthritis.

Keywords: hyaluronic acid; hydrogel; cancer; drug delivery; click chemistry; biomaterial

1. Introduction

Hydrogels are three-dimensional, hydrated polymeric networks, formed by crosslinked hydrophilic polymers with a high affinity for water and biological fluids, capable of absorbing from 10% up to thousands of times their dry weight in water [1].

In recent years, thanks to their unique properties such as biocompatibility, biodegradability, flexibility, softness, etc., hydrogels have been widely investigated for biomedical applications like cell therapy, tissue engineering, drug delivery, and diagnostics [2]. For example, hydrogels made of pectin, carboxymethylcellulose and propylene glycol or polyethylene glycol (PEG) and propylene glycol are used as wound dressings [3,4], keratin- or polyvinyl alcohol-based hydrogels as scaffolds for cell growth [5,6], PEG-based hydrogel (DEXTENZA®), recently approved by the Food and Drug Administration, as ophthalmic inserts, etc. [7].

Among biopolymers, hyaluronic acid (HA) represents one of the most used in the design of hydrogels for biomedical applications due to its biocompatibility, native biofunctionality, biodegradability, non-immunogenicity, and versatility.

HA is a natural linear polysaccharide that consists of alternating units of D-glucuronic acid and N-acetyl-D-glucosamine, connected by β-1,3- and β-1,4-glycosidic bonds.

HA is a non-sulfated glycosaminoglycan that is widely found in the epithelial and connective tissues of vertebrates and it is the major component of the extracellular matrix (ECM) [8]. It is synthesized by hyaluronan synthase at the plasma membrane and it is then extruded to the extracellular matrix [9]. HA is found in a wide range of molecular weights from 20,000 up to several million Daltons, depending on the enzyme that catalyzes its synthesis.

Around 30% of HA present in the body is rapidly degraded by hyaluronidases and oxidative species, while the remaining 70% is catabolized by liver and lymphatic vessels endothelial cells, with tissue half-lives going from minutes in the bloodstream to weeks in cartilage [10]. Upon physiological conditions, HA is a polyanion associated with extracellular cations (Na^+, Ca^{2+}, Mg^{2+}, K^+) known as hyaluronan [11].

HA plays important physiological and biological roles in the human body. In the extracellular matrix of most tissues it contributes to maintain the tissue's mechanical integrity, homeostasis, viscoelasticity and lubrication thanks to its high molecular weight and its capacity to absorb a high quantity of water [12]. Furthermore, it also plays an important role in intracellular functions; in fact, it is able to regulate, due to its binding to cell surface specific receptors (such as CD44 or RHAMM), cell adhesion, migration, proliferation, and differentiation and, consequently, processes like inflammation, wound healing, tissue development, morphogenesis, tumor progression, and metastasis [13].

For these reasons, in recent years, hydrogels built from HA have been developed and investigated for biomedical applications like tissue regeneration, tissue engineering, drug delivery, gene therapy, diagnostics, etc.

Nowadays several HA-based hydrogels are already used in medicine as dermal fillers, viscosupplements, wound dressings, etc., and the market is continuously increasing worldwide. They are now progressing in their design to be responsive to several triggers, to have various features like stability, complex structures, and biochemical cues. The aim of the present review is to highlight and discuss recent advances made in the last years on the design of chemical and physical HA-based hydrogels and their application for biomedical purposes, in particular, drug delivery.

2. Physical and Chemical Hydrogels

Hydrogels can be classified into "physical" and "chemical" gels, depending on the type of bond that is formed between the polymer chains from which they derive.

Hydrogels are called "reversible" or "physical" if the networks are formed as a result of weak physical interactions between the macromolecular chains such as ionic, H-bonding, Van der Waals interactions, hydrophobic forces, or molecular entanglements [14].

Physical hydrogels can be synthesized by warming or cooling polymer solution, mixing solution of polyanion and polycation, combining polyelectrolyte with multivalent ions of opposite charge, etc. [1].

Physical hydrogels are often heterogeneous, unstable, and reversible; in fact, they are not able to maintain their structural integrity and dissolve easily by changing environmental factors like temperature, pH, etc.

Instead, hydrogels are called "permanent" or "chemical" if the polymeric chains are connected by covalent bonds [15]. For this reason, these materials, after swelling, retain their structural integrity, even if it is possible a degradation when particular bonds, sensitive to chemical or enzymatic hydrolysis, are present in the structure.

Chemical hydrogels can be generated by crosslinking polymers with radiations, chemical crosslinkers, polyfunctional compounds, free radical generating compounds, etc. [1]. Consequently, these systems have a better chemical, mechanical, and thermal stability compared to physical hydrogels.

Even though HA, due to its conformation and molecular weight, can form molecular networks in solution, it is not able to form physical gel alone. For this reason, chemical modifications, covalent crosslinking, and gelling agents are needed in order to obtain HA hydrogels.

HA turns out to be a functional and suitable polymer for chemical modification with reactive species due to its chemical structure; in particular, the chemical modifications concern three functional groups: the carboxylic acid group, the hydroxyl group, and the amino group (after deacetylation) [16].

This section reviews the different modified HA macromers and chemical techniques described in the literature in the last years used for the design of physical and chemical HA-based hydrogels.

2.1. Chemical Hydrogels

Chemical crosslinking turns out to be a versatile method to obtain hydrogels with excellent chemical, mechanical and thermal stability. However, this approach presents some limitations like the use of metal catalysts, photoinitiators, low reaction yield, etc. [17]. With regard to the chemical approach, HA-based hydrogels can be obtained via condensation reactions, enzymatic crosslinking, disulfide crosslinking, click chemistry, polymerization, etc. HA can be directly crosslinked by divinyl sulfone [18], glutaraldehyde [19], carbodiimide [20], bisepoxide [21], etc.; however, direct crosslinking cannot be considered suitable for hydrogels design since it requires harsh reaction condition, toxic by-products can be formed and the crosslinking agents used are cytotoxic. Nowadays, one of the most promising strategies for hydrogels preparation turns out to be click chemistry due to its high specificity, high yield, bioorthogonality, and mild reaction conditions [22].

2.1.1. Diels Alder Reaction (Click Chemistry)

In recent years, a particular interest has been addressed to the Diels–Alder reaction between furan and maleimide moieties for hydrogels design due to its selectivity, efficiency, and thermoreversibility [23].

In this regard, Fisher et al. recently developed a HA-based hydrogel with tunable properties to use as a platform to investigate breast cancer cells invasion. The hydrogel was obtained via a Diels–Alder click reaction between furan modified HA and bismaleimide functional peptides with the aim of mimicking ECM [24]. A similar approach was reported by Yu et al. in order to obtain a 3D patterned hydrogel. In this work Diels–Alder click chemistry has been used in order to get a HA-based hydrogel that can be subsequently subjected to thiol-ene photocoupling allowing its spatiotemporal patterning [25].

2.1.2. Azide-Alkyn Huisgen Cycloaddition (Click Chemistry)

The Huisgen reaction is a cycloaddition between an azide and an alkyne to produce triazoles which requires the presence of a catalyst (Cu^+) as reported by Rostovtsev et al. [26]. In recent years it has become one of the most used strategies for hydrogels preparation thanks to its high yield, efficiency, excellent bioorthogonality, fast reaction rate, etc. [27,28]. For example, Manzi et al. fabricated nanohydrogels based on derivatives of HA and riboflavin obtained by Cu^+ catalyzed Huisgen cycloaddition [29].

Despite the various advantages offered by this reaction, the use of copper as a catalyst can be problematic since it is a cytotoxic element. However, recently, it has been observed that cyclooctyne functionalized molecules are able to react rapidly with azide without the presence of copper [30]. This alternative reaction, called strain-promoted azide-alkyne cycloaddition, is currently more used for hydrogels design since it presents biosafety as well as the advantages of the previous reaction. On this matter, Fu et al. fabricated an injectable HA-PEG based hydrogel [31]. In particular, cyclooctyne modified HA was synthesized by reacting HA with 2-(aminoethoxy)cyclooctyne (Figure 1); subsequently, it was reacted with azide functionalized PEG in order to obtain the hydrogel. Interestingly, the resulting hydrogel showed fast gelation time, excellent mechanical properties, and high stability.

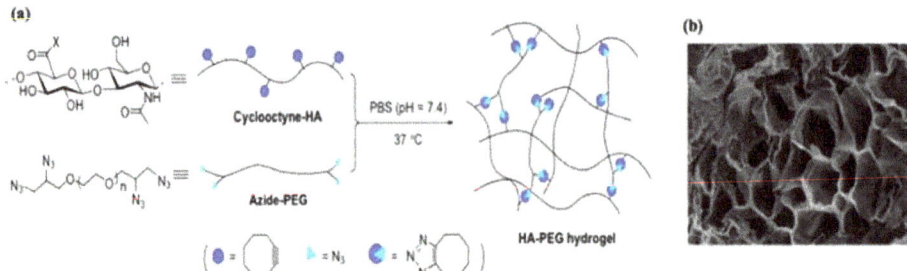

Figure 1. Preparation of the HA-PEG hydrogel (**a**), SEM image of the hydrogel (**b**) [31]. Reproduced with permission from Elsevier, 2017.

2.1.3. Thiol-ene Photocoupling (Click Chemistry)

The thiol-ene reaction consists of a radical addition (induced by light) between a thiol and enes which has a high yield, efficiency, specificity and a fast reaction rate [32]. This method is particularly attractive for hydrogels preparation because it is solvent free and allows the hydrogels spatiotemporal control; for this reason, it is particularly investigated for the design of hydrogels to use as scaffolds for tissue engineering and cell culture or as drug delivery systems [33,34]. Different vinyl groups are employed for thiol-ene click chemistry like norbornene [35], vinyl sulfone [36], maleimide, etc. The thiol-norbornene reaction is characterized by greater specificity compared to the use of other functional groups. For example, Gramlich et al. employed this method for the synthesis of a photopatterned HA-based hydrogel by reacting norbornene modified HA (NorHA) with dithiothreitol (Figure 2) [37]. Hydrogels with an elastic modulus ranging from 1000 Pa to 70,000 Pa were obtained by varying the quantity of crosslinker. Furthermore, they reported that a secondary thiol-norbornene reaction can be performed to the hydrogel by reducing the initial amount of crosslinker.

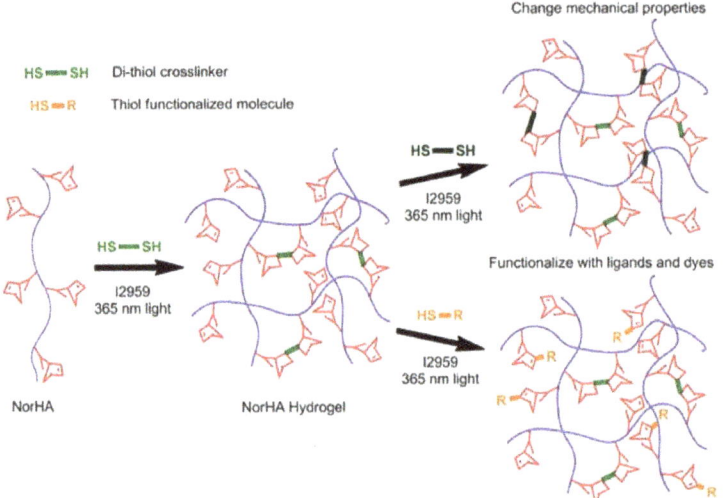

Figure 2. Synthesis scheme of hydrogel [37]. Reproduced with permission from Elsevier, 2013.

In this context, we also find the thiol-Michael addition which, however, is characterized by lower orthogonality. In this regard, Khetan et al. designed and prepared a 3D hydrogel via a two step crosslinking process: firstly, via a thiol-Michael addition between methacrylate-maleimide functionalized HA and thiols of peptides and, subsequently, via methacrylates photopolymerization [38].

2.1.4. Aldehyde-Hydrazide Coupling (Click Chemistry)

The aldehyde-hydrazide reaction has currently attracted interest in hydrogels design due to its high efficiency, cytocompatibility, simplicity, reversibility, and mild reaction conditions [39–41]. In particular, covalent hydrazone crosslinked hydrogels seem to be a promising approach for tissue engineering. In this regard, Chen et al. recently developed an injectable HA-pectin based hydrogel, by reacting HA adipic dihydrazide with biofunctionalized pectin-dialdehyde, and investigated its use as a scaffold for cartilage tissue engineering (Figure 3) [42]. Interestingly, the resulting hydrogel exhibited a fast gelation rate, good mechanical properties, biocompatibility, and cytocompatibility that make it a potential platform suitable for tissue regeneration. To further improve the structural integrity of hydrazone crosslinked hydrogels, Wang et al. recently reported the design and the preparation of an elastin-like protein/HA-based hydrogel by combining two different crosslinking processes (covalent and thermal) [43]. Firstly, the hydrogel was obtained via an aldehyde-hydrazide coupling between hydrazine modified elastin-like protein and aldehyde modified HA; the use of a thermoresponsive protein allowed a secondary thermal crosslinking that improved its structural integrity and stability. The resulting hydrogel showed shear-thinning and self-healing properties, easy injectability and protection of cells from the mechanical stress of injection and for these reasons can be considered a promising candidate for stem cells delivery.

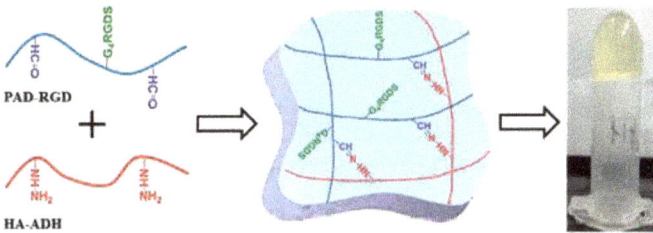

Figure 3. Hydrogels synthetic scheme [42]. Reproduced with permission from Elsevier, 2017.

2.1.5. Enzymatic Crosslinking

Enzymatic crosslinking represents an interesting approach for HA-based hydrogels preparation because it is characterized by mild reaction condition, fast gelation rate and leads to obtaining hydrogels with excellent mechanical properties [44,45]. Among different enzymes, horseradish peroxidase (HRP) turns out to be one of the most employed; it is usually employed in combination with hydrogen peroxide and the reaction can be summarized as follows: $2Ph + H_2O_2 \rightarrow 2Ph\cdot + H_2O$ [46]. In literature are reported various tyramine modified HA-based hydrogels which are formed as a result of an enzymatic crosslinking process that occurs through oxidation of tyramine which causes the formation of di-tyramine bonds [47]. In this regard, Xu et al. designed and fabricated HA-tyramine hydrogels by crosslinking tyramine moieties of HA in the presence of HRP and hydrogen peroxide (Figure 4) [48]. By varying the amounts of the enzyme and hydrogen peroxide, hydrogels with different mechanical strength were formed and were investigated in order to obtain a stable scaffold for stem cells culture. Interestingly, it was observed that the hydrogel with an elastic modulus of 350 Pa supported the proliferation of stem cells. A similar approach was reported by Raia et al. that enzymatically crosslinked tyramine functionalized HA and silk fibroin in order to increase the mechanical strength and the stability of tyramine-HA-based hydrogels [49]. By changing polymers concentration, hydrogels with tunable properties were obtained, resulting in versatile platforms that can be employed for various applications in tissue engineering.

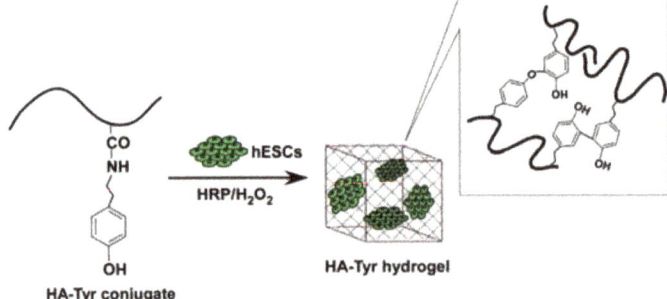

Figure 4. Schematic representation of hydrogels preparation and of encapsulation of human embryonic stem cells (hESCs) [48]. Reproduced with permission from Elsevier, 2015.

2.1.6. Disulfide Crosslinking

In the last years, disulfide crosslinked hydrogels have attracted growing attention because this crosslinking method presents various advantages such as biosafety, ease of execution, reversibility and permits to obtain hydrogels with *in-situ* gelation properties and responsiveness to reductant stimuli. Generally, disulfide bonds are formed via oxidation of thiols induced by air or oxidating agents like Cu(II)SO$_4$ [50]. Disulfide crosslinked HA hydrogels are currently investigated for tissue regeneration thanks to their degradability since they can be cleaved enzymatically by hyaluronidase and by physiological reductants like glutathione and cysteine [51]. For example, Bian et al. proposed self-crosslinking HA-based hydrogels as scaffolds for cell culture (Figure 5) [52]. They were prepared through exposition to air of different thiolated HA derivatives which were obtained by varying the degree of thiol substitution and molecular weights of HA. Gelation rate, mechanical properties, swelling degree, and degradation were investigated and the resulting hydrogel showed excellent biocompatibility, degradation behavior and, consequently, a great potential for applications in tissue engineering.

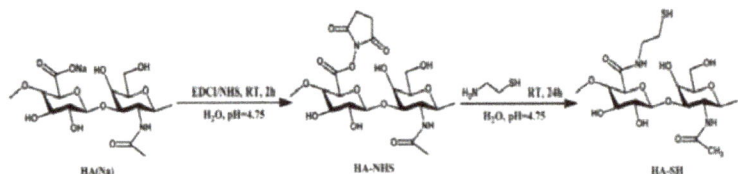

Figure 5. Synthesis scheme of thiol modified HA [52]. Reproduced with permission from Elsevier, 2016.

However, disulfide crosslinking presents some disadvantages like long reaction times, the presence of strong oxidants, etc. To overcome these limitations, an interesting strategy for disulfide crosslinked HA hydrogels preparation has been recently proposed by Velasco et al. [53]. Herein, the authors investigated the effects of the presence of various electron-withdrawing groups at the β position of thiol modified HA (cysteine, *N*-acetyl-L-cysteine). Interestingly, HA functionalized with cysteine or *N*-acetyl-L-cysteine showed fast gelation rate at physiological pH, while HA-thiol did not form any gel in the same conditions. Furthermore, the resulting hydrogels showed excellent mechanical properties and hydrolytic stability.

2.1.7. Crosslinking by Radical Polymerization

Hydrogels can be formed via radical polymerization of monomers in the presence of crosslinking agents and an initiator like a redox pair or a photoinitiator [54]. Methacrylates represent the most common groups used for HA-based hydrogels preparation and they can be introduced to HA by reacting it with glycidyl methacrylate or methacrylic anhydride [55,56]. An advantage of methacrylated HA-based hydrogels is that it is possible to tune their properties by varying HA molecular weight, the concentration of the functional monomer, the degree of substitution, etc. [57]. In this regard, Tavsanli et al. developed silk/HA-based hydrogels and investigated their mechanical properties [58]. The hydrogels were prepared by reacting methacrylated HA (MeHA) and silk fibroin (SF) in aqueous solution in the presence of N,N,N',N'-tetramethylethylenediamine (TEMED), ammonium persulfate (APS), and N,N-dimethylacrylamide (DMMA) which has the function of connecting methacrylated HA macromers via their vinyl groups (Figure 6). Interestingly, the resulting hydrogels showed bicompatibility, excellent mechanical properties and stability thanks to the presence of SF since its β-sheet domains act as physical crosslinks.

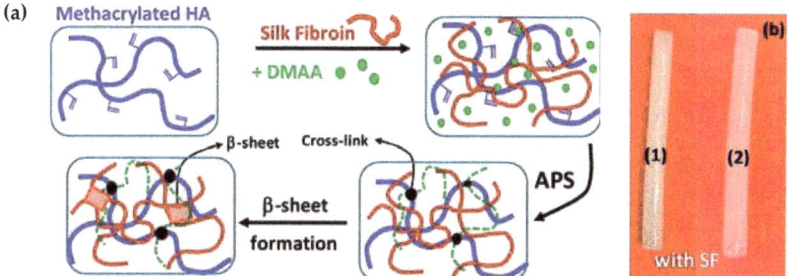

Figure 6. Schematic formation of HA-SF based hydrogel (a) and photographs of hydrogels with SF (b) [58]. Adapted with permission from Elsevier, 2019.

2.1.8. Crosslinking by Condensation Reactions

Condensation reactions are often applied for hydrogels synthesis. Considering the chemical structure of HA, among the different condensation reactions, esterification turns out to be one of the most commonly employed for hydrogels design. In this regard, Larrañeta et al. recently developed an attractive eco-friendly strategy for the synthesis of HA-based hydrogels [59]. For this purpose, Gantrex S97 was used as crosslinking agent and the hydrogels were obtained via esterification between the hydroxyl groups of HA and the carboxylic groups of Gantrex S97 (Figure 7). Since the reaction takes place in solid phase inside a microwave or an oven, the process can be considered green because it does not need organic solvents or toxic substances. Furthermore, the release capabilities and the antimicrobial properties were investigated. Interestingly, the resulting hydrogel showed a sustained release and anti-infective properties resulting in a promising candidate for the design of drug delivery systems and wound dressings.

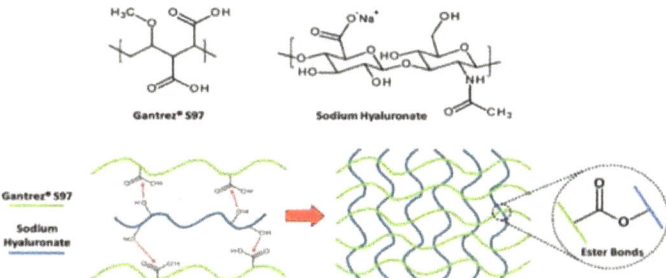

Figure 7. Schematic crosslinking mechanism between sodium hyaluronate and Gantrez® S97 [59]. Reproduced with permission from Elsevier, 2018.

2.2. Physical Hydrogels

In recent years, non-covalent bonds and supramolecular interactions have been widely investigated for hydrogels design thanks to their singular features. First of all, since these interactions are reversible, the non-covalent assembly allows to obtain hydrogels with tunable properties and responsivity to various cues like light, pH, temperature, etc. [60,61]. In contrast to covalent crosslinking, physical crosslinking leads to the formation of less mechanically and chemically stable hydrogels. However, this aspect can be considered an advantageous feature since it can be exploited in order to obtain hydrogels with shear-thinning and self-healing properties [17].

In this context, inclusion complexation represents one of the most used strategies for the preparation of physical gels. It can be considered the result of supramolecular interactions and structural complementarity between two molecules called "host" and "guest" [62]. Cyclodextrins are one of the most widely employed hosts which have hydrophobic cavities with a high affinity for hydrophobic guests. Several guest molecules employed in pair with cyclodextrins have been reported in literature and among these the most representative is adamantane. In this regard, Rodell et al. designed a self-assembling HA hydrogel based on supramolecular interactions between adamantane functionalized HA and β-cyclodextrin functionalized HA [63]. Hydrogel formation occurred rapidly by mixing host and guest molecules in aqueous solution. Physical properties were investigated and it has been observed that were dependent on the crosslink density and structure that can be modified by varying host and guest concentrations, molar ratio, etc. The obtained hydrogel displayed shear-thinning properties resulting in a promising injectable system. Another investigated pair for inclusion complexation broadly reported in literature is represented by α- or β-cyclodextrin and azobenzenes since *trans*-azobenzene has a high binding affinity for α- or β-cyclodextrin, while *cis*-azobenzene has a low binding affinity for them. On this subject, Rosales et al. recently developed a supramolecular HA-based hydrogel using HA functionalized with β-cyclodextrin and azobenzene [64]. It has been shown that it is possible to modulate hydrogel properties with light; in fact, upon irradiation (λ = 365 nm), isomerization of azobenzene occurs changing the binding affinity between host/guest molecules and, consequently, the network connectivity and the elastic modulus of the hydrogel. Furthermore, the release capabilities were investigated, highlighting the possibility to tune drugs release profile with light exposure. A similar approach was reported by Rowland et al. using cucurbit [8] uril and cysteine-phenylalanine as host/guest pair in order to obtain a supramolecular HA-based hydrogel [65]. Another interesting non-covalent approach for HA-based hydrogels design is represented by functionalization of HA with hydrophobic molecules in order to render it amphiphilic and consequently determine the macromers self assembly in nanogels. In this regard, Montanari et al. designed HA-based hydrogels via self-assembly of macromers in water after the functionalization of HA with cholesterol [66]. In particular, the self-assembly of macromers occurs due to the hydrophobic interactions between the cholesterol cores and the hydrophilic interactions between the shells formed by HA.

Moreover, the use of gelling agents in combination with HA can be considered a valid strategy for HA physical hydrogels design. For example, Jung et al. recently reported the preparation of a thermosensitive hydrogel based on HA and Pluronic F-127 [67]. Pluronic F-127 is a triblock copolymer able to form rapidly thermoresponsive hydrogels which, however, are unstable in physiological conditions due to their low mechanical strength. To overcome this problem, in this study HA was mixed with Pluronic F-127 in water in order to obtain a hydrogel with improved structural integrity and stability due to the hydrophobic interactions that occur between acetyl groups of HA and methyl groups of Pluronic F-127. Interestingly, the resulting hydrogel not only showed an increased mechanical strength but also a sustained drug release, reducing the typical burst release observed in Pluronic F-127-based hydrogels.

3. HA-Based Hydrogels for Biomedical Applications

Currently, HA-based hydrogels are widely investigated for biomedical purposes like drug delivery, tissue engineering, regenerative medicine thanks to their biocompatibility, biodegradability, non–immunogenicity, responsivity to various cues, and tunable properties [68–70]. This section reviews the main biomedical applications of HA-based hydrogels reported in literature in the last few years, focusing in particular on drug delivery.

3.1. Drug Delivery

HA-based hydrogels are particularly interesting for drug delivery since, in addition to above cited features, allow to have a controlled and targeted drug release in response to different triggers that turns out to be attractive when aiming for targeted therapy [71,72].

3.1.1. Stimuli-Responsive Hydrogels

Various smart hydrogels responsive to different environmental factors such as pH, temperature, light, biochemical molecules have been developed as drug delivery systems. With regard to stimuli-responsive platforms, physical crosslinking is preferred since supramolecular interactions are reversible and consequently results easier to tune hydrogels properties.

In this context, Highley et al. recently proposed an interesting strategy for the design of a near infrared light (NIR)/temperature responsive platform [73]. In this study, the platform was prepared in a microfluidic mixing device by combining gold nanorods with a HA supramolecular hydrogel obtained via the inclusion complexation of β-cyclodextrin and adamantane. The presence of nanorods caused heating in response to NIR irradiation causing consequently the breakage of supramolecular interactions and the networks disruption. The release capability of the resulting platform in response to different NIR exposures was evaluated, and interestingly it has been observed that the drug release can be modulated by varying two parameters: irradiation time, and light intensity; specifically, the quantity of the molecule released from the platform increased with increasing power and irradiation time.

Inclusion complexation employing azobenzene/cyclodextrin as host/guest pair has been broadly investigated for photoresponsive hydrogels design since the supramolecular host/guest interactions can be disrupted upon *trans-cis* photoisomerization of azobenzene induced by ultraviolet (UV) light [74]. An interesting example of a photoresponsive drug delivery platform has been described by Rosales et al. [64]. Thus, HA was functionalized with azobenzene and β-cyclodextrin in order to obtain self-assembled hydrogels. The resulting hydrogels showed reversible changes in crosslink density and, consequently, in mesh size, upon UV exposures. These changes were exploited to modulate drug release profiles and, therefore, the release capability upon different UV irradiations was evaluated. In particular, a fluorescently labeled protein was loaded as a model drug and it has been observed that upon irradiation hydrogels released a double amount of protein compared to the non irradiated ones.

Even if physical crosslinking is preferred for smart hydrogels preparation, also the chemical approach has been recently investigated. In this regard, Kwon et al. reported the preparation of pH-sensitive hydrogels based on hydroxyethyl cellulose and hyaluronic acid and investigated their potential use as transdermal delivery systems for the treatment of skin lesions [75]. In this study, the hydrogels were synthesized via Michael addition between HA and hydroxyethyl cellulose by using divinyl sulfone as crosslinking agent and their physicochemical properties were investigated. Hydrogels were then loaded with isoliquiritigenin, which has antimicrobial activity, and its release efficiency has been investigated by in vitro measurements at different values of pH. Experimental data showed that the quantity of isoliquiritigenin released increased with increasing pH beyond 7 due to electrostatic repulsions between the carboxylate groups of HA that cause consequently an increase of mesh size.

3.1.2. HA-Based Hydrogels for Targeted Cancer Treatment

As already reported, HA regulates different cellular functions such as cell adhesion, differentiation, migration, proliferation, etc., which arise as a result of HA binding to specific membrane surface receptors, called hyaldherins, like CD44, LYVE-1, and RHAMM [76]. In particular, CD44 is the main receptor involved in cellular proliferation, differentiation, and migration pathways and consequently in tumor progression and metastasis; moreover, it is overexpressed in various types of tumors like melanoma, chondrosarcoma, breast, gastrointestinal, prostate, bladder, lung, and pancreatic cancers, and different studies have reported a relationship between CD44 expression and poor prognosis [77]. For these reasons, HA has recently emerged as a promising molecule for the design of anticancer drug delivery systems for active targeting of malignant tumors [78]. Comprehensive reviews by Huang et al. and Choi et al. supply an interesting description of HA-based drug delivery systems developed for targeted cancer treatment [79,80].

In the last years, several HA-based hydrogels have been studied for the delivery of different antitumor drugs such as doxorubicin, paclitaxel, cisplatin, etc., in order to improve their antitumor activity and reduce their systemic side effects [81,82]; some of the most interesting and recent examples will now be presented.

Aiming at preparing a suitable drug delivery platform for the targeted release of doxorubicin, Yang et al. prepared various HA-based nanogels via copolymerization of methacrylated HA with di(ethylene glycol) diacrylate [83]. Nanogels with a diameter of about 70 nm and a spherical shape were obtained, which were then loaded with doxorubicin by an incubation method. In vitro studies showed a CD44-dependent cellular uptake and consequently a greater internalization of nanogels in tumor cell lines that overexpress CD44 receptor (Figure 8).

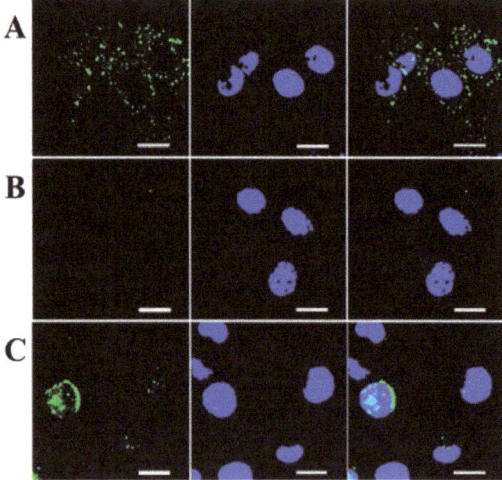

Figure 8. Confocal laser scanning microscopy of (**a**) A549, (**b**) NIHT3T, and (**c**) H22 cells incubated with FITC-labeled HA nanogels [83], The scale bar =10µm. Reproduced with permission from Elsevier, 2015.

Furthermore, the nanogels showed higher accumulation in the tumor site and a superior antitumor activity compared with the free doxorubicin, resulting in a promising drug delivery system for cancer therapy.

A noteworthy further example of doxorubicin delivery platform has been reported by Jhan et al. [84]. In this study, injectable thermosensitive hydrogels based on Pluronic F-127 and HA-doxorubicin nanocomplexes were prepared via physical mixing and their physiochemical properties were investigated. The doxorubicin release profile was studied in vitro, while nanogels antitumor activity both in vivo and in vitro. Experimental data showed a pH sensitive and sustained release of doxorubicin from hydrogels with a faster release rate at tumoral pH. Moreover, hydrogels showed an excellent cytotoxic activity against tumor cell lines that overexpress CD44 receptor and a high affinity targeting to the lymphonodes, resulting in promising injectable formulations for the treatment of local and metastatic tumors.

Furthermore, in this context, an efficient approach for metastatic breast cancer treatment has been recently described by Chen et al. [85]. In particular, the authors prepared saporin loaded epidermal growth factor receptor (EGFR) and CD44 dual targeted HA nanogels by combining inverse nanoprecipitation and tetrazole-alkene photocoupling. Nanogels with a diameter of about 160 nm and a spherical shape were obtained and evaluated for the treatment of metastatic breast cancer. In vitro studies showed an excellent internalization of nanogels in 4T1 breast cancer cell line that overexpresses both EGFR and CD44. Furthermore, in vivo studies in metastatic 4T1-luc breast tumor bearing mice displayed that the nanogels enhanced the therapeutic efficacy of saporin, showing an excellent inhibition of tumor growth and lung metastasis.

Currently intraperitoneal (IP) chemotherapy is emerging as an efficient strategy for the treatment of solid tumors present in the peritoneal cavity [86]. However, the delivery systems suitable for the IP chemotherapy should have some requirements like biocompatibility, biodegradability, non-immunogenicity and the capacity to control the drug release. Since HA hydrogels have these features, they are now also studied for the design of drug delivery platforms for IP chemotherapy. In this regard, Cho et al. recently reported the design of in situ crosslinkable HA-based gels and evaluated their potential use as IP carriers of platinum for the treatment of ovarian cancer [87]. Firstly, they prepared platinum loaded nanoparticles that were incorporated in HA-based hydrogels obtained via the aldehyde-hydrazide coupling. The obtained platforms showed sustained platinum release, good anti-tumor activity and a long permanence in the peritoneal cavity resulting attractive for IP chemotherapy of ovarian cancer.

Unfortunately, one problem that can occur sometimes when using hydrogels as drug delivery systems is the burst release [88]; with the attempt to reduce the burst release of drugs from hydrogels, Zhang et al. proposed an innovative strategy for HA-based hydrogels design [89]. In this regard, they prepared multilayer hydrogel capsules based on chitosan, HA and doxorubicin via the ionotropic crosslinking method. Release studies concerning these hydrogels showed a pH-sensitive, controlled release of doxorobucin with a notable reduction of the burst release due to their particular structure; in fact, the multilayer structure reduced the drug concentration gradient between the capsules external layer and the surrounding environment limiting the release of doxorubicin adsorbed on the surface of the hydrogels.

3.1.3. HA-Based Hydrogels for Osteoarthritis Treatment

Osteoarthritis is an inflammatory, chronic joint disorder characterized by progressive cartilage erosion. Currently, osteoarthritis treatment is limited to anti-inflammatory drugs administration, viscosupplementation and, if necessary, prosthesis graft at the last stage [90].

As already reported, HA performs multiple biological functions: at the articular level, thanks to its viscoelasticity, it acts as a lubricant, increasing the viscosity of the synovial fluid, and as a cushioning, allowing the separation of the articular surfaces under load.

HA presents also chondroprotective and anti-inflammatory effects [91]. Furthermore, some studies reported the overexpression of CD44 receptor on human articular chondrocytes [92]. For these reasons, HA-based hydrogels are widely investigated and used as viscosupplements and delivery platforms for osteoarthritis treatment.

In this regard, Jung et al. recently reported the preparation of an injectable thermosensitive hydrogel via physical mixing of HA and Pluronic F-127 [67]. As previously reported, Pluronic F-127 is a gelling agent able to rapidly form thermoresponsive hydrogels that however are instable in physiological conditions due to their low mechanical strength. To overcome this problem, in this study,

HA was physically mixed with Pluronic F-127 in order to obtain a hydrogel with improved structural integrity and stability due to the hydrophobic interactions that occur between HA and Pluronic. The hydrogel was then loaded with piroxicam and evaluated for the treatment of osteoarthritis. In Vitro release studies showed a 10 days sustained and slow release of piroxicam from HA-Pluronic F-127 hydrogel, while Pluronic F-127 based hydrogels displayed a faster release behavior (Figure 9). Furthermore, in vivo pharmacokinetic studies reported an increase of drug bioavailability and half-life in comparison to a commercial Paclitaxel formulation.

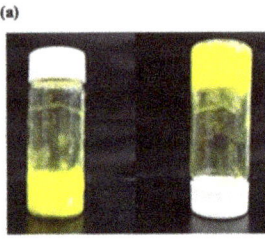
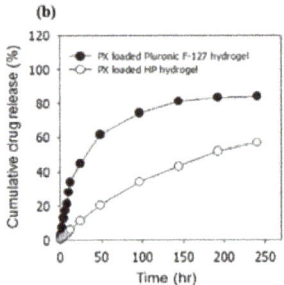

Figure 9. Photographs of the hydrogel (**a**) and in vitro Paclitaxel release from Pluronic F-127 and Pluronic F-127/HA-based hydrogels (**b**) [67]. Reproduced with permission from Elsevier, 2016.

In addition to the classical therapeutic approaches, nowadays gene silencing of signal molecules, proteins, enzymes, that play an important role in osteoarthritis degenerative events, is emerging as a promising strategy for osteoarthritis treatment.

In this regard, Cai et al. recently developed a HA-based hydrogel loaded with gapmer antisense oligonucleotides that was studied for silencing target gene expression in osteoarthritis [93]. In particular, the hydrogel was prepared via Schiff reaction between aldehyde modified HA and chitosan, and subsequently, it was loaded with a gapmer oligonucleotide, obtaining a high encapsulation efficiency (~97%), in order to reduce COX-2 expression. In vitro studies showed a sustained release of COX-2 gapmer up to five days with a low burst release and, furthermore, a 10–14 days long COX-2 gene silencing activity in osteoarthritis chondrocytes. A similar approach was recently reported by Garcia et al. in order to obtain a HA-based hydrogel for the delivery of chondrocytes and antisense oligonucleotides [94]. In this case hydrogels made of HA and fibrin were loaded with an antisense oligonucleotide in order to modulate the expression of genes that codify for ADAMTS (A Disintegrin and Metallo Proteinase with Thrombospondin Motifs) enzymes which showed to play a key role in causing proteoglycans loss in osteoarthritis [95]; chondrocytes were also incorporated in the scaffolds in order to have both regenerative and therapeutic effects. In Vitro studies showed 14-day long sustained release and an efficient and long genes inhibition in both incorporated and resident chondrocytes. These features make this platform a potential formulation for osteoarthritis treatment.

4. Conclusions

In recent decades, HA has emerged as an attractive molecule for hydrogels design thanks to its biocompatibility, native biofunctionality, biodegradability, non-immunogenicity, and versatility. Nowadays, several HA-based hydrogels are already used in medicine as dermal fillers, viscosupplements, wound dressings, etc., and the market is continuously increasing worldwide.

Since HA is not able to form gels alone, new crosslinking methods, like click chemistry reactions, disulfide crosslinking, enzymatic crosslinking, or supramolecular assembly methods like inclusion complexation, functionalization with lipophilic molecules, etc., have been widely investigated resulting in efficient strategies for chemical and physical hydrogels design. However, these current synthetic strategies present several advantages as well as some limitations. For example, various chemical crosslinking techniques often require organic solvents, metal catalysts, reaction by-product can be formed, etc. Thus, in this respect, research is aimed at developing new advantageous synthetic strategies.

HA-based hydrogels turn out to be versatile platforms ranging from passive and static matrices to smart, stimuli-responsive platforms with tunable properties and consequently they showed to have great potential as drug delivery systems, scaffolds for tissue engineering and regenerative medicine, and so on. In particular, their tunability is exploited for the design of platforms for controlled and targeted drug delivery; in this regard, a notable attention is given to inclusion complexation employing cyclodextrin and azobenzene as a host/guest pair, which allows obtaining photoresponsive drug delivery systems. Furthermore, since HA receptors were found to be overexpressed on various tumor cells and on chondrocytes, different HA-based hydrogels have been broadly developed for these purposes, showing promising results for targeted cancer and osteoarthritis therapies.

Nowadays, one of the main goals is the design of intelligent hydrogels with various features like stability, complex structures, biochemical cues and responsive to several triggers that, surely, will find a place into clinical practice.

Funding: The authors thank the Department of Pharmacy, Health and Nutritional Sciences, UNICAL Department of Excellence funded according the Law 232/2016 and the project POR Calabria FESR/FSE 2014-2020.

Conflicts of Interest: The authors declare no conflict of interest.

References

1. Hoffman, A.S. Hydrogels for biomedical applications. *Adv. Drug Deliv. Rev.* **2012**, *64*, 18–23. [CrossRef]
2. Seliktar, D. Designing cell-compatible hydrogels for biomedical applications. *Science* **2012**, *336*, 1124–1128. [CrossRef] [PubMed]
3. ConvaTec Website. Available online: https://www.convatec.it/ (accessed on 12 June 2019).
4. Covidien Website. Available online: https://www.covidien.com/ (accessed on 12 June 2019).
5. Blanchard, C.R.; Timmons, S.F.; Smith, R.A. Keratin-Based Hydrogel for Biomedical Applications and Method of Production. U.S. Patent 6,379,690 B2, 30 April 2002.
6. Kumar, A. Hydrogel scaffolds for tissue engineering. U.S. Patent 2013/0236971 A1, 12 September 2013.
7. Ocular Therapeutix Website. Available online: https://www.ocutx.com/products/dextenza/ (accessed on 12 June 2019).
8. Fraser, J.R.E.; Laurent, T.C.; Laurent, U. Hyaluronan: Its nature, distribution, functions and turnover. *J. Intern. Med.* **1997**, *242*, 27–33. [CrossRef] [PubMed]
9. Prehm, P. Hyaluronate is synthesized at plasma membranes. *Biochem. J.* **1984**, *220*, 597–600. [CrossRef] [PubMed]
10. Fallacara, A.; Baldini, E.; Manfredini, S.; Vertuani, S. Hyaluronic acid in the third millennium. *Polymers* **2018**, *10*, 701. [CrossRef]
11. Laurent, T.C.; Fraser, J. Hyaluronan. *FASEB J.* **1992**, *6*, 2397–2404. [CrossRef]
12. Dicker, K.T.; Gurski, L.A.; Pradhan-Bhatt, S.; Witt, R.L.; Farach-Carson, M.C.; Jia, X. Hyaluronan: A simple polysaccharide with diverse biological functions. *Acta Biomater.* **2014**, *10*, 1558–1570. [CrossRef]
13. Toole, B.P. Hyaluronan: From extracellular glue to pericellular cue. *Nat. Rev. Cancer* **2004**, *4*, 528. [CrossRef]
14. Ahmed, E.M. Hydrogel: Preparation, characterization, and applications: A review. *J. Adv. Res.* **2015**, *6*, 105–121. [CrossRef]
15. Caló, E.; Khutoryanskiy, V.V. Biomedical applications of hydrogels: A review of patents and commercial products. *Eur. Polym. J.* **2015**, *65*, 252–267. [CrossRef]
16. Schanté, C.E.; Zuber, G.; Herlin, C.; Vandamme, T.F. Chemical modifications of hyaluronic acid for the synthesis of derivatives for a broad range of biomedical applications. *Carbohydr. Polym.* **2011**, *85*, 469–489. [CrossRef]
17. Appel, E.A.; del Barrio, J.; Loh, X.J.; Scherman, O.A. Supramolecular polymeric hydrogels. *Chem. Soc. Rev.* **2012**, *41*, 6195–6214. [CrossRef] [PubMed]
18. Ibrahim, S.; Kang, Q.K.; Ramamurthi, A. The impact of hyaluronic acid oligomer content on physical, mechanical, and biologic properties of divinyl sulfone-crosslinked hyaluronic acid hydrogels. *J. Biomed. Mater. Res. Part A* **2010**, *94*, 355–370. [CrossRef] [PubMed]

19. Crescenzi, V.; Francescangeli, A.; Taglienti, A. New gelatin-based hydrogels via enzymatic networking. *Biomacromolecules* **2002**, *3*, 1384–1391. [CrossRef] [PubMed]
20. Kuo, J.W.; Swann, D.A.; Prestwich, G.D. Chemical modification of hyaluronic acid by carbodiimides. *Bioconj. Chem.* **1991**, *2*, 232–241. [CrossRef]
21. Segura, T.; Anderson, B.C.; Chung, P.H.; Webber, R.E.; Shull, K.R.; Shea, L.D. Crosslinked hyaluronic acid hydrogels: A strategy to functionalize and pattern. *Biomaterials* **2005**, *26*, 359–371. [CrossRef]
22. Jiang, Y.; Chen, J.; Deng, C.; Suuronen, E.J.; Zhong, Z. Click hydrogels, microgels and nanogels: Emerging platforms for drug delivery and tissue engineering. *Biomaterials* **2014**, *35*, 4969–4985. [CrossRef]
23. Gandini, A. The furan/maleimide Diels–Alder reaction: A versatile click–unclick tool in macromolecular synthesis. *Prog. Polym. Sci.* **2013**, *38*, 1–29. [CrossRef]
24. Fisher, S.A.; Anandakumaran, P.N.; Owen, S.C.; Shoichet, M.S. Tuning the microenvironment: Click-crosslinked hyaluronic acid-based hydrogels provide a platform for studying breast cancer cell invasion. *Adv. Funct. Mater.* **2015**, *25*, 7163–7172. [CrossRef]
25. Yu, F.; Cao, X.; Li, Y.; Chen, X. Diels–Alder click-based hydrogels for direct spatiotemporal postpatterning via photoclick chemistry. *ACS Macro Lett.* **2015**, *4*, 289–292. [CrossRef]
26. Rostovtsev, V.V.; Green, L.G.; Fokin, V.V.; Sharpless, K.B. A stepwise huisgen cycloaddition process: Copper (I)-catalyzed regioselective "ligation" of azides and terminal alkynes. *Angew. Chem. Int. Ed.* **2002**, *41*, 2596–2599. [CrossRef]
27. Pahimanolis, N.; Sorvari, A.; Luong, N.D.; Seppälä, J. Thermoresponsive xylan hydrogels via copper-catalyzed azide-alkyne cycloaddition. *Carbohydr. Polym.* **2014**, *102*, 637–644. [CrossRef] [PubMed]
28. Gong, T.; Adzima, B.J.; Baker, N.H.; Bowman, C.N. Photopolymerization reactions using the photoinitiated Copper (I)-Catalyzed Azide-Alkyne Cycloaddition (CuAAC) reaction. *Adv. Mater.* **2013**, *25*, 2024–2028. [CrossRef] [PubMed]
29. Manzi, G.; Zoratto, N.; Matano, S.; Sabia, R.; Villani, C.; Coviello, T.; Matricardi, P.; Di Meo, C. "Click" hyaluronan based nanohydrogels as multifunctionalizable carriers for hydrophobic drugs. *Carbohydr. Polym.* **2017**, *174*, 706–715. [CrossRef] [PubMed]
30. Laughlin, S.T.; Baskin, J.M.; Amacher, S.L.; Bertozzi, C.R. In vivo imaging of membrane-associated glycans in developing zebrafish. *Science* **2008**, *320*, 664–667. [CrossRef]
31. Fu, S.; Dong, H.; Deng, X.; Zhuo, R.; Zhong, Z. Injectable hyaluronic acid/poly (ethylene glycol) hydrogels crosslinked via strain-promoted azide-alkyne cycloaddition click reaction. *Carbohydr. Polym.* **2017**, *169*, 332–340. [CrossRef]
32. Hoyle, C.E.; Lee, T.Y.; Roper, T. Thiol–enes: Chemistry of the past with promise for the future. *J. Polym. Sci. Part A Polym. Chem.* **2004**, *42*, 5301–5338. [CrossRef]
33. Sawicki, L.A.; Kloxin, A.M. Design of thiol–ene photoclick hydrogels using facile techniques for cell culture applications. *Biomater.Sci.* **2014**, *2*, 1612–1626. [CrossRef]
34. Yang, C.; Mariner, P.D.; Nahreini, J.N.; Anseth, K.S. Cell-mediated delivery of glucocorticoids from thiol-ene hydrogels. *J. Controll. Release* **2012**, *162*, 612–618. [CrossRef]
35. Fairbanks, B.D.; Schwartz, M.P.; Halevi, A.E.; Nuttelman, C.R.; Bowman, C.N.; Anseth, K.S. A versatile synthetic extracellular matrix mimic via thiol-norbornene photopolymerization. *Adv. Mater.* **2009**, *21*, 5005–5010. [CrossRef]
36. Lutolf, M.; Hubbell, J. Synthetic biomaterials as instructive extracellular microenvironments for morphogenesis in tissue engineering. *Nat. Biotechnol.* **2005**, *23*, 47. [CrossRef]
37. Gramlich, W.M.; Kim, I.L.; Burdick, J.A. Synthesis and orthogonal photopatterning of hyaluronic acid hydrogels with thiol-norbornene chemistry. *Biomaterials* **2013**, *34*, 9803–9811. [CrossRef]
38. Khetan, S.; Guvendiren, M.; Legant, W.R.; Cohen, D.M.; Chen, C.S.; Burdick, J.A. Degradation-mediated cellular traction directs stem cell fate in covalently crosslinked three-dimensional hydrogels. *Nat. Mater.* **2013**, *12*, 458. [CrossRef]
39. Yan, S.; Wang, T.; Feng, L.; Zhu, J.; Zhang, K.; Chen, X.; Cui, L.; Yin, J. Injectable in situ self-cross-linking hydrogels based on poly (L-glutamic acid) and alginate for cartilage tissue engineering. *Biomacromolecules* **2014**, *15*, 4495–4508. [CrossRef]
40. Tian, W.; Zhang, C.; Hou, S.; Yu, X.; Cui, F.; Xu, Q.; Sheng, S.; Cui, H.; Li, H. Hyaluronic acid hydrogel as Nogo-66 receptor antibody delivery system for the repairing of injured rat brain: In vitro. *J. Controll. Release* **2005**, *102*, 13–22. [CrossRef]

41. Ito, T.; Fraser, I.P.; Yeo, Y.; Highley, C.B.; Bellas, E.; Kohane, D.S. Anti–inflammatory function of an in situ cross–linkable conjugate hydrogel of hyaluronic acid and dexamethasone. *Biomaterials* **2007**, *28*, 1778–1786. [CrossRef]
42. Chen, F.; Ni, Y.; Liu, B.; Zhou, T.; Yu, C.; Su, Y.; Zhu, X.; Yu, X.; Zhou, Y. Self–crosslinking and injectable hyaluronic acid/RGD–functionalized pectin hydrogel for cartilage tissue engineering. *Carbohydr. Polym.* **2017**, *166*, 31–44. [CrossRef]
43. Wang, H.; Zhu, D.; Paul, A.; Cai, L.; Enejder, A.; Yang, F.; Heilshorn, S.C. Covalently adaptable elastin-like protein–hyaluronic acid (ELP–HA) hybrid hydrogels with secondary thermoresponsive crosslinking for injectable stem cell delivery. *Adv. Funct. Mater.* **2017**, *27*, 1605609. [CrossRef]
44. Kurisawa, M.; Lee, F.; Wang, L.S.; Chung, J.E. Injectable enzymatically crosslinked hydrogel system with independent tuning of mechanical strength and gelation rate for drug delivery and tissue engineering. *J. Mater. Chem.* **2010**, *20*, 5371–5375. [CrossRef]
45. Tran, N.Q.; Joung, Y.K.; Lih, E.; Park, K.M.; Park, K.D. Supramolecular hydrogels exhibiting fast in situ gel forming and adjustable degradation properties. *Biomacromolecules* **2010**, *11*, 617–625. [CrossRef]
46. Roberts, J.J.; Naudiyal, P.; Lim, K.S.; Poole–Warren, L.A.; Martens, P.J. A comparative study of enzyme initiators for crosslinking phenol–functionalized hydrogels for cell encapsulation. *Biomater. Res.* **2016**, *20*, 30. [CrossRef]
47. Rizzuto, F.; Spikes, J.D. The eosin-sensitized photooxidation of substituted phenylalanines and tyrosines. *Photochem. Photobiol.* **1977**, *25*, 465–476. [CrossRef]
48. Xu, K.; Narayanan, K.; Lee, F.; Bae, K.H.; Gao, S.; Kurisawa, M. Enzyme–mediated hyaluronic acid–tyramine hydrogels for the propagation of human embryonic stem cells in 3D. *Acta Biomater.* **2015**, *24*, 159–171. [CrossRef]
49. Raia, N.R.; Partlow, B.P.; McGill, M.; Kimmerling, E.P.; Ghezzi, C.E.; Kaplan, D.L. Enzymatically crosslinked silk–hyaluronic acid hydrogels. *Biomaterials* **2017**, *131*, 58–67. [CrossRef]
50. Su, J. Thiol–mediated chemoselective strategies for in situ formation of hydrogels. *Gels* **2018**, *4*, 72. [CrossRef]
51. Choh, S.-Y.; Cross, D.; Wang, C. Facile synthesis and characterization of disulfide–cross–linked hyaluronic acid hydrogels for protein delivery and cell encapsulation. *Biomacromolecules* **2011**, *12*, 1126–1136. [CrossRef]
52. Bian, S.; He, M.; Sui, J.; Cai, H.; Sun, Y.; Liang, J.; Fan, Y.; Zhang, X. The self–crosslinking smart hyaluronic acid hydrogels as injectable three–dimensional scaffolds for cells culture. *Coll. Surf. B Biointerfaces* **2016**, *140*, 392–402. [CrossRef]
53. Bermejo-Velasco, D.; Azémar, A.; Oommen, O.P.; Hilborn, J.N.; Varghese, O.P. Modulating Thiol pKa promotes disulfide formation at physiological pH: An elegant strategy to design disulfide cross–linked hyaluronic acid hydrogels. *Biomacromolecules* **2019**, *20*, 1412–1420. [CrossRef]
54. Hennink, W.E.; van Nostrum, C.F. Novel crosslinking methods to design hydrogels. *Adv. Drug Deliv. Rev.* **2012**, *64*, 223–236. [CrossRef]
55. Ibrahim, S.; Kothapalli, C.; Kang, Q.; Ramamurthi, A. Characterization of glycidyl methacrylate–crosslinked hyaluronan hydrogel scaffolds incorporating elastogenic hyaluronan oligomers. *Acta Biomater.* **2011**, *7*, 653–665. [CrossRef]
56. Poldervaart, M.T.; Goversen, B.; De Ruijter, M.; Abbadessa, A.; Melchels, F.P.; Öner, F.C.; Dhert, W.J.; Vermonden, T.; Alblas, J. 3D bioprinting of methacrylated hyaluronic acid (MeHA) hydrogel with intrinsic osteogenicity. *PloS ONE* **2017**, *12*, e0177628. [CrossRef]
57. Burdick, J.A.; Chung, C.; Jia, X.; Randolph, M.A.; Langer, R. Controlled degradation and mechanical behavior of photopolymerized hyaluronic acid networks. *Biomacromolecules* **2005**, *6*, 386–391. [CrossRef]
58. Tavsanli, B.; Okay, O. Mechanically robust and stretchable silk/hyaluronic acid hydrogels. *Carbohydr. Polym.* **2019**, *208*, 413–420. [CrossRef]
59. Larrañeta, E.; Henry, M.; Irwin, N.J.; Trotter, J.; Perminova, A.A.; Donnelly, R.F. Synthesis and characterization of hyaluronic acid hydrogels crosslinked using a solvent–free process for potential biomedical applications. *Carbohydr. Polym.* **2018**, *181*, 1194–1205. [CrossRef]
60. Zheng, Z.; Hu, J.; Wang, H.; Huang, J.; Yu, Y.; Zhang, Q.; Cheng, Y. Dynamic softening or stiffening a supramolecular hydrogel by ultraviolet or near–infrared light. *ACS Appl. Mater. Interfaces* **2017**, *9*, 24511–24517. [CrossRef]

61. Rombouts, W.H.; de Kort, D.W.; Pham, T.T.; van Mierlo, C.P.; Werten, M.W.; de Wolf, F.A.; van der Gucht, J. Reversible temperature–switching of hydrogel stiffness of coassembled, silk–collagen–like hydrogels. *Biomacromolecules* **2015**, *16*, 2506–2513. [CrossRef]
62. Chen, G.; Jiang, M. Cyclodextrin–based inclusion complexation bridging supramolecular chemistry and macromolecular self–assembly. *Chem. Soc. Rev.* **2011**, *40*, 2254–2266. [CrossRef]
63. Rodell, C.B.; Kaminski, A.L.; Burdick, J.A. Rational design of network properties in guest–host assembled and shear–thinning hyaluronic acid hydrogels. *Biomacromolecules* **2013**, *14*, 4125–4134. [CrossRef]
64. Rosales, A.M.; Rodell, C.B.; Chen, M.H.; Morrow, M.G.; Anseth, K.S.; Burdick, J.A. Reversible control of network properties in azobenzene–containing hyaluronic acid–based hydrogels. *Bioconj. Chem.* **2018**, *29*, 905–913. [CrossRef]
65. Rowland, M.J.; Atgie, M.; Hoogland, D.; Scherman, O.A. Preparation and supramolecular recognition of multivalent peptide–polysaccharide conjugates by cucurbit [8] uril in hydrogel formation. *Biomacromolecules* **2015**, *16*, 2436–2443. [CrossRef]
66. Montanari, E.; D'arrigo, G.; Di Meo, C.; Virga, A.; Coviello, T.; Passariello, C.; Matricardi, P. Chasing bacteria within the cells using levofloxacin–loaded hyaluronic acid nanohydrogels. *Eur. J. Pharm. Biopharm.* **2014**, *87*, 518–523. [CrossRef]
67. Jung, Y.-S.; Park, W.; Park, H.; Lee, D.-K.; Na, K. Thermo–sensitive injectable hydrogel based on the physical mixing of hyaluronic acid and Pluronic F–127 for sustained NSAID delivery. *Carbohydr. Polym.* **2017**, *156*, 403–408. [CrossRef]
68. Huang, G.; Huang, H. Application of hyaluronic acid as carriers in drug delivery. *Drug Deliv.* **2018**, *25*, 766–772. [CrossRef]
69. Hemshekhar, M.; Thushara, R.M.; Chandranayaka, S.; Sherman, L.S.; Kemparaju, K.; Girish, K.S. Emerging roles of hyaluronic acid bioscaffolds in tissue engineering and regenerative medicine. *Int. J. Biol. Macromol.* **2016**, *86*, 917–928. [CrossRef]
70. Liu, Z.; Tang, M.; Zhao, J.; Chai, R.; Kang, J. Looking into the future: Toward advanced 3D biomaterials for stem-cell-based regenerative medicine. *Adv. Mater.* **2018**, *30*, 1705388. [CrossRef]
71. Dosio, F.; Arpicco, S.; Stella, B.; Fattal, E. Hyaluronic acid for anticancer drug and nucleic acid delivery. *Adv. Drug Deliv. Rev.* **2016**, *97*, 204–236. [CrossRef]
72. Li, J.; Mooney, D.J. Designing hydrogels for controlled drug delivery. *Nat. Rev. Mater.* **2016**, *1*, 16071. [CrossRef]
73. Highley, C.B.; Kim, M.; Lee, D.; Burdick, J.A. Near–infrared light triggered release of molecules from supramolecular hydrogel–nanorod composites. *Nanomedicine* **2016**, *11*, 1579–1590. [CrossRef]
74. Yamaguchi, H.; Kobayashi, Y.; Kobayashi, R.; Takashima, Y.; Hashidzume, A.; Harada, A. Photoswitchable gel assembly based on molecular recognition. *Nat. Commun.* **2012**, *3*, 603. [CrossRef]
75. Kwon, S.S.; Kong, B.J.; Park, S.N. Physicochemical properties of pH–sensitive hydrogels based on hydroxyethyl cellulose–hyaluronic acid and for applications as transdermal delivery systems for skin lesions. *Eur. J. Pharm. Biopharm.* **2015**, *92*, 146–154. [CrossRef]
76. Mattheolabakis, G.; Milane, L.; Singh, A.; Amiji, M.M. Hyaluronic acid targeting of CD44 for cancer therapy: From receptor biology to nanomedicine. *J. Drug Target.* **2015**, *23*, 605–618. [CrossRef]
77. Chen, C.; Zhao, S.; Karnad, A.; Freeman, J.W. The biology and role of CD44 in cancer progression: Therapeutic implications. *J. Hematol. Oncol.* **2018**, *11*, 64. [CrossRef]
78. Rao, N.V.; Yoon, H.Y.; Han, H.S.; Ko, H.; Son, S.; Lee, M.; Lee, H.; Jo, D.-G.; Kang, Y.M.; Park, J.H. Recent developments in hyaluronic acid–based nanomedicine for targeted cancer treatment. *Expert Opin. Drug Deliv.* **2016**, *13*, 239–252. [CrossRef]
79. Choi, K.Y.; Han, H.S.; Lee, E.S.; Shin, J.M.; Almquist, B.D.; Lee, D.S.; Park, J.H. Hyaluronic acid–based activatable nanomaterials for stimuli-responsive imaging and therapeutics: Beyond CD44-mediated drug delivery. *Adv. Mater.* **2019**, 1803549. [CrossRef]
80. Huang, G.; Huang, H. Hyaluronic acid–based biopharmaceutical delivery and tumor–targeted drug delivery system. *J. Controll. Release* **2018**, *278*, 122–126. [CrossRef]
81. Fu, C.; Li, H.; Li, N.; Miao, X.; Xie, M.; Du, W.; Zhang, L.-M. Conjugating an anticancer drug onto thiolated hyaluronic acid by acid liable hydrazone linkage for its gelation and dual stimuli–response release. *Carbohydr. Polym.* **2015**, *128*, 163–170. [CrossRef]

82. Bajaj, G.; Kim, M.R.; Mohammed, S.I.; Yeo, Y. Hyaluronic acid–based hydrogel for regional delivery of paclitaxel to intraperitoneal tumors. *J. Controll. Release* **2012**, *158*, 386–392. [CrossRef]
83. Yang, C.; Wang, X.; Yao, X.; Zhang, Y.; Wu, W.; Jiang, X. Hyaluronic acid nanogels with enzyme–sensitive cross–linking group for drug delivery. *J. Controll. Release* **2015**, *205*, 206–217. [CrossRef]
84. Jhan, H.-J.; Liu, J.-J.; Chen, Y.-C.; Liu, D.-Z.; Sheu, M.-T.; Ho, H.-O. Novel injectable thermosensitive hydrogels for delivering hyaluronic acid–doxorubicin nanocomplexes to locally treat tumors. *Nanomedicine* **2015**, *10*, 1263–1274. [CrossRef]
85. Chen, J.; He, H.; Deng, C.; Yin, L.; Zhong, Z. Saporin–loaded CD44 and EGFR dual–targeted nanogels for potent inhibition of metastatic breast cancer in vivo. *Int. J. Pharm.* **2019**, *560*, 57–64. [CrossRef]
86. Dakwar, G.R.; Shariati, M.; Willaert, W.; Ceelen, W.; De Smedt, S.C.; Remaut, K. Nanomedicine–based intraperitoneal therapy for the treatment of peritoneal carcinomatosis—Mission possible? *Adv. Drug Deliv. Rev.* **2017**, *108*, 13–24. [CrossRef] [PubMed]
87. Cho, E.J.; Sun, B.; Doh, K.-O.; Wilson, E.M.; Torregrosa-Allen, S.; Elzey, B.D.; Yeo, Y. Intraperitoneal delivery of platinum with in–situ crosslinkable hyaluronic acid gel for local therapy of ovarian cancer. *Biomaterials* **2015**, *37*, 312–319. [CrossRef] [PubMed]
88. Qiu, Y.; Park, K. Environment–sensitive hydrogels for drug delivery. *Adv. Drug Deliv. Rev.* **2001**, *53*, 321–339. [CrossRef]
89. Zhang, W.; Jin, X.; Li, H.; Wei, C.-X.; Wu, C.-W. Onion–structure bionic hydrogel capsules based on chitosan for regulating doxorubicin release. *Carbohydr. Polym.* **2019**, *209*, 152–160. [CrossRef]
90. Goldring, M.B.; Berenbaum, F. Emerging targets in osteoarthritis therapy. *Curr. Opin. Pharmacol.* **2015**, *22*, 51–63. [CrossRef] [PubMed]
91. Dougados, M. Sodium hyaluronate therapy in osteoarthritis: Arguments for a potential beneficial structural effect. *Semin. Arthr. Rheum.* **2000**, *30*, 19–25. [CrossRef]
92. Ishida, O.; Tanaka, Y.; Morimoto, I.; Takigawa, M.; Eto, S. Chondrocytes are regulated by cellular adhesion through CD44 and hyaluronic acid pathway. *J. Bone Mineral Res.* **1997**, *12*, 1657–1663. [CrossRef]
93. Cai, Y.; López-Ruiz, E.; Wengel, J.; Creemers, L.B.; Howard, K.A. A hyaluronic acid–based hydrogel enabling CD44–mediated chondrocyte binding and gapmer oligonucleotide release for modulation of gene expression in osteoarthritis. *J. Controll. Release* **2017**, *253*, 153–159. [CrossRef]
94. Garcia, J.P.; Stein, J.; Cai, Y.; Riemers, F.; Wexselblatt, E.; Wengel, J.; Tryfonidou, M.; Yayon, A.; Howard, K.A.; Creemers, L.B. Fibrin–hyaluronic acid hydrogel–based delivery of antisense oligonucleotides for ADAMTS5 inhibition in co–delivered and resident joint cells in osteoarthritis. *J. Controll. Release* **2019**, *294*, 247–258. [CrossRef]
95. Verma, P.; Dalal, K. ADAMTS-4 and ADAMTS-5: Key enzymes in osteoarthritis. *J. Cell. Biochem.* **2011**, *112*, 3507–3514. [CrossRef]

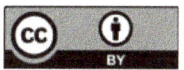

© 2019 by the authors. Licensee MDPI, Basel, Switzerland. This article is an open access article distributed under the terms and conditions of the Creative Commons Attribution (CC BY) license (http://creativecommons.org/licenses/by/4.0/).

MDPI
St. Alban-Anlage 66
4052 Basel
Switzerland
Tel. +41 61 683 77 34
Fax +41 61 302 89 18
www.mdpi.com

Pharmaceutics Editorial Office
E-mail: pharmaceutics@mdpi.com
www.mdpi.com/journal/pharmaceutics

www.ingramcontent.com/pod-product-compliance
Lightning Source LLC
LaVergne TN
LVHW071953080526
838202LV00064B/6739